DATE DUE

Demco, Inc. 38-293

ADVANCES

IN

GYNECOLOGICAL
ENDOCRINOLOGY

ADVANCES
IN
GYNECOLOGICAL ENDOCRINOLOGY

*The Proceedings of the Plenary Sessions of the
8th World Congress of Gynecological Endocrinology*

Florence, Italy, December 2000

**A. R. Genazzani,
F. Petraglia and P. G. Artini**

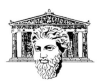

The Parthenon Publishing Group
International Publishers in Medicine, Science & Technology

A CRC PRESS COMPANY
BOCA RATON   LONDON   NEW YORK   WASHINGTON, D.C.

Library of Congress Cataloging-in-Publication Data

Advances in gynecological endocrinology / edited by A.R. Genazzani, F. Petraglia, and P.G. Artini.
    p. ; cm.
    Includes bibliographical references and index.
    ISBN 1-84214-071-X (alk. paper)
    1. Generative organs, Female--Cancer.
I. Genazzani, Andrea R. II. Petraglia, F.
III. Artini, P.G.
    [DNLM: 1. Genital Diseases, Female--therapy. 2. Endocrine Diseases--complications. 3. Endocrine Diseases--diagnosis. 4. Endocrine Diseases--therapy.
5. Genital Diseases, Female--complications.
6. Genital Diseases, Female--diagnosis,
WP 505 A244 2001]
RC280,G5 A35 2001
618.1--dc21
                        2001036110

British Library Cataloguing in publication Data
Advances in gynecological endocrinology
    1. Endocrine gynecology
    I. Genazzani, Andrea II. Petraglia, F.
III. Artini, P. G. 618.1

ISBN 184214071X

Published in the USA by
The Parthenon Publishing Group Inc.
One Blue Hill Plaza
PO Box 1564, Pearl River
New York 10965, USA

Published in the UK and Europe by
The Parthenon Publishing Group
23–25 Blades Court
Deodar Road
London SW15 2NU, UK

Copyright © 2002
The Parthenon Publishing Group

Typeset by Siva Math Setters, Chennai, India
Printed and bound by Bookcraft (Bath) Ltd., Midsomer Norton, UK

Contents

List of principal contributors

P.-N. Barri
Department of Obstetrics and
    Gynecology
Institut Universitari Dexeus
Paseo de la Bonanova 67
08017 Barcelona
Spain

Z. Blumenfeld
Reproductive Endocrinology
    and Infertility Section
Department of Obstetrics and
    Gynecology
Technion-Faculty of Medicine
Rambam Medical Center
31096 Haifa
Israel

M. L. Brandi
Department of Internal Medicine
University of Florence
Viale Pieraccini 6
50139 Florence
Italy

H. G. Burger
Prince Henry's Institute of
    Medical Research
PO Box 5152
Clayton
Victoria 3168
Australia

M. Busacca
Second Department of Obstetrics
    and Gynecology
Clinic L. Mangiagalli
Via Commenda 12
20122 Milan
Italy

E. M. Coutinho
CEPARH
Rua Caetano Moura 35
Salvador
40210-341 Bahia
Brazil

G. Creatsas
Second Department of Obstetrics &
    Gynecology
Aretaieion Hospital
76 Vasilissis Sophias Avenue
11528 Athens
Greece

P. G. Crosignani
Department of Obstetrics
    and Gynecology
University of Milan
Via Commenda 12
20122 Milan
Italy

G. D'Ambrogio
Reproductive Medicine &
    Child Development
Division of Gynecology
    and Obstetrics
University of Pisa
Via Roma 35
56100 Pisa
Italy

S. Daya
Department of Obstetrics
    and Gynecology
McMaster University
1200 Main Street West
Hamilton, Ontario
Canada L8N 3Z5

L. Devoto
Department of Obstetrics and Gynecology
University of Chile
Faculty of Medicine
PO Box 226-3
Santiago
Chile

J. Donnez
Department of Gynecology
Cliniques Universitaires St-Luc
Avenue Hippocrate 10
1200 Brussels
Belgium

F. Facchinetti
Department of Obstetrics and Gynecology
University of Modena
Via del Pozzo 71
41100 Modena
Italy

P. Fénichel
Department of Reproductive Medicine
Hospital de L'Archet, BP 79
Nice 06202
France

A. R. Genazzani
Reproductive Medicine & Child
    Development
Division of Gynecology and Obstetrics
University of Pisa
Via Roma 35
56100 Pisa
Italy

T. Gürgan
Department of Obstetrics and Gynecology
Hacettepe University Faculty of Medicine
Sihhiye
Ankara 06100
Turkey

P. C. Ho
Department of Obstetrics and Gynecology
University of Hong Kong
6/F Professorial Block
Queen Mary Hospital

Pokfulam Road
Hong Kong
China

A. J. W. Hsueh
Department of Gynecology and Obstetrics
Stanford University School of Medicine
300 Pasteur Drive, A344
Stanford, CA 94305-5317
USA

F. Labrie
Oncology and Molecular Endocrinology
    Research Center
Laval University Medical Center (CHUL)
2705 Laurier Boulevard
Quebec City G1V 4G2
Canada

A. Lanzone
Department of Obstetrics and Gynecology
Universita Cattolica del Sacro Cuore
Largo Agostino Gemelli 8
00168 Rome
Italy

M. Massobrio
Department of Obstetrics and Gynecology
University of Torino
Ospedale S. Anna
Via Ventimiglia 3
10128 Torino
Italy

L. Mastroianni, Jr
Department of Obstetrics and Gynecology
University of Pennsylvania
    Medical Center
3400 Spruce Street
Philadelphia, PA 19104
USA

G. B. Melis
Department of Obstetrics, Gynecology
    and Human Reproduction
University of Cagliari
Via Ospedale 46
9124 Cagliari
Italy

J. M. Mendez Ribas
Department of Gynecology
Hospital de Clinicas
Cordoba Avenue 2351
1120 Buenos Aires
Argentina

A. Milewicz
Department of Endocrinology and
    Diabetology
University of Medicine
50-367 Wroclaw
Patseura 4
Poland

R. Pasquali
Department of Endocrinology
S. Orsola-Malpighi Hospital
Via Massarenti 9
40138 Bologna
Italy

F. Petraglia
Department of Obstetrics
    and Gynecology
University of Siena
Policlinico Le Scotte
Viale Bracci
53100 Siena
Italy

M.-P. Piccinni
Department of Internal Medicine
Immunoallergology Unit
Viale Morgagni 85
50134 Firenze
Italy

Ch. V. Rao
Department of Obstetrics and Gynecology
University of Louisville
438 MDR Building
Louisville, KY 40292
USA

E.-M. Rutanen
Department of Obstetrics and Gynecology
Helsinki University Central Hospital
Box 140, Haartmaninkatu 2

00029 Helsinki
Finland

A. E. Schindler
Department of Obstetrics
    and Gynecology
University of Essen
Hufelandstr. 55
D-45122 Essen
Germany

H. P. G. Schneider
Department of Obstetrics
    and Gynecology
University of Münster
Von-Esmarch-Str. 56
D-48149 Münster
Germany

M. M. Seibel
Fertility Center of New England
333 Elm Street, 3rd Floor
Dedham, MA 02026
USA

M. Serio
Department of Endocrinology
University of Florence
Viale Pieraccini 6
50139 Florence
Italy

T. Simoncini
Department of Reproductive Medicine
    and Child Development
Division of Obstetrics and Gynecology
University of Pisa
Via Roma 67
56100 Pisa
Italy

N. O. Siseles
Climacteric Section
Department of Obstetrics
    and Gynecology
University of Buenos Aires
Av. Santa Fe 3802
Buenos Aires 1425
Argentina

P. G. Spinola
Maternidade Climério de Oliveira
Federal University of Bahia
Rua do Limoeiro, No. 1
Salvador
40.055-150 Bahia
Brazil

M. Stomati
Department of Reproductive Medicine
   and Child Development
Division of Obstetrics and Gynecology
University of Pisa
Via Roma 67
56100 Pisa
Italy

J. F. Strauss III
Center for Research on Reproduction &
   Womens Health
1354 BRBII, 421 Curie Boulevard
Philadelphia, PA 19104
USA

J. Studd
Academic Department of Obstetrics and
   Gynaecology
Chelsea & Westminster Hospital
369 Fulham Road
London SW10 9NH
UK

M. Szamatowicz
Clinic of Gynecology
University Medical School
Marii Sklodowskiej-Curie 24a,
15-276 Bialystok
Poland

S. L. Tan
Department of Obstetrics and Gynecology
McGill University
Royal Victoria Hospital

Women's Pavilion
687 Pine Avenue West
Montreal H3A 1A1
Quebec, Canada

B. C. Tarlatzis
1st Department of Obstetrics
   and Gynecology
Aristotle University of Thessaloniki
9 Agias Sofias St
Thessaloniki 54623
Greece

A. Tempone
Department of Gynecology
University of Buenos Aires
Olleros 2020
1426 Buenos Aires
Argentina

A. Volpe
Institute of Obstetrics
   and Gynecology
Policlinico de Modena
Via del Pozza 71
41100 Modena
Italy

O. Ylikorkala
Department of Obstetrics
   and Gynecology
Helsinki University Central Hospital
Box 140, Haartmaninkatu 2
00029 Helsinki
Finland

J. Yu
Department of Obstetrics & Gynecology
Fudan University Medical Centre
#419 Fang Xie Road
Shanghai 200011
P.R. China

The impact of the genomic revolution on gynecological endocrinology

1

K. M. Wasson and A. J. W. Hsueh

Shifting scientific paradigms

Classically, the characterization of novel reproductive endocrine genes was a time-intensive endeavor, utilizing multiple strategies including degenerate polymerase chain reaction (PCR), low stringency hybridization, expression or differential cloning, protein purification schemes, or domain interactions[1]. With the development of the Human Genome Project, the genomic revolution began[2], and led the way in the development of scientific technologies and the augmentation of searchable public databases, both of which have been beneficial to the entire research community. The classical approaches to novel gene discovery are now being replaced by *in silico* (computer-based research) approaches that drastically reduce the time spent performing wet-bench research.

A labyrinth of genome and molecular databases exists[3–5], which provides computer-literate scientists with the resources to substitute preliminary wet-bench research with dry-bench computer research. Researchers now perform virtual PCR and cloning techniques that expedite novel gene discoveries. For example, computational analysis programs such as BLAST (Basic Local Alignment Search Tool; http://www.ncbi.nlm.nih.gov/blast/blast.cgi) perform statistically relevant pairwise comparisons of known nucleotide and protein sequences annotated in public databases. Such comparisons enable scientists to elucidate novel genes based on evolutionarily conserved sequences or on the limited similarity of specific protein motifs[1].

Hsu *et al.*[6] utilized the evolutionarily conserved sequences of putative glycoprotein hormone receptors in *Drosophila* and the sea anemone as the search query in the expression sequence tag (EST) databases. This approach led to the identification of two novel genes that encoded leucine-rich repeat-containing, G protein-coupled receptors (LGRs). Hsu *et al.*[7] performed further searches of EST databases and identified two additional members of this LGR family based on evolutionary conservation. Although these receptors are expressed in multiple tissues, the functional significance of these receptors and their respective ligands remains unknown.

Hsu[8] utilized the structural homology among the members of the insulin/relaxin family as the search query in the EST databases. Members of this protein family display low overall sequence identity but share the characteristic B-C-A domain structure of insulin. Hsu[8] found two novel genes whose deduced amino acid sequences contained the characteristic B-C-A domain structure but had low sequence identity to relaxin. These genes were named relaxin insulin-like factor (RIF)-1 and (RIF)-2; however, again, the functions remain unknown.

Laitinen *et al.*[9] utilized the GDF-9 sequence as the search query in the EST database to identify putative novel GDF-9-like sequences. GDF-9 is an oocyte-specific protein essential for normal follicle development. An EST cDNA that encoded a putative protein was isolated from the mouse two-cell embryo library and named GDF-9B. Laitinen *et al.* showed that GDF-9B colocalizes with GDF-9 in mouse oocytes and both are expressed during folliculogenesis. Whether GDF-9B is essential for follicle development remains unclear.

Bae et al.[10] utilized the human myeloid cell leukemia (Mcl)-1 cDNA sequence as the search query in the EST database to identify putative novel Mcl-1-like sequences. Mcl-1 is an antiapoptotic Bcl-2 family protein, which contains Bcl-2 homology (BH) domains 1, 2, and 3 and a C-terminal transmembrane region. Three independent partial nucleotide sequences were isolated from an ovary tumor library, and a germinal center B-cell library, that were homologous to Mcl-1 cDNA except for the deletion of 248 nucleotides from the C-terminus. Deletion of these nucleotides resulted in the loss of BH1, BH2 and the transmembrane domains, thus causing the conversion from promoting antiapoptotic functions to promoting proapoptotic functions.

Future of research

These brief examples demonstrate the ease with which novel ovarian genes are now being discovered, and the role of molecular databases in this process. Previously, individual laboratories would focus on only one or a few genes; however, with the development of large-scale methods of genomic analysis, the one gene/one laboratory approach is giving way to global expression profiling. The global response of cells or tissues to induced disease states or specific treatments is now measured on DNA microarrays that provide a view of the activity of several thousand genes during one experiment. This technology was used to determine that at least eight single nucleotide polymorphisms exist in the BRCA-1 gene, a breast and ovarian cancer gene[11]. Once the entire human genome becomes publicly available, further discovery of single nucleotide polymorphisms will easily be made.

Integration of wet-bench global expression data with dry-bench computational analyses and existing physiological data poses new challenges for scientists in the 21st century. A simple search of PubMed using 'ovary and NOT CHO' as keyword search criteria generates over 2 300 peer-reviewed articles published in 2000, and over 59 000 articles in all of PubMed. Critical analysis of these articles and integration with genomic data provides a daunting task for even the most seasoned ovarian researcher[12].

The Ovarian Kaleidoscope database

To assist the ovarian research community in the managing of physiological and genomic data, we have developed a searchable database called the Ovarian Kaleidoscope database (OKdb) (http://ovary.stanford.edu). The OKdb provides a unified online gateway for information about ovarian-specific genes[13].

The OKdb is a resource for the ovarian research community providing timely information on physiological and genomic data in a user-friendly, Window-based environment. It differs from most curated databases because the creation of individual gene records is not restricted to the database developers. Scientists with expertise on specific ovarian genes are encouraged to submit their information to the database. Usernames are utilized and password-authenticated access to each gene record provides a secure environment for the author to establish and maintain records for each submitted gene.

New gene submission is easily done via a window-driven menu. The submitter provides as much information as is known for the gene of interest. The submission form asks for information on general cellular functions and localization, ovary-specific functions and localization, and regulation of gene expression (Table 1). Submitters simply mark appropriate dialog boxes for each category. Comment boxes for each category allow submitters to add relevant text supported by PubMed. Simply providing the PubMed identification (PMID) number of the citation creates a direct link to the PubMed abstract. When available, Genbank accession numbers for human, rat, mouse, sheep and cattle will provide links to the Genbank entries, and

Table 1 Categories for gene submission and searches in the Ovarian Kaleidoscope database (OKdb)

General functions	Ovarian-specific functions
cell signaling/cell adhesion	follicle recruitment
hormone/growth factor/cytokine	follicle growth and/or maturation
receptor	follicle atresia
cell adhesion	ovulation
signal transduction	steroidogenesis
channels/transport proteins	luteinization
intracellular signal transduction	luteolysis
microtubule-associated/motors	primordial germ cell development
gene expression	oocyte growth and/or maturation
transcription factor	unknown
translation factor	
RNA synthesis and turnover	Expression regulation factors
protein synthesis and turnover	follicle-stimulating hormone
metabolism and trafficking	luteinizing hormone
metabolism/energy conversion	human chorionic gonadotropin
intracellular trafficking	steroids
proteases	growth factors/cytokines
protease	eicosanoids
protease inhibitor	other factors
cell life and death	
apoptosis	Ovarian cell localization
cell cycle regulation	oocyte
DNA synthesis and repair	cumulus cells
oncogene	granulosa cells
tumor suppressor	theca cells
cell structure/motility	luteal cells
chromosome structure	stromal cells
cytoskeleton	surface epithelium
cell motility	other cells
extracellular matrix	
	Follicle stage localization
Cellular localization	primordial
cytoplasmic	primary
cell surface	secondary
secreted	antral
nuclear	preovulatory
mitochondrial	corpus luteum
	other stages

Online Mendelian Inheritance in Man (OMIM) record numbers will provide links to the OMIM entries. Thus utilized, with supporting links to relevant publications and databases, the OKdb provides a gateway to genomic and physiological data for ovarian-specific genes.

A search command for gene records can be based on any of the criteria used for inputting the gene information (Table 1). The database is also searchable by specific gene names. Until now, rapid access to a large ovarian-specific gene record database has not been available. Recent estimates suggest that there are approximately 20 000 ovarian genes[13]; however, only a small percentage of those have been fully characterized and their functions identified. The recent development of the OKdb provides a manageable number of genes for the initial construction (presently over 530 records). Because the OKdb allows submitters to continually incorporate new reports and data of ovary-specific genes, it is anticipated that this resource will provide a valuable tool for current and future research[12].

Conclusion

Major advances in genomics are expected to revolutionize the fields of biomedicine, including gynecological endocrinology.

Acknowledgments

We thank Caren Spencer for editorial assistance. The OKdb server is maintained by Ursula Vitt with individual records submitted by national and international researchers. The web service for the OKdb is supported by the Specialized Cooperative Centers Program in Reproduction Research, NICHD, NIH.

References

1. Hsu SY, Hsueh AJ, Discovering new hormones, receptors, and signaling mediators in the genomic era. *Mol Endocrinol* 2000;14:594–604
2. Collins FS, Patrinos A, Jordan E, *et al*. New goals for the U.S. Human Genome Project: 1998–2003. *Science* 1998;282:682–9
3. Borsani G, Ballabio A, Banfi S. A practical guide to orient yourself in the labyrinth of genome databases. *Hum Mol Genet* 1998;7:1641–8
4. Baxevanis AD. The molecular biology database collection: an online compilation of relevant database resources. *Nucleic Acids Res* 2000;28: 1–7
5. Baasiri RA, Glasser SR, Steffen DL, *et al*. The breast cancer gene database: a collaborative information resource. *Oncogene* 1999;18: 7958–65
6. Hsu SY, Liang SG, Hsueh AJ. Characterization of two LGR genes homologous to gonadotropin and thyrotropin receptors with extracellular leucine-rich repeats and a G protein-coupled, seven-transmembrane region. *Mol Endocrinol* 1998;12:1830–45
7. Hsu SY, Kudo M, Chen T, *et al*. The three subfamilies of leucine-rich repeat-containing G protein-coupled receptors (LGR): identification of LGR6 and LGR7 and the signaling mechanism for LGR7. *Mol Endocrinol* 2000; 14:1257–71
8. Hsu SY. Cloning of two novel mammalian paralogs of relaxin/insulin family proteins and their expression in testis and kidney. *Mol Endocrinol* 1999;13:2163–74
9. Laitinen M, Vuojolainen K, Jaatinen R, *et al*. A novel growth differentiation factor-9 (GDF-9) related factor is co-expressed with GDF-9 in mouse oocytes during folliculogenesis. *Mech Dev* 1998;78:135–40
10. Bae J, Leo CP, Hsu SY, *et al*. MCL-1S, a splicing variant of the antiapoptotic BCL-2 family member MCL-1, encodes a proapoptotic protein possessing only the BH3 domain. *J Biol Chem* 2000;275:25255–61
11. Hacia JG, Brody LC, Chee MS, *et al*. Detection of heterozygous mutations in BRCA1 using high density oligonucleotide arrays and two-colour fluorescence analysis. *Nat Genet* 1996; 14:441–7
12. Wasson KM, Hsueh AJW. Ovarian Gene Database. *J Soc Gynecol Invest* 2001;8:537–9
13. Leo CP, Vitt U, Hsueh AJW. The ovarian kaleidoscope database (OKdb) – an online resource for the ovarian research community. *Endocrinology* 2000;141:3052–4

Evaluation and therapy of postmenarcheal menstrual disorders

2

J. M. Méndez Ribas

Introduction

For the past 14 years, the Clinicas Hospital in Buenos Aires has provided an integrated service for adolescents. The team is made up of gynecologists, pediatricians, social workers, psychologists and psychiatrists. Male and female adolescents, between 10 and 19 years old, attend, with an average of 600 consultations per month. An interdisciplinary approach is used.

Girls with menstrual disorders attend the clinic.

On the recommendation of the mental health team, we categorize adolescents according to their psychological maturity, in relation to their degree of independence from their parents. Group A retain the psychological perspective of childhood. They mainly consult for menstrual disorders, delayed puberty, or disturbance of body image (obesity, anorexia nervosa). This group is usually accompanied by their mothers. On the other hand, Group B are adolescents who are prematurely introduced into the adult world. Their reasons for consultation include genital infections, unplanned pregnancies and contraception difficulties, and they generally come alone.

Those with menstrual disorders we arbitrarily assign to Group A.

Almost 50% of female adolescents attending hospital have menstrual disorders, but this number is reduced to 26% if only healthy out-patients are taken into consideration.

Thus, it may be observed that in our studied population 74% have postmenarcheal regular menses. Our results are comparable

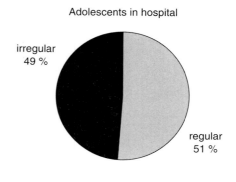

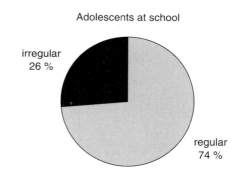

Figure 1 Postmenarcheal menstrual disorders

with international data (Figure 1). Almost 45% of girls with menstrual disorders spontaneously acquire regular menses within a postmenarcheal period of 3 years (range 2–10 years) (Figure 2). These results should be taken into consideration before hormonal therapy is started.

Of more than 13 000 who have consulted for gynecological problems, 26% presented with cycle disorders, while 8.2 % had secondary

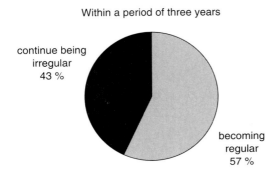

Within a period of three years

continue being irregular 43 %

becoming regular 57 %

Figure 2 Spontaneous evolution of irregular menstrual cycles

amenorrhea. Cycle inhibition was mainly caused by:

hyperandrogenism

psychophysical distress

hyperprolactinemia

anorexia/bulimia nervosa

thyroid dysfunction

premature ovarian failure

Oligomenorrhea

Oligomenorrhea is the most frequent menstrual disorder among adolescents, and its differential diagnosis should be elaborated based on careful questioning that takes into account the whole complex process of adolescence.

By means of basal temperature and progesterone levels on day 30–36 of menstrual cycle, we may distinguish ovulatory from anovulatory oligomenorrhea. If ovulation takes place, the adolescent remains under observation. Anovulation tends to fall into two groups.

Group A has the following features: normal phenotype; normal luteinizing hormone/follicle-stimulating hormone (LH/FSH) relation; regular sized ovaries. If the patient belongs to group A, we investigate habits of life that could influence anovulation such as unsuitable diet, excess of physical activity and emotional disorders.

Group B has the following features: signs of hyperandrogenism; LH > FSH relation; enlarged ovaries; insulin resistance. After thorough questioning and physical examination, we obtain one blood sample on day 3 of the menstrual cycle to determine levels of LH, FSH, thyroid-stimulating hormone (TSH) and androgens (testosterone, androstenedione, 17-OH-progesterone), and also ovarian volume is sonographically measured. If the patient belongs to group B, different causes of hyperandrogenism are then taken into consideration:

polycystic ovarian syndrome (PCOS)

PCOS with insulinic resistance, obesity and acanthosis nigricans

late adrenal syndrome

peripheral hirsutism

Therapy is applied based on clinical findings, in particular LH/FSH relation. This is how we categorize the patients for treatment:

(1) normal LH/FSH relation with regular sized ovaries

estradiol valerate 2 µg (11 days)

estradiol valerate 2 µg + levonorgestrel 0.2 mg (10 days)

(2) normal LH/FSH relation with signs of hyperandrogenism

estradiol valerate 2 µg (11 days)

estradiol valerate 2 µg + cyproterone 1 mg (10 days)

(3) LH > FSH relation with enlarged ovaries and hyperandrogenism:

ethinylestradiol 35 µg + cyproterone 2 mg

(4) insulin resistance

diet

physical activity

metformin 500 mg daily

(5) high levels of 17-OH-progesterone

prednisone 2–4 mg daily

(6) peripheral hirsutism with high levels of dehydrotestosterone

finasteride 5 mg daily

Secondary amenorrhea

Eating disorders

We have a team who specialize in this typically adolescent's condition made up of a psychiatrist, a psychologist, a nutritionist and a gynecologist.

The gynecologist is alert to this diagnosis when a girl consults for amenorrhea, and investigates eating habits and determines body mass index. Treatment is initiated by the mental health team and the nutritional counseling team, and, when it is appropriate, the gynecologist prescribes hormone replacement therapy.

Low doses of estrogens are initially provided so as to evaluate tolerance and acceptance, until reaching levels of 30–50 µg of ethinylestradiol. In order to complete therapy, bone densitometry is measured. Our tables are coordinated to the girl's age. We evaluate the need to add alendronate and calcium therapy, depending on decalcification rate due to hypoestrogenemia.

Hypothyroidism

A clinical examination of the gland is routinely performed. Basal TSH is measured to detect subclinical hypothyroidism. If this result is indefinite, a thyrotropin releasing hormone/TSH test is indicated.

Hyperprolactinemia

If high prolactin has biological activity and causes amenorrhea and/or galactorrhea, we exclude the following causes:

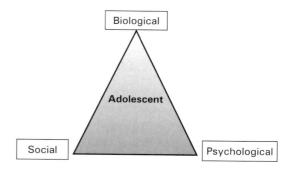

Figure 3 The adolescent within a biopsychosocial process

psychopharmacological therapy

distress

hypothyroidism

hypothalamic–pituitary tumors

organic sellar pathology (by means of magnetic resonance)

Hyperprolactinemia is treated with carbegoline 0.25 mg twice a week.

Premature ovarian failure

Although it is very rare under the age of 18, we have assisted 15 cases: six due to premature menopause; four to dysgenetic ovaries; three to follicular insufficiency; and two to resistant ovaries.

In order to define its etiology, a genetic study is performed (short or long arm alteration of X chromosome), and investigation of anti-FSH antibodies. In translaparoscopic ovarian biopsy we observe the follicles, estroma and vessels. Consequent on these results, we evaluate prognosis and select appropriate HRT.

In conclusion, the adolescent must be treated within a biopsychosocial process, the components of which are in constant interaction (Figure 3). Ultimately, success of treatment depends on this coordination.

Hormonal substitution in young women with gonadal dysgenesis

3

G. Creatsas

Introduction

Gonadal dysgenesis and Turner's syndrome are characterized by a significant number of anomalies. Short stature and amenorrhea as well as other phenotype anomalies (stigmata) depend on the severity of the disease as well as the genotype pattern. Short stature is recognized during childhood, while amenorrhea is seen during puberty. It is the responsibility of the pediatrician to diagnose this condition early, following notification by the parents.

The presence of functional ovarian tissue as well as follicular development and ovulation depend on the severity of the syndrome. However, the majority of cases lack follicular presence and ovulation. A limited number of mosaic cases present scanty ovulation so that it is possible for the young woman to present some kind of menstrual bleeding or menstruation.

The absence of follicles leads to estrogen deficiency. Young women with gonadal dysgenesis carry all the short- and long-term negative effects of estrogen depletion (Table 1). Even in cases of mosaicism, estrogen serum levels are low and symptoms of estrogen depletion are prominent. Hypogonadism during adolescence may also be found in cases of thalassemia major, castrated young women after chemotherapy, and in cases of radiotherapy or surgical treatment for ovarian malignancy. Gonadectomy is also performed in gonadal dysgenetic XY females to prevent malignant degeneration of gonads (Table 2).

Table 1 Estrogen deficiency symptoms

Lipid metabolism anomalies and cardiovascular disease
Juvenile osteoporosis
Uterine atrophy
Vulval dryness
Vaginal atrophy
Atrophic cystitis
Vasomotor symptoms
Psychological problems
Long-term effects in the central nervous system
Skin dryness

Table 2 Causes of primary amenorrhea

Anatomic origin (congenital anomalies)
Hypothalamic abnormalities:
   thalassemia major
Gonadal dysgenesis
XY female genotype requiring
   gonadectomy
Malignancy requiring gonadectomy

Hormonal substitution

Hormonal substitution is required in all cases of gonadal dysgenesis, and must be started as soon as possible, in combination with growth hormone which assists attainment of the optimal final height. There are various reports on different regimens for the use of human growth hormone, either alone or in combination with estrogen substitution and oxandrolone administration[1,2]. There are various forms of estrogen replacement therapy (ERT).

ERT should be followed by progestogen administration, to prevent endometrial hyperplasia. It should be mentioned that endometrial carcinoma has been reported even in cases of gonadal dysgenesis in those who have never received HRT. Micronized progesterone may be used instead of progestogens. HRT is further tailored after two or three cycles, according to the ultrasonographic findings of endometrial thickness and uterine volume, the clinical characteristics of menstrual function, and the development of secondary sexual characteristics. Later on, HRT is also adjusted according to the bone mass content.

At the beginning of therapy, a high dose of ERT is advised in order to overcome estrogen deficiency symptoms, to inhibit fast bone loss, and to enhance the development of secondary sexual characteristics (Table 3). The type of estrogen to be used is chosen depending on each individual case. No significant differences are found between the use of conjugated estrogens and transdermal estradiol. However, higher doses are suggested when the transdermal route is used. Other forms of ERT are also in use, such as implants and combined oral contraceptives. The latter, due to their low estrogen concentration, only have a minimal long-term beneficial effect on bone mass, and their use is advised during the second and third decades. The selective estrogen receptor modulators (SERMs) and the phytoestrogens should be considered as future or alternative methods of treatment.

A very important problem is the low bone mass seen in these patients during a period of bone growth acceleration and development. Osteopenia and juvenile osteoporosis are found in almost all cases[3]. Starting HRT early prevents fast bone loss and juvenile osteoporosis during adolescence, when the bone matrix is normally formed. Chronic estrogen deficiency, as found in utreated gonadal dysgenetic cases, is associated with failure of elevation of somatomedin C, normally seen during adolescence.

Cardiovascular anomalies are also very common in children with Turner's syndrome, occurring in more than 30% of these cases,

Table 3 End points of hormone replacement therapy in cases of gonadal dysgenesis

Regulation of menstrual pattern
Induction of secondary sexual characteristics
Optimal final height
Prevention of cardiovascular disease
Prevention of juvenile osteoporosis
Increased endometrial thickness
Increased uterine volume
Future fertility
Increased vaginal thickness
Facilitation of sexual intercourse
Improvement in psychological status
Patient satisfaction with treatment

and usually complicated by the presence of hyperlipedemia[4]. It is now clear that ERT exerts a beneficial effect on lipid metabolism[5,6]. Also, the high plasma levels of endothelin 1–21 (a potent vasoconstrictor factor), found in hypoestrogenic cases and implicated in cardiovascular disease, are shown to be reduced by up to 31% in gonadal dysgenetic patients after ERT[7].

The menstrual pattern is also related to ERT and progesterone use. Adolescents are likely to see at least a sample of bleeding and would like to have the experience of a normal period when talking to peers. Also, HRT assists the increase of uterine volume and endometrial preparation required for future fertility options with ovum donation. Furthermore, HRT increases vaginal thickness and facilitates intercourse. Several of the above effects may be neutralized when a progestogen is added. However, progestogens or micronized progesterone are necessary during ERT to prevent endometrial hyperplasia and atypia. Even when a progesterone is applied, endometrial thickness should be periodically checked by ultrasonography, and the endometrial pattern by regular biopsies. Medroxyprogesterone acetate is the progestogen most often in use.

Young patients under HRT should be carefully screened for the so-called negative effects of treatment. Ultrasonography is considered a useful tool for breast check-up following clinical examination. Mammography and uterine biopsies are considered second-choice examinations, to be used in older women with gonadal dysgenesis, under long-term HRT. Magnetic resonance imaging could be a useful tool. Analysis of the metabolic profile, together with a cardiovascular check-up, should be included in the follow-up of the patients.

There are many reports on the effect of estrogens on the central nervous system. It is believed that HRT assists these patients to overcome early functional brain problems related to estrogen depletion.

Two major problems associated with the presence of gonadal dysgenesis and Turner's syndrome are social and psychological problems. Short stature and amenorrhea as well as 'stigmata' should be discussed with a psychologist. Finally, the problem of compliance should be discussed briefly, since some patients discontinue therapy. To increase compliance, a careful explanation should be given to adolescents and their parents. Compliance is optimal when simple HRT schemes are used and when information is provided in detail. The myths surrounding HRT should be discussed and overcome. It should be stated that there is no high risk of breast cancer. It should also be pointed out that the benefits of HRT outweigh the risks. Parents should reassure the child and assist in the understanding of HRT. It should be emphasized that a Pap smear is to be carried out every year, regardless of the sexual activity of the adolescent. Finally, as has been mentioned, the breasts should be checked by both the physician and the young woman herself, and strong advice should be given to avoid smoking.

Conclusion

It is concluded that the management of gonadal dysgenesis should be undertaken in pediatric and adolescent gynecological centers, where the problem should be examined in collaboration with a pediatric geneticist, a pediatric gynecologist, an endocrinologist and a psychologist, in order to provide the best possible management and follow-up.

References

1. Knudtzon J, Aarskog D, the Norwegian Study Group. Results of 2 years of growth hormone treatment followed by combined growth hormone and estradiol in Turner's syndrome. *Horm Res* 1993;39:7–17
2. Ranke MB, Grauer ML. Adult height in Turner's syndrome. Results of a multinational survey in 1993. *Horm Res* 1994;42:90–4
3. Guleki B, Davies M, Jacobs H. Effect of treatment on established osteoporosis in young women with amenorrhea. *Clin Endocrinol* 1994;41:275–81
4. Mitsibounas DN, Kosmaidou Z, Kontoleon P, *et al*. Hyperlidemia and presence of thyroid autoantibodies in girls with Turner's syndrome or mosiac variance. *J Adolesc Gynecol* 1997;10:133–9
5. Creatsas G, Arefetz N, Adamopoulos PN, *et al*. Transdermal estradiol plus oral medroxyprogesterone acetate replacement therapy in primary amenorrheic adolescents. Clinical, hormonal and metabolic aspects. *Maturitas* 1994;18:105–14
6. Gisternino M, Nahoul K, Borrola M, *et al*. Transdermal estradiol substitution therapy for the induction of puberty in female hypogonadism. *J Endocr Invest* 1991;14:481–8
7. Creatsas G, Malamitsi-Puchner A, Hassan E. Endothelin plasma levels in primary amenorrheic adolescents before and after estrogen treatment. *J Soc Gynecol Invest* 1996;3:350–3

Adrenal dysfunction evaluation and hyperandrogenic states in young postpubertal patients

4

A. Tempone

Introduction

The adrenal glands play an important role during pubertal growth and development. Steroidogenesis in the adrenal glands and ovaries have common enzymatic pathways and therefore the pathophysiology of associated conditions to establish the real source may be unclear. Adrenal hyperandrogenism in most cases is associated with ovarian hyperandrogenism. Postpuberal anovulation appears to be common to both syndromes. In precocious puberty (pubic hair before 8 years), the association of adrenal hyperandrogenism with glucose intolerance and insulin resistance or low insulin sensitivity has been observed[1].

The adrenocorticotropic hormone (ACTH) test is useful to determine enzymatic defects, and the adrenal response is mainly evaluated through the determination of the delta-4/5-17-OH-progesterone, androstendione and pregnenolone curves. Dehydroepiandrosterone (DHEA) and dehydroepiandrosterone sulfate (DHEAS) play important physiological roles during puberty and their dysfution in the postpuberal period may result in adrenal hyperandrogenism. Within 3–5 years after menarche, a spontaneous change occurs from anovulatory to ovulatory cycles[2,3]. If an anovulatory state persists during this period, an increased pulse of luteinizing hormone (LH) and high delta-4-androstendione and testosterone levels[4] are is observed in most cases. Low fertility has been associated with increased levels of androgens during puberty[5].

Very recently, anovulation after precocious puberty was described, associated with ovarian hyperandrogenism related to reduced fetal growth, which would indicate its possible prenatal origin[1]. In some patients with precocious puberty an association between hyperinsulinemic state, ovarian hyperandrogenism and dyslipemia has been described[6–8].

Decreased insulin-like-growth factor binding protein (IGFBP-1) and sex hormone-binding globulin (SHBG) concentrations occur during the physiological pubertal development period with hyperinsulinemia, dyslipemia and ovarian hyperandrogenism, but there are not necessarily any clinical signs of androgen excess. A comparison between early postmenarche (3 years after menarche), late postmenarche and healthy female controls under the ACTH stimulation test showed an increased response to 17-OH-progesterone during the late postmenarche period in some of the precocious puberty group[1].

Mechanisms of hyperandrogenism

LH (bioactive–immunoactive) levels are two to three-fold elevated in approximately 70% of women with hyperandrogenic anovulation, due to increased amplitude and frequency of pulses of LH in comparison with follicle-stimulating hormone (FSH)[9]. This fact reflects in part the consequence of acyclic estrogen production unopposed by progesterone, sensitizing the pituitary to gonadotropin-releasing hormone (GnRH), enhancing GnRH-stimulated LH synthesis and increasing the amount of releasable pituitary LH[10]. The temporary reversal of LH hypersecretion in hyperandrogenic women in response to endogenous or exogenous progesterone also shows hypothalamic–pituitary sensitivity to estrogen negative and positive feedback[11]. This suggests that hyperandrogenic anovulation is the result rather than the cause of chronic anovulation due to some neuroendocrine abnormalities.

The GnRH analog test, by measuring gonadotropin and steroid response to a single injection of GnRH analog given to stimulate pituitary and gonadal secretion[12,13], shows an exaggerated early LH response and a reduced FSH response in patients with hyperandrogenic anovulation[14]. This type of 'masculinized' secretory pattern of LH also occurs in women with congenital adrenal virilizing disorders, (classical congenital adrenal hyperplasia (CAH) and adrenal virilizing carcinoma), which suggests that prenatal androgen exposure irreversibly alters neuroendocrine function[15]. The findings of persistent LH hypersecretion in adult female monkeys exposed prenatally to androgen supports this hypothesis[16].

An exaggerated response to 17-OH-progesterone and androstenedione when GnRH testing hyperandrogenic anovulatory women suggests increased activity of the 17-hydroxylase/17,20-lyase enzyme complex[12], promoting androgen excess in comparison with normal women. In spite of this fact it remains unclear whether ovarian 17-hydroxylase/17,20-lyase hyperactivity is the cause or the result of hyperandrogenism, because sex steroids, inhibin, insulin and insulin-like growth factors may modulate the function of this enzyme. Reduced insulin levels have been shown to diminish the exaggerated 17-OH-progesterone response to GnRH analog testing[17].

Almost 50% of hyperandrogenic anovulatory women have increased serum DHEA and DHEAS levels[18,19]. The ACTH test in some of these patients may show adrenal 17-hydroxylase/17,20-lyase hyperactivity through exaggerated secretion of delta-4-steroids (17-OH-progesterone and androstenedione) and delta-5-steroids (17-OH-pregnenolone 5 (17-OH-P 5) and DHEA)[13].

The adrenal hyperactivity of 17-hydroxylase/17,20-lyase stimulates ovarian hyperandrogenism directly, by similar enzymatic abnormality, and indirectly, because DHEA is a sustrate for ovarian testosterone synthesis.

Control of adrenal androgen secretion

In comparison with other species, the human adrenal gland is unusual in its large secretion of androgens: DHEA, DHEAS, androstenedione. Whereas the secretion of cortisol is regulated by ACTH, aldosterone is modulated by angiotensin and potassium; the control of adrenal androgen secretion is not as well understood. Adrenal androgens may play a role in a variety of physiologic functions including obesity, diabetes, atherosclerosis, immunologic regulation, carcinogenesis, reproduction, metabolism and osteoporosis[20–22].

Adrenal steroids are derived from pregnenolone. A number of steps in the steroidogenic pathway, including the rate-limiting step of conversion from cholesterol to pregnenolone, are catalyzed by cytochrome P450 enzymes, a term given to a family of heme-containing enzymes with characteristic spectral absorbance at 450 nm. These enzymes are part of a mitochondrial electron transport chain involving NADPH, which mediates steroid conversions such as hydroxylation[23]. Other types of cytochrome P450 steroidogenic enzymes are 17α-hydroxylase and C17–20 desmolase, which constitute a single enzyme; 21-hydroxylase; 11-hydroxylase; and 18-hydroxylase. The conversion of 21-carbon steroids (glucocorticoids and progestins) to 19-carbon steroids (androgens) is catalyzed by C17–20 desmolase. Steroids are converted from delta-5 to delta-4, and DHEA to androstenedione, by the microsomal non-P450 enzyme 3β-hydroxysteroid dehydrogenase-isomerase (3β-HSD). The sulfation of DHEA is mediated by steroid sulfotransferase, and the reverse reaction is mediated by steroid sulfatase. DHEA, found in the highest concentration in human circulation, can also be synthesized from sulfated precursors, such as cholesterol sulfate and pregnenolone sulfate[24]. DHEA may also be converted to androstenediol, an adrenal steroid which is unusual in that it has inherent estrogenic bioactivity. Androstenediol binds to SHBG and estrogen receptors[25].

ACTH is widely accepted as a regulating factor for adrenal androgen secretion under certain physiologic and pharmacologic conditions, as shown by studies of ACTH stimulation and dexamethasone suppression. However, whereas ACTH causes an increase in cortisol secretion, its effect on adrenal androgen secretion is variable[26]. Dexamethasone administration has been found to decrease cortisol and adrenal androgen secretion, but often to varying degrees[27]. Although ACTH has a role in the modulation of adrenal secretion, there is evidence that indicates that there are other mechanisms or substances which either act in synergy or interact with ACTH in the regulation of adrenal secretion.

Physiological adrenal androgen production

Fetal adrenal

The cortex of the fetal adrenal gland is the source of large quantities of androgens and estrogen precursors, and, at birth, weighs approximately the same as the adult adrenal gland because of a large fetal zone, which occupies 80% of its volume. However, the fetal adrenal, in the presence of ACTH, prolactin and growth hormones, involutes after birth, showing a sharp decrease in DHEA concentrations, which are four times higher at birth than cortisol concentrations. The decrease of DHEA secretion persists until adrenarche and is unaccompanied by similar changes in cortisol metabolism[28].

Adrenarche

Adrenarche precedes gonadarche in both sexes. From the ages of 6 to 8 years onwards, ahead of any increase in circulating gonadotropin levels, adrenal androgen concentration and excretion begin to increase. This occurs while cortisol concentration, production and secretion remain stable and constant. DHEA, DHEAS, and androstenedione increase during adrenarche. The increase in DHEA/cortisol ratio continues during puberty[29].

Puberty

GnRH activation of the pituitary–gonadal axis by pubertal secretion produces an elevation in the concentrations of testosterone and estradiol. At this time DHEA, DHEAS and androstenedione also increase. These changes are independent of basal ACTH concentration[30]. The increase in DHEA levels appears to be related to bone age, in contrast to the absence of corresponding changes in concentration of cortisol and ACTH. Acute ACTH stimulation during puberty produces a disproportionate elevation in androstenedione/cortisol and DHEA/cortisol ratios, which suggests an increased adrenal sensitivity to ACTH with still no clear etiology[31].

Serum SHBG decreases gradually with age before the clinical onset of puberty[32]. At the same time, serum non-SHBG-bound (bioavailable) testosterone and estradiol increase with age. Therefore, with advancing age there is a progressive increase in the exposure of all tissue to androgens in normal subjects before the onset of puberty. The same applies to serum non-SHBG bound estradiol levels before puberty. In conclusion, low doses of bioavailable androgen and estrogen play an important role before puberty in tissue maturation[33].

Association with adrenal androgen dysfunction

Insulin-like growth factor-1

Steroidogenesis abnormalities are consistent with exaggerated P450c17α activity resulting in increased 17-hydroxylase and/or 17,20 lyase activity and androgen excess. However, the cause of increased activity remains unknown[32,33].

Although a polymorphism has been found in the CYP17 gene promoter, which codes the P450c17α enzyme, prevalence of alleles A1 and A2 in hyperandrogenic women are similar to normal controls[34] and no evidence of other potential functional variants within CYP17 have been demonstrated in gene screening. Others factors may be implicated in the dysregulation of P450c17α. In the regulation of adrenal and ovarian steroideogenesis, growth factors may be relevant, having a role in functional androgen excess.

Growth hormone (GH) and insulin-like growth factor-1 (IGF-1) modulate ovarian function. All elements of the IGF system are present in the ovary; IGF-1 appears to amplify LH-mediated upregulation of P450c17α mRNA, enzyme levels and androgen synthesis[35]. Both IGF-1 and IGF-2 stimulate androgen production in human adrenocortical cells, activating the type 1 IGF receptor[36]. Insulin, which plays a very important role in the development of androgen excess, possibly enhances P450c17α activity[37].

Two different tests could be applied to try to distinguish the origin of ovarian or adrenal androgens: the GnRH analog test and the ACTH test. Various publications feature this type of test, with interpretation of the adrenal response to 1–24 ACTH and ovarian response to GnRH agonist, and the correlation of different steroid response ratios and precursor ratios to evaluate adrenal enzymatic activity, and serum IGF-1, IGFBP-3, GH, insulin, insulin/glucose ratio in hyperandrogenic patients vs. normal controls. Escobar-Morreale et al.[38] and other authors have described that the delta androstenedione/delta-progesterone ratio signifies overall P450c17α activity, delta-17-OH-progesterone/progesterone ratio represents delta-4-17-hydroxylase activity, the delta-androstenedione/delta 17-OH-progesterone and delta-androstenedione/delta-cortisol ratios were used to assess delta-4-17, 20-lyase activity, the delta-17-OH-progesterone/delta-cortisol ratio signifies 21α- and 11β-hydroxylase activity, and the delta-11-deoxycortisol/delta-cortisol ratio reflects 11β-hydroxylase activity.

From these data we conclude that the possible involvement of the IGF-1 axis in the pathogenesis remains controversial[39]. When free androgen and free testosterone remain elevated after gonadal suppression, these patients appear to have a mainly adrenal component in their androgen excess, having a two-fold increase in serum IGF-1 concentration, in comparison with patients with ovarian hyperandrogenism and idiopathic hirsutism or controls. IGFBP-3 concentrations are decreased in ovarian hyperandrogenism[39].

Estrogens and growth factors

Adrenal hyperandrogenism is a prevalent feature in many women with polycystic ovary syndrome (PCOS). Although a lot of studies have been carried out, its pathogenesis remains unclear. Hyperestrogenism and hyperinsulinism were studied in most of the investigations in relation to this syndrome. Very interesting results were obtained by Carmina et al.[40] who demonstrated in patients with PCOS that all androgen levels were elevated as well as unbound estradiol, insulin, and non-IGFBP-1 bound IGF-1 in comparison with matched ovulatory controls. A positive correlation was observed between estrogen and basal ACTH stimulated delta-5 adrenal androgens.

Insulin showed a strong correlation with the delta-4 pathway and androstenedione in particular. Serum IGF-1 was correlated with basal DHEAS only. Androstenedione was increased under hyperinsulinemic conditions by the activity of 17,20-lyase. It is suggested that estrogen may have a greater influence on enhancing delta-5 androgen secretion, and insulin a greater effect on the delta-4 pathway. IGF-2 does not correlate with androgen concentration, suggesting it may have a paracrine or direct role in adrenal androgen regulation[41]. These extra-adrenal hormones may induce adrenal hyperandrogenism in different ways. The use of steroids ratios to evaluate true enzymatic activities should be used with some caution.

In summary the data support a role for the IGF axis in the development of hirsutism, particularly, but not exclusively, in young women with functional adrenal hyperandrogenism. Whether the IGF axis effects a primary event or has a permissive role in the development of this disorder remains to be elucidated.

Corticotropin-releasing hormone

Corticotropin-releasing hormone (CRH) has been found to be a potent adrenal secretagogue in adolescents with hyperandrogenism after precocious puberty. In patients who have been pretreated with dexamethasone, CRH infusion produces a modest rise in serum ACTH, a consistent increment of cortisol, and striking increase in DHEA, DHEAS, and andro-stenedione. These marked responses are unlikely to be attributable solely to ACTH[42,43].

Ibañez et al.[44] have described the immediate CRH effects on adrenal androgen release in healthy young men, postulating CRH as a candidate for the role of endogenous adjuvant adrenal androgen secretagogue. CRH receptors are present in the zona reticularis, which develops at the interphase of adrenal cortex and medulla[45]. Adrenomedullary chromaffin cells are present in the whole adrenal cortex and have been shown recently by Ehrhart-Bornstein et al.[46] to secrete CRH and ACTH, among others neuropeptides. Secretory chromaffin cells are potent stimulators of adrenocortical steroideogenesis. It is acceptable that the main source of CRH during the adrenarche period could be the adrenal medulla. CRH and ACTH are secreted by the hypothalamic–pituitary axis possibly in parallel within the zona reticularis.

Petraglia et al.[47] in rats and Olster and Ferin[48] in ovariectomized rhesus monkeys showed the inhibition of GnRH by CRH from the hypothamic–pituitary circulation. In summary, CRH has been found to be a potent adrenal androgen secretagogue in adolescent girls with hyperandrogenism after precocious puberty.

Molecular basis of adrenal dysfunction

When patients have signs of suspicious adrenal androgen hyperfunction (clinical and laboratory), the ACTH test is indicated to evaluate the delta-4/delta-5 enzymatic defect. 21-Hydroxylase deficiency and 3β-hydroxysteroid dehydrogenase deficiency are among the most common causes. Recent molecular advances have provided the genetic basis for the phenotypic variability in CAH, a means for accurately genotyping family members of CAH patients including prenatal prediction of the fetus genotype, and have helped to focus the hormonal criteria for the spectrum of CAH disorders. In addition, biochemical advances have allowed the therapeutic monitoring of these patients.

Current treatment methods, however, may not be optimal for achieving normal genetic height and appropiate weight in CAH patients, and more effective approaches to CAH therapy remain to be explored[49]. As an example, CYP21B and CYP21A gene were mapped within the HLA complex[50], and a mutation reported in the CYP21B gene from the alleles of patients from five populations. Type II 3β-HSD gene structure and a mutation in type II 3β-HSD were described in 3β-HSD deficiency[51].

Conclusion

Adrenal androgen hyperactivity is the most common clinical and metabolic condition associated with patients with oligomenorrhea, anovulation, hirsutism or fertility problems from probably the fetal period through adolescence up to the adult period. In part, the pattern of adrenal secretion is regulated by ACTH, analogous to the control of cortisol. In various instances, including adrenarche, puberty, aging and severe illness, androgen adrenal secretion and cortisol diverge for reasons that are still unclear. Intra-adrenal factors may modulate adrenal androgen secretion. These include the availability of cofactors of steroideogenesis enzymes, and the intrinsic properties of enzymes or adrenal cells. These mechanism may be modified in turn by exogenous factors to the gland.

There is evidence for a regulatory role of GH, IGF-1, gonadotropins, non-bound and bound estrogens and androgens, insulin, CRH, prostaglandins, etc., and pituitary or extrapituitary subtances may also have a role in the control of adrenal androgen secretion. There is evidence for the inability of ACTH to maintain a normal adrenal androgen/cortisol ratio in adrenal suppressed patients. The heterogeneous nature of adrenal hyperandrogenism means that further studies are required to understand more fully this complex syndrome.

References

1. Ibañez L, Potau N, Virclis R, *et al*. Postpuberal outcome in girls diagnosed of premature pubarche during childhood. *J Clin Endrocrinol Metab* 1993;76:1599–603
2. Apter D. Serum steroids and pituitary hormones in female puberty. *Clin Endocrinol (Oxf)* 1980;12:107–20
3. Metcalf MG, Skidmore DS, Lowry GF, *et al*. Incidence of ovulation in the years after the menarche. *J Endocrinol* 1983;97:213–9
4. Venturoli S, Porcus E, Fabbri R, *et al*. Longitudinal evaluation of the different gonadotropin pulsatile patterns in anovulatory cycles of young girls. *J Clin Endocrinol Metab* 1992;74:836–41
5. Apter D, Vihko R. Endocrine determinants of fertility: serum androgen concentration during follow up of adolescents into the 3rd decade of life. *J Clin Endocrinol Metab* 1990;71:836–41
6. Ibañez L, Potau N, Zampolli M, *et al*. Hyperinsulinemia, and decreased insulin-like growth factor binding protein-1 are common features in prepubertal and pubertal girls with a history of premature pubarche. *J Clin Endocrinol Metab* 1997;82:2283–8
7. Ibañez L, Potau N, Chacon P, *et al*. Hyperinsulinemia, dyslipaemia and cardiovascular risk in girls with a history of premature pubarche. *Diabetologia* 1998;41:1057–63
8. Ibañez L, Potau N, Francois J, *et al*. Precocious pubarche, hyperinsulinism, and ovarian hyperandrogenism in girls: relation to reduced fetal growth. *J Clin Endocrinol Metab* 1998;83:3558–62
9. Rebar RW. Gonadotropin secretion in PCOD. *Semin Reprod Endocrinol* 1984;23:223
10. Speroff L, *et al. Clinical Gynecology Endocrinology and Infertility*, 5th edn. Baltimore: Williams & Wilkins, 1994
11. Rebar RW, Judd HL, Yen SS, *et al*. Characterization of the inappropiate gonadotropin secretion in polycystic ovary syndrome. *J Clin Invest* 1976;57:1320–9
12. Ehrmann DA, Barnes RB, Rosenfield RL. Polycystic ovary syndrome as a form of functional ovarian hyperandrogenism due to dysregulation of androgen secretion. *Endocr Rev* 1995;16:322–53
13. Ehrmann DA, Rosenfield RL, Barnes RB, *et al*. Detection of functional ovarian hyperandrogenism in women with androgen excess. *N Engl J Med* 1992;327:157–62
14. Rosenfield RL, Barnes RB, Cara JF. Dysregulation of cytochrome P450c17a as the cause of polycystic ovarian syndrome. *Fertil Steril* 1990;53:785–91
15. Barnes RB, Rosenfield RL, Ehrmann DA, *et al*. Ovarian hyperandrogenism as a result of congenital adrenal virilizing disorders: Evidence for perinatal masculinization of neuroendocrine function in women. *J Clin Endocrinol Metab* 1994;79:1328–33
16. Dumesic DA, Abbott DH, Eisner JR, *et al*. Prenatal exposure of female rhesus monkeys to testosterone propionate increases serum luteinizing hormone levels in adulthood. *Fertil Steril* 1997;67:155–63
17. Jacubowicz DJ, Nestler JE. 17α-hydroxyprogesterone responses to leuprolide and serum androgen in obese women with and without polycystic ovary syndrome after dietary weight loss. *J Clin Endocrinol Metab* 1997;82:556–60
18. Hoffman DL, Klove K, Lobo RA. The prevalence and significance of elevated DHEA-S levels in anovulatory women. *Fertil Steril* 1984;42:76–81
19. Maroulis GB, *et al*. Diagnostic test in hirsutism. In Mahesh VB, Greenblatt RB, eds. *Hirsutism and Virilism: Pathogenesis, Diagnosis*

and Management. Boston: John Wright PSG, 1983:295

20. Barrett-Connor, Kaaw KT. Absence of an inverse relation of dehydroepiandrosterone sulfate with cardiovascular mortality in postmenopausal women. *N Engl J Med* 1987;317:711

21. Mortola J, Yen SS. The effects of oral DHA on endocrine and metabolic parameters in post-menopausal women. *J Clin Endocrinol Metab* 1990;71:696–704

22. Parker L. What is the biological role of adrenal androgen? In *Adrenal Androgens in Clinical Medicine*. San Diego: Academic Press, 1989:483

23. Miller WL. Molecular biology of steroid hormone synthesis. *Endocr Rev* 1988;9:295–318

24. Lieberman S, Greenfield NJ, Wolfson A. A heuristic proposal for understanding steroidogenic processes. *Endocr Rev* 1984;5:128–48

25. Kalimi M, *et al.* Physicochemical characterization of DHEA binding in rat liver. *Biochem Biophys Res Commun* 1988;156:22

26. Nieschlag E, Loriaux DL, Ruder HJ, *et al.* The secretion of DHEA and DHEAS in man. *J Endocrinol* 1973;57:123–34

27. Branchaud C, Goodyer CG, Hall CS, *et al.* Steroidogenic activity of hACTH and related peptides on the human neocortex and fetal adrenal cortex in organ culture. *Steroids* 1978; 31:557–72

28. De Peretti E, Forest MG. Patterns of plasma DHAS levels in humans from birth to adulthood: evidence for testicular production. *J Clin Endocrinol Metab* 1978;47:572–7

29. Babalola A, Ellis G. Serum DHAS in a normal pediatric population. *Clin Biochem* 1985; 18:184–9

30. Apter D, Pakarinen A, Hammond GL, *et al.* Adrenocortical function in puberty. *Acta Paediatr Scand* 1979;68:599–604

31. Genazzani A, Pintor C, Facchinetti F, *et al.* Changes throughout puberty in adrenal secretion after ACTH. *J Steroid Biochem* 1979;11: 571–7

32. Belgorosky A, Rivarola MA. Progressive decrease in serum sex hormone-binding globulin from infancy to late prepuberty in boys. *J Clin Endocrinol Metab* 1986;63:510–2

33. Belgorosky A, Rivarola MA. Progressive increase in non SHBG bound-testosterone and estradiol from infancy to late prepuberty in girls. *J Clin Endocrinol Metab* 1988;67:234–7

34. Escobar-Morreale HF, Serrano-Gotarredona J, Garcia-Robles R, *et al.* Lack of an ovarian function influence on the increased adrenal androgen secretion present in women with functional ovarian hyperandrogenism. *Fertil Steril* 1997;67:654–62

35. Ehrmann DA, Barns RB, Rosenfield RL. Polycystic ovary syndrome as a form of functional ovarian hyperandrogenism due to dysregulation of androgen secretion. *Endocr Rev* 1995;16:322–53

36. Techatraisk K, Conway ES, Ramsby E, *et al.* Frequency of a polymorphism in the regulatory region of the 17ª-hydroxylase (CYP 17) gene in hyperandrogenic states. *Clin Endocrinol* 1997;46:131

37. Mesiano S, Katz SL, Lee JY, *et al.* Insulin-like growth factors augment steroid production and expression of steroideogenesis enzymes in human fetal adrenal cortical cells: implications for adrenal androgen regulation. *J Clin Endocrinol Metab* 1997;82:1390–6

38. Escobar-Morreale HF, Serrano-Gotarredona J, Garcia-Robles R, *et al.* Abnormalities in the serum insulin-like growth factor-1 axis in women with hyperandrogenism. *Fertil Steril* 1998;70:1090–100

39. Nestler JE, Jakubowicz DL. Decrease in ovarian cytochrome P450c17 alpha activity and serum free testosterone after reduction of insulin secretion in polycystic ovary syndrome. *N Engl J Med* 1996;335:617–23

40. Carmina E, Gonzales F, Vidali A, *et al.* The contribution of estrogen and growth factors to increased adrenal androgen secretion in PCO syndrome. *Hum Reprod* 1999;14:307

41. Smith R, Mesiano S, Chan EC, *et al.* Corticotropin-releasing hormone directly and preferentially stimulates dehydroepiandrosterone sulfate secretion by human fetal adrenal cortical cells. *J Clin Endocrinol Metab* 1998;83:2916–20

42. Bridges NA, Hindmarsh PC, Pringle PJ, *et al.* Cortisol, androstenedione (A4), dehydro-epiandrosterone sulphate (DHEAS) and 17 hydroxyprogesterone (17OHP) responses to low doses of (1–24)ACTH. *J Clin Endocrinol Metab* 1998;83:3750–3

43. Ambrosi B, Barbetta L, Re T, *et al.* The one microgram adrenocorticotropin test in the assessment of hypothalamic-pituitary-adrenal function. *Eur J Endocrinol* 1998;139:575–9

44. Ibanez L, Potau N, Marcos MV, de Zegher F. Corticotropin-releasing hormone: a potent androgen secretagogue in girls with hyperandrogenism after precocious pubarche. *J Clin Endocrinol Metab* 1999;84:4602–6

45. Grombach MK, Styne DM. Puberty: ontogeny, neuroendocrinology, physiology and disorders. In Wilson JD, Foster DN, Krokenberg HM, Larsen PR, eds. Williams Textbook of Endocrinology, 9th edition. Philadelphia: WB Saunders Co., 1998;1548–50

46. Ehrhart-Bornstein M, Hinson JP, Bornstein SR, *et al.* Intraadrenal interactions in the regulation of adrenocortical steroidogenesis. *Endocr Rev* 1998;19:101–43

47. Petraglia F, Sutton S, Vale W, Plotsky P. Corticotropin-releasing factor decreases plasma luteinizing hormone levels in female rats by inhibiting gonadotropin-releasing hormone release into hypophysial-portal circulation. *Endocrinology* 1987;120:1083–8

48. Olster DH, Ferin M. Corticotropin-releasing hormone inhibits gonadotropin secretion in the ovariectomized rhesus monkey. *J Clin Endocrinol Metab* 1987;65:262–7

49. Songya P. Congenital Adrenal Hyperplasia, Diagnosis Evaluation Update *Endocrinol Metab Clin N Am* 1997;1997

50. Azzis R, Wells G, Zacur HA, *et al.* Abnormalities of 21-hydroxylase gene ratio and adrenal steroideogenesis in hyperandrogenic women. *J Clin Endocrinol Metab* 1991;73:1327–31

51. Labrie F, *et al.* Structure, function and tissue-specific gene expression of 3B-HSD/5ene-4ene isomerase enzymes. *J Steroid Biochem Mol Biol* 1992;43:805

Differential steroidogenic effect of pituitary hormones in primate corpus luteum

5

L. Devoto, P. Kohen, O. Castro, A. Palomino and M. Vega

Introduction

Luteal steroidogenesis requires precise regulation to sustain ovarian cyclicity and development of endometrial receptivity. Progesterone derived from the corpus luteum (CL) and subsequently from the trophoblast is essential for maintenance of gestation. Primate CL retains the ability to produce estrogens, distinguishing it from the CL of domestic animals and rodent species. However, the exact nature of the essential action of estrogen during the luteal phase has not been well defined.

The observation that human luteal cells express specific receptors for luteinizing hormone (LH), follicle-stimulating hormone (FSH), human prolactin (hPRL) and growth hormone (GH) suggests a physiological role of these peptides in luteal function[1–4]. Nevertheless, the production of steroid hormones is largely dependent on pituitary-derived LH, acting through the cyclic adenosine monophosphate (cAMP) second messenger signaling system to regulate genes essential for hormone synthesis and luteal development. Even though LH is essential for the development and maintenance of the primate CL, luteal regression is not due to changes in LH pulse frequency or amplitude[5]. This suggests that the actions of LH are regulated by intraluteal factors. Indeed, the effects of LH and human chorionic gonadotropin (hCG) on luteal cells' steroidogenesis are modified by a variety of molecules encompassing growth factors, peptide and steroid hormones, nitric oxide, cytokines and insulin-like growth factor (IGF) binding proteins[6].

On the other hand, luteal phase inadequacy has been implicated as a cause of both infertility and early pregnancy loss. However, incidence rates vary depending on the populations studied and the method of diagnosis employed. Published estimates suggest that luteal phase inadequacy affects 25–35% of those presenting with habitual abortion[7]. Understanding the mechanisms that govern the steroidogenic changes that occur during the human luteal phase is important for defining therapeutic strategies that might either assist or prevent fertility.

Effect of FSH in human luteal steroidogenesis

It is well established that estradiol synthesis by granulosa cells of the ovarian follicle is stimulated by FSH. Unique to the CL of many primates, including the human, is the secretion of a significant amount of androgens and estradiol. It is well known that androgens are an essential substrate for estrogen biosynthesis. The enzyme catalyzing androgen synthesis, 17α hydrolase/17,20 lyase (P450$_{c17}$), is located in luteal cells near the periphery of the gland along the vascular tract. In contrast, luteal cells stained for aromatase (P450$_{arom}$) are observed throughout the luteal parenchyma[8]. Moreover, large luteal cells in culture release significantly greater amounts of estrogens than small cells in the presence of androstenedione or testosterone, suggesting greater aromatization capability of large luteal cells[9].

These immunohistochemical and functional characteristics of the human luteal cells are consistent with the two-cell model of luteal estradiol biosynthesis. Interestingly, FSH did not stimulate estradiol synthesis by luteal cells in culture or sustain luteal steroidogenesis *in vivo*[10]. Thus, although the two-cell system for estrogen production is retained after luteinization of the follicle, the role of FSH in the stimulation of androgen aromatization is not conserved. The action of FSH is evidently subserved by LH and IGF-1, which can sustain estradiol synthesis by luteal cells in culture[11].

Effect of prolactin in human luteal steroidogenesis

Biochemical studies have shown that prolactin receptors are located in human luteal cells. The examination of the 24-hour pattern of serum hPRL levels throughout the menstrual cycle displays a clear trend of increasing hPRL from the early follicular to late luteal phase[12]. However, the role of hPRL in normal ovarian function is poorly understood. Systemic suppression of pituitary hPRL secretion during the luteal phase with bromocriptine yields conflicting results with both normal cycles and luteal insufficiency[13,14].

Hyperprolactinemia can interrupt normal ovarian function through a variety of mechanisms. Hyperprolactinemic patients have low gonadotropin pulses resulting in absence of, or inadequate, follicular development and luteal steroidogenesis. In addition, luteinization of granulosa cells and progesterone production by luteal cells *in vitro* may be negatively affected by very high concentrations of prolactin[15].

The fact that ovulation induction can be successfully achieved with pulsatile gonadotropin-releasing hormone or human menopausal gonadotropin and hCG in hyperprolactinemic patients argues for a neuroendocrine, rather than an ovarian-dependent, suppression of steroidogenesis.

Effect of growth hormone in luteal steroidogenesis

Growth hormone is a pituitary hormone necessary for growth and development. It is, however, also involved in sexual differentiation and pubertal maturation. Many of the effects of GH are mediated by insulin-like growth factor (IGF)-1, which is predominantly synthesized in the liver. However, IGFs and IGF-binding proteins are produced in luteal tissue, and may act in a paracrine-autocrine manner[16,17]. Moreover, IGF-1 synergizes with LH and FSH to stimulate growth, differentiation and steroidogenesis of ovarian follicular cells.

There are species differences in the effects of GH in reproductive biology. In most species, including the human being, GH receptor is expressed within the CL, where GH may elicit a direct stimulation on luteal steroidogenesis. However, IGF-1 antibody diminishes the GH-induced steroidogenic effect in cultured human luteal cells, suggesting that IGF-1 mediates the positive GH action on steroid biosynthesis. On the other hand, the direct effects of GH on luteal cell progesterone synthesis are moderate compared with those of IGF-1[18]. This information suggests that GH could influence luteal steroidogenesis through different systems and mechanisms.

Effect of LH/hCG in luteal steroidogenesis

Pituitary-derived LH is essential for steroid biosynthesis and luteal development. During the cycle of conception, trophoblastic production of hCG prevents the regression of the CL. LH/hCG binds to and activates a specific glycoprotein hormone receptor on the membrane of the steroidogenic cells, initiating a cAMP second messenger signaling system that regulates processes essential for steroid synthesis, including the uptake of lipoprotein-carried cholesterol, cholesterol translocation to the inner mitochondrial membrane and the expression of several steroidogenic enzymes, comprising cytocrome side-chain cleavage ($P_{450\ scc}$) and 3β-hydroxy-steroid dehydrogenase (3β-HSD).

Numerous investigators have demonstrated the presence of LH/hCG receptor mRNA and protein within the CL. It was found that LH receptor did not display significant changes throughout the life span of the CL[1]. This finding suggests that steroidogenic function and regression of the CL are determined by factors downstream of the LH/hCG receptor. Cholesterol is converted into pregnenolone in the cholesterol side-chain cleavage reaction, which is catalyzed by $P_{450\ scc}$. This enzyme complex is primarily driven by LH; however, it shows a relatively constant expression within the CL throughout the luteal phase. In spite of the fact that 3β-HSD mRNA changes in response to trophic hormones, levels of this enzyme are probably in excess of that needed to convert pregnenolone to progesterone. Consequently, it is unlikely that these enzymes affect the amount of progesterone produced by the CL[19].

The steroidogenic acute regulatory protein (StAR) governs the rate-limiting step in steroidogenesis, which is the translocation of cholesterol from the outer to the inner mitochondrial membrane[20]. Thus, to understand the significant steroidogenic changes that occur during the human luteal phase, it is important to define StAR gene expression within the CL. The process of luteinization is associated with a dramatic up-regulation of StAR in granulosa-lutein cells. We confirmed the findings of Chung et al.[21] and Duncan et al.[22] that the 1.6 transcript is the dominant StAR mRNA expressed in the human CL throughout the luteal phase. Moreover, our data illustrate that StAR mRNA is most abundant during the early- and mid-luteal phases and declines significantly in the late-luteal phase.

Western blot analysis showed that the mature StAR (30 kDa) mitochondrial protein was the most abundant species within the CL throughout the luteal phase. The mature StAR (30 kDa) protein decreased significantly during the late-luteal phase, following the pattern of StAR mRNA. The levels of the 37 kDa preprotein changed in a similar pattern. In addition, a high correlation coefficient between the 30 kDa StAR protein within the CL and plasma concentration of progesterone was detected. This finding is consistent with the hypothesis that StAR protein plays a key role in regulating luteal progesterone output.

Taken together, these data indicate that changes in the level of StAR mRNA, whose expression is controlled by LH, most probably account for the cyclic pattern of progesterone production. Although the agents causing regression of the CL in a non-fertile cycle are not fully defined, intraluteal growth factors, and cytokines that modify the action of LH, are candidate molecules to govern the reduction of StAR expression and the fall in progesterone production.

Acknowledgements

This work was supported in part by Fondecyt Grant 1-99-0042.

References

1. Duncan WC, McNeilly AS, Fraser HM, et al. Luteinizing hormone receptor in the human corpus luteum: lack of down-regulation during maternal recognition of pregnancy. *Human Reprod* 1996;11:2291–7
2. Bramley TE, Stirling D, Swantson IA, et al. Specific binding sites for gonadotrophin-releasing hormone, LH/chorionic gonadotrophin, low-density lipoprotein, prolactin and FSH in homogenates of human corpus luteum. II. Concentrations throughout the luteal phase of the menstrual cycle and early pregnancy. *J Endocrinol* 1987;113:317
3. Ben-David M, Schenker JG. Human ovarian receptors to human prolactin: implications in fertility. *Fertil Steril* 1982;38:182–6
4. Sharara FI, Nieman LK. Identification and cellular localization of growth hormone receptor gene expression in the human ovary. *J Clin Endocrinol Metabolism* 1994;79:670–2

5. Hutchison JS, Zeleznik AJ. Effects of different gonadotropin pulse frequencies on corpus luteum function during the menstrual cycle of the rhesus monkey. *Endocrinology* 1986;119:1965–71

6. Devoto L, Vega M, Kohen P, *et al.* Endocrine and paracrine-autocrine regulation of the human corpus luteum during the mid-luteal phase. *J Reprod Fertil,* 2000;55(Supp):13–20

7. Brodie LB, Wentz AC. An update on the clinical relevance of luteal phase inadequacy. *Seminar in Reprod Endocrinol* 1989;7(2):138–9

8. Sanders SL, Stouffer RL. Localization of steroidogenic enzymes in macaque luteal tissue during the menstrual cycle and simulated early pregnancy: Immunohistochemical evidence supporting the two-cell model for estrogen production in the primate corpus luteum. *Biol Reprod* 1997;56:1077–87

9. Ohara A, Mori T, Taii S, *et al.* Functional differentiation in steroidogenesis of two types of luteal cells isolated from mature human corpora lutea of menstrual cycle. *J Clin Endocrinol Metab* 1987;65:1192–200

10. Devoto L, Vega M, Navarro V, *et al.* Regulation of steroid hormone synthesis by human corpora lutea: failure of follicle-stimulating hormone to support steroidogenesis *in vivo* and *in vitro. Fertil Steril* 1989;51:628–33

11. Johnson C, Devoto L, Retamales I, *et al.* Localization of insulin-like growth factor (IGF-I) and IGF-I receptor expression in human corpora lutea: role on estradiol secretion. *Fertil Steril* 1996;65:489–94

12. Brumsted JR, Riddick DH. Prolactin and the human menstrual cycle. *Seminar Reprod Endocrinol* 1992;10(3):220–7

13. Del Pozo E, Goldstein M, Friesen H, *et al.* Lack of action of prolactin suppression on the regulation of the human menstrual cycle. *Am J Obstet Gynecol* 1975;123:719

14. Schultz KD, Geiger W, Del Pozo E, *et al.* Pattern of sexual steroids, prolactin and gonadotropic hormones during prolactin inhibition in normally cycling women. *Am J Obstet Gynecol* 1978;132:561

15. Soto EA, Tureck RW, Strauss JF III. Effects of prolactin on progestin secretion by human granulosa cells in culture. *Biol Reprod* 1985;32:541–5

16. Apa R, Di Simone N, Ronsisvalle E, *et al.* Insulin-like growth factor (IGF)-I and IGF-II stimulate progesterone production by human luteal cells: role of IGF-I as mediator of growth hormone action. *Fertil Steril* 1996;66(2):235–9

17. Fraser HM, Lunn SF, Kim H, *et al.* Changes in insulin-like growth factor binding protein-3 messenger ribonucleic acid in endothelial cells of the human corpus luteum: A possible role in luteal development and rescue. *J Clin Endocrinol Metab* 2000;85:1672–7

18. Devoto L, Kohen P, Castro O, *et al.* Multihormonal regulation of progesterone synthesis in cultured human midluteal cells. *J Clin Endocrinol Metab* 1995;80:1566–70

19. Strauss JF III, Penning TM. Synthesis of the sex steroid hormones: molecular and structural biology with application to clinical practice. In Fauser BCJM, Rutherford AJ, Strauss JF III, *et al.*, eds. *Molecular Biology in Reproductive Medicine.* New York: Parthenon Publishing, 1999:201–32

20. Strauss JF III, Kallen CB, Christenson LK, *et al.* The steroidogenic acute regulatory protein (StAR): a window into the complexities of intracellular cholesterol trafficking. *Recent Prog Horm Res* 1999;54:369–95

21. Chung PH, Sandhoff TW, McLean MP. Hormone and Prostaglandin F2α regulation of messenger ribonucleic acid encoding steroidogenic acute regulatory protein in human corpora lutea. *Endocrine* 1998;8:153–160

22. Duncan WC, Cowen GM, Illingworth J. Steroidogenic enzyme expression in human corpora lutea in the presence and absence of exogenous human chorionic gonadotropin (HCG). *Molec Human Reprod* 1999;5:291–8

Does a genetic factor cause increased thecal androgen secretion in polycystic ovary syndrome?

6

J. F. Strauss III, J. R. Wood, L. K. Christenson and J. M. McAllister

Introduction

Polycystic ovary syndrome (PCOS) is a common endocrine disorder, which affects 5–10% of premenopausal women[1]. The reproductive and endocrine abnormalities in women with PCOS include anovulation/oligo-ovulation, infertility, hirsutism and acne resulting from increased levels of bioavailable testosterone, due at least in part to increased production of androgens by the ovaries[1]. The presence of multiple follicular cysts (≥ 8 follicles with diameters of less than 10 mm) on the ovary, while indicative of the syndrome, is not intrinsically linked to the metabolic disturbances of PCOS, as women with polycystic ovary morphology can have normal androgen levels and regular ovulatory cycles[2,3]. Consequently, the currently recommended diagnostic criteria for PCOS are elevated serum androgen levels or symptoms of hyperandrogenism, and ovulatory dysfunction (≤ 6 menses/year), after exclusion of other diseases such as adrenal 21-hydroxylase deficiency, hyperprolactinemia and androgen-secreting neoplasms[4].

Women with PCOS also have an increased incidence of insulin resistance and obesity resulting in an increased risk of type 2 diabetes mellitus[5]. The role of insulin, insulin-like growth factors (IGF), insulin/IGF receptors and IGF-binding proteins in the etiology of PCOS has been widely studied, as discussed below. Likewise, because the hypothalamic–pituitary–ovarian axis plays an essential role in the stimulation of thecal androgen biosynthesis, and because suppression of luteinizing hormone (LH) secretion can ameliorate the symptoms of hyperandrogenism, LH secretion and receptor function have been scrutinized in PCOS patients[6]. Additionally, while it is apparent that there is a genetic component to PCOS[1], the mechanisms for the reproductive and metabolic dysfunctions related to this disorder remain unclear.

Although there is general agreement that the primary site of androgen synthesis resulting in the hyperandrogenemia of PCOS is the ovary, specifically the theca cells of the multiple cystic follicles, the molecular and cellular mechanisms that underlie the increase in thecal androgen production are not known. Moreover, there is still debate as to whether the excess thecal androgen synthesis is the result of an intrinsic theca cell abnormality or a secondary consequence of endocrine dysfunction in other organs, e.g. increased LH levels or increased insulin levels. Here we will discuss the current understanding of the molecular basis of the hyperandrogenemia associated with PCOS, the cardinal feature of this syndrome, and review strategies to identify underlying genetic factors that lead to increased thecal androgen synthesis.

Hyperandrogenemia

A prospective study of the first-degree relatives of women diagnosed with PCOS revealed that nearly 50% of the sisters whose phenotype could be ascertained had elevated total or bioavailable testosterone[1]. Analysis of the levels of bioavailable testosterone of the sisters of PCOS women suggests a bimodal distribution, with one peak approximating that of a normal, age and body mass index-matched control population with regular menses and a second peak at a higher mean bioavailable testosterone level. Two significant conclusions emerged from this study: (1) hyperandrogenemia clusters in families; and (2) hyperandrogenemia appears to be a dominant genetic trait.

Ovarian androgen production takes place primarily in the theca cells of antral follicles. Gilling-Smith *et al.*[7] reported that primary cultures of freshly isolated theca cells from PCOS ovaries produce more dehydroepiandrosterone, progesterone, 17α-hydroxyprogesterone (17OH-progesterone) and androstenedione than theca cells isolated from normal ovaries. It is important to note that not only overproduction of androgens but also progestins in PCOS theca cells was observed in this study. This would suggest that an abnormality in the key enzyme governing androgen formation, 17α-hydroxylase/ 17,20 lyase (CYP17), could not account for the differences between the normal and PCOS theca cells. However, because the cells were studied almost immediately after isolation from the ovaries, it was not possible to determine whether their steroidogenic activity reflected a primary ovarian defect as opposed to the memory of their prior *in vivo* exposure to gonadotropins.

Using a novel system of propagating human theca cells in long-term culture isolated from size-matched follicles from ovaries of normal and PCOS women, we have shown that enhanced production of progesterone, 17OH-progesterone, and testosterone is a persistent biochemical phenotype of PCOS theca cells[8]. The differences in steroidogenic output between normal and PCOS theca cells was accentuated by treatment with the adenyl cyclase activator forskolin. The concentration of forskolin required to achieve half-maximal stimulation of steroid output by both normal and PCOS cells was identical, thus indicating that the differences in steroid output in the presence of forskolin were not due to differences in adenyl cyclase activity. Because these theca cells could be maintained through multiple population doublings, the increased steroidogenic activity of PCOS theca cells compared to normal theca cells is unlikely to reflect the influence of *in vivo* hormonal stimulation, i.e. increased LH levels associated with PCOS. Consequently, these observations are consistent with the notion that dysregulation of androgen biosynthesis is an intrinsic property of PCOS theca cells. However, a long-lasting metabolic imprint received *in vivo* can still not definitively be excluded.

There are several genes that are critical for androgen synthesis including the steroidogenic acute regulatory protein (StAR), P450 side-chain cleavage enzyme (CYP11A), CYP17, 3β-hydroxysteroid dehydrogenase (3β-HSD) and 17β-HSD[8]. Studies in which PCOS and normal theca cells were incubated with various radiolabeled steroid precursors, and the metabolism of the tracers monitored, demonstrate that PCOS theca cells have increased 3β-HSD, CYP17 and 17β-HSD activities[8].

Northern blot analysis showed that CYP17 and CYP11A mRNAs were more abundant in PCOS theca cells than normal theca cells, while there were similar levels of StAR mRNA in both PCOS and normal theca cells[8]. It appears that the 17β-HSD that reduces androstenedione to testosterone in theca cells, is not the type I or 'estrogenic' enzyme that catalyzes the formation of estradiol in granulosa cells or the type III or 'androgenic' enzyme that catalyzes the formation of testosterone from androstenedione in Leydig cells[9]. Consistent with Northern blot analyses, transient transfection experiments indicated that the CYP17 promoter is more active in PCOS theca cells than in normal theca cells, while the StAR promoter was not differentially regulated in PCOS and normal theca cells[10]. In addition, the activity of a promoter construct containing multiple cAMP response elements (CREs) was similar in control and forskolin-treated normal and PCOS theca cells. Thus, a defect in the signaling cascade that activates

Table 1 Stable biochemical and molecular characteristics of polycystic ovary syndrome theca cells

Biochemical phenotype	mRNA, promoter and enzymatic activity
↑ Progesterone synthesis	↑ 3β-HSD activity
	↑ CYP11A mRNA
	StAR mRNA – no change
	StAR promoter activity – no change
↑ 17OH-progesterone and androstenedione synthesis	↑ 17α-hydroxylase activity
	↑ CYP17 mRNA
	↑ CYP17 promoter activity
↑ Testosterone synthesis	↑ 17β-HSD activity

17OH-progesterone, 17α-hydroxyprogesterone; 3β-HSD, 3β-hydroxysteroid dehydrogenase; CYP11A, P450 side-chain cleavage enzyme; STAR, steroidogenic acute regulatory protein; CYP17, 17α-hydroxylase/17,20 lyase; 17β-HSD, 17β-hydroxysteroid dehydrogenase

the transcription factor cAMP-response element binding protein (CREB) cannot explain the differences in transcriptional activity of the CYP17 promoter in normal and PCOS theca cells. These experiments suggest selective transcriptional regulation of genes encoding specific steroidogenic enzymes, but not all components of the steroidogenic machinery in PCOS theca cells, leading to increased production of progestins and androgens (Table 1). Therefore, it is unlikely that the hyperandrogenemia of PCOS is due to variation or mutation of a gene encoding a single steroidogenic enzyme, as suggested by other investigators[11].

Insulin resistance

Careful comparisons of age- and weight-matched PCOS and normal women provides compelling evidence that PCOS women are at increased risk of developing the classic symptoms of type 2 diabetes, including glucose intolerance, hyperinsulinemia, and peripheral insulin resistance[5]. Sensitivity of target tissues to insulin is decreased in obese PCOS women, i.e. glucose disposal is decreased and glucose production is increased[12,13]. Adipocyte uptake of glucose is impaired because of a decrease in GLUT4 glucose transporters[14]. In addition, insulin secretion by pancreatic β-cells is impaired[15]. These abnormalities are not found in all women with PCOS, but they are more likely to be detected in women with more profound reproductive disturbances.

The elevated insulin levels associated with insulin resistance of PCOS could contribute to hyperandrogenemia in several ways. Insulin suppresses hepatic production of sex hormone-binding globulin (SHBG), and the decline in SHBG exacerbates the hyperandrogenemia[16]. Insulin can also act as a co-gonadotropin, enhancing the actions of both follicle-stimulating hormone (FSH) and LH, including the stimulatory effects of LH on thecal androgen synthesis[1]. The actions of insulin can be mediated via the insulin receptor or, in the case of significantly elevated insulin concentrations, on the IGF receptor. However, the enigma of insulin resistance in some tissues, e.g. skeletal muscle and adipose tissue, with preservation of insulin action in others, e.g. ovary, liver, requires consideration. One simple explanation is that insulin resistance resulting from a defect in insulin signaling via the insulin receptor leads to high insulin levels which activate the ovarian IGF receptor. However, excessive insulin levels as found in individuals with inactivating mutations in the insulin receptor, are not characteristic of PCOS[1]. Thus, so-called 'spillover' activation of the IGF receptor is unlikely to be a major factor in the thecal androgen excess of PCOS. Alternatively, there may be abnormalities in specific insulin receptor signaling pathways. There is now abundant evidence that insulin can trigger different intracellular signaling cascades after it binds to its receptor, some involved in metabolic effects, others involved in cell growth and differentiation[5]. Therefore, a defect in only one signaling pathway could account for selective insulin resistance. A genetic or biochemical alteration that leads to this scenario in PCOS has yet to be identified. Although inactivating mutations in the insulin receptor gene are associated with PCOS, these are rare and thus mutations in the structural insulin receptor gene are not a common cause of the disorder. However, there is evidence for altered phosphorylation of the β-subunit of the insulin receptor in some but not all women with PCOS[5], which might reflect abnormal activity of a protein kinase or phosphatase.

A genetic basis for PCOS?

Based on the studies showing familial clustering of hyperandrogenemia, we favor the idea that the increased steroidogenic activity of PCOS theca cells is genetic. Given that expression of multiple genes involved in steroidogenesis appear to be affected in the PCOS theca cells, it will be important to characterize the full repertoire of differentially expressed genes. Differential gene expression can be analyzed using several techniques including cDNA array analysis, differential display, serial analysis of gene expression (SAGE) and suppression subtractive hybridization (SSH)[17-20]. We are using cDNA arrays, SAGE[21] and, most recently, SSH in our studies of PCOS[22]. In addition to these molecular approaches, the genetic analysis of PCOS families, i.e. affected sibling pair analysis and transmission disequilibrium test, is continuing as an independent approach to identifying the causative factor(s) of PCOS[23,24]. However, the later approach requires a large number of families and is currently only useful in the evaluation of candidate genes. Unfortunately, to date there has been little consensus among groups pursuing the gene-tics of PCOS with respect to potential PCOS genes. This is not too surprising given that different ascertainment criteria have been used, the sample sizes are still quite small, and the candidate genes examined represent but a tiny fraction of the human genome.

Strategies for identifying PCOS genes

What is the most likely nature of the 'PCOS gene(s)'? Given the evidence for familial clustering of hyperandrogenemia, the suggestion that it is a dominant trait, and the evidence

for abnormalities in transcription of multiple genes involved in thecal steroidogenesis, we predict that the PCOS genes are factors, receptors or intracellular signaling molecules that regulate the activity of transcription factors that control expression of the suite of dysregulated genes.

How can the putative regulatory factors predicted to be abnormal in PCOS be characterized? We have proposed a strategy encompassing SSH and chromatin immuno-precipitation (ChIP) analysis to identify differentially transcribed genes using long-term cultures of proliferating PCOS and normal theca cells[22]. These complementary technologies will hopefully provide essential information that will lead to the identification of the common regulatory features in these genes differentially expressed in PCOS theca cells and then the proximate cause of the augmented transcriptional activity, which presumably underlies the fundamental reproductive and metabolic abnormalities of PCOS. This strategy could also be applied to comparison of differential gene expression in other cells or tissues of interest in PCOS, e.g. granulosa cells, skeletal muscle, adipocytes, endometrium. It should be noted that the success of this strategy using cultured cells is based on the assumption that the molecular phenotype of the normal and PCOS cells is maintained in long-term culture and reflects the original genetic background, or that tissue culture conditions have an equal influence on the expressed genetic programs of normal and PCOS cells. Alternatively, primary cells which can be collected easily and in large quantities and thus would not require long-term culturing may provide a good source for comparison and alleviate the aforementioned considerations associated with cell culture.

Suppression subtractive hybridization

SSH combines two independent procedures, subtractive hybridization and suppressive polymerase chain reaction (PCR), to effectively limit detection of common genes and enhance detection of rare transcripts[20]. Since

SSH subtracts out genes common to both PCOS and normal theca cells, the labor intensive job of screening and sequencing hundreds of clones, which is required for SAGE and microarray analysis, is significantly reduced. Unlike microarray analysis, SSH is not limited to known cDNAs and expressed sequence tags, and therefore provides an unbiased approach to the identification of both previously described and novel genes. The enhancement of rare transcripts in SSH increases the probability of detecting genes, which may be missed using SAGE or differential display. Furthermore, the SSH technique produces fewer false positive clones than differential display when comparing two sample types with only a small number of differentially expressed genes[20]. Thus, we feel that the SSH technique, as well as the stringent screening process described below, will prove to be an efficient and reliable method of identifying genes differentially regulated in PCOS compared to normal theca cells.

Real-time reverse transcriptase-polymerase chain reaction (RT-PCR) will confirm if the genes identified by SSH are indeed represented at quantitatively different levels in PCOS and normal theca cells. Any novel sequences that are obtained will be studied in greater detail to identify the temporal changes in theca cell expression and the function of the protein. While differential expression of the genes encoding steroidogenic enzymes mentioned above (CYP11A, 3β-HSD, CYP17) in PCOS theca cells is expected, our preliminary analyses detected genes encoding cytokine-induced proteins, which are more abundantly expressed in PCOS theca cells than normal theca cells. These findings suggest that the differential gene expression in PCOS cells extends beyond the steroidogenic enzymes.

Chromatin immunoprecipitation

ChIP allows for the *in vivo* trapping of histones and other DNA-associated proteins, including transcription factors, to their target regulatory elements in multiple genes

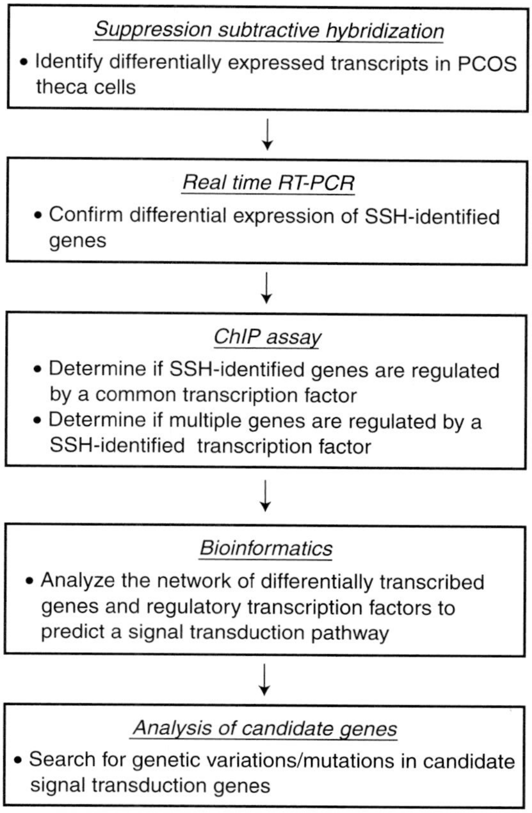

Figure 1 Schematic representation of the strategies utilized to elucidate the etiology of excess androgen production in polycystic ovary syndrome (PCOS) theca cells. RT-PCR, reverse trancscriptase–polymerase chain reaction; SSH, suppression subtractive hybridization; ChIP, chromatin immunoprecipitation

simultaneously[25,26]. The recent findings that acetylation of histones 3 and 4 by coactivators is an essential part of transcription, and the development of antiacetylated histone antibodies allowed the immunoprecipitation of transcriptionally active genes[27].

ChIP could be used as an alternative approach to detect transcriptionally active genes associated with the PCOS phenotype. The true power of this technique will be to analyze the transcriptional activity of specific genes that are identified by the SSH method. Moreover, if the increased transcription of genes in PCOS theca cells can be attributed to specific transcription factor(s), this technique can be used to identify all genes that are directly regulated by that transcription factor using an antibody to the transcription factor in the ChIP assay.

One advantage of the ChIP assay over SSH, SAGE, differential display and microarray analysis is that the ChIP procedure only identifies genes that are transcriptionally active, while these latter methods can only detect differences in mRNA levels which can be influenced by changes in mRNA stability as well as transcription. However, ChIP analysis using an antiacetylated histone antibody does not eliminate genes that are common to both normal and PCOS cells. Nevertheless, application of a methodology similar to SSH using ChIP genomic libraries prepared from PCOS and normal theca cells might be able to identify differentially transcribed genes. As previously noted, the ChIP methodology is best suited to the analysis of specific genes already identified or for the identification of genes regulated by a specific transcription factor suspected to be involved in the etiology of PCOS. However, with this information together with bioinformatics tools that can identify common regulatory elements in genes selected from the SSH/ChIP screen, the network of transcription factors and intracellular signaling molecules involved in expression of these genes can be disclosed, revealing new candidate genes.

Conclusions

Two lines of evidence suggest a genetic basis for the hyperandrogenemia of PCOS: (1) family studies demonstrate familial clustering of hyperandrogenemia in sisters and provide evidence that the hyperandrogenemia is a dominant trait; and (2) theca cells from PCOS ovaries display a stable biochemical phenotype of increased steroidogenesis and increased transcription of specific genes encoding steroidogenic enzymes. The propagating cultures of human theca cells derived from PCOS and normal ovaries maintained in culture through multiple population doublings represent a powerful tool for the identification of differentially expressed genes in PCOS, and ultimately the genetic factors that are responsible for the altered gene expression.

We have outlined a strategy (Figure 1) using two complementary approaches, SSH and ChIP assays, to catalog differentially expressed genes, document their transcriptional activity and subsequently verify the involvement of specific transcription factors in the control of gene expression. This strategy should define the network of dysregulated genes in PCOS theca cells and clarify the signal transduction cascades(s) that lead to altered transcriptional activity, directing us to the proximate cause of PCOS.

References

1. Legro RS, Spielman R, Urbanek M, *et al.* Phenotype and genotype in polycystic ovary syndrome. *Rec Prog Horm Res* 1998;53:217–56
2. Polson DW, Adams J, Wadsworth J, *et al.* Polycystic ovaries – a common finding in normal women. *Lancet* 1988;1(8590):870–2
3. Franks S. Polycystic ovary syndrome [published erratum appears in *N Engl J Med* 1995;333: 1435]. *N Engl J Med* 1995;333:853–61
4. Dunaif A, Givens J, Haseltine F, *et al. The Polycystic Ovary Syndrome*. Cambridge: Blackwell Scientific, 1992
5. Dunaif A. Insulin resistance and the polycystic ovary syndrome: mechanism and implications for pathogenesis. *Endocr Rev* 1997;18:774–800
6. Waldstreicher J, Santoro NF, Hall JE, *et al.* Hyperfunction of the hypothalamic-pituitary axis in women with polycystic ovarian disease: indirect evidence for partial gonadotroph desensitization. *J Clin Endocrinol Metab* 1988; 66:165–72
7. Gilling-Smith C, Willis DS, Beard RW, *et al.* Hypersecretion of androstenedione by isolated thecal cells from polycystic ovaries. *J Clin Endocrinol Metab* 1994;79:1158–65
8. Nelson VL, Legro RS, Strauss III JF, *et al.* Augmented androgen production is a stable steroidogenic phenotype of propogated theca cells from polycystic ovaries. *Mol Endocrinol* 1999;13:946–57

9. Qin K, Rosenfield RL, Legro RS, *et al*. 17β-Hydroxysteroid dehyrogenase type 5 (17β-HSD5) expression is increased in ovarian theca cells isolated with polycystic ovary syndrome (PCOS). Presented at the *Proceedings of the Endocrine Society, 82nd Annual Meeting*. Toronto, Ontario, Canada, 2000;399

10. Wickenheisser JK, Quinn PG, Nelson VL, *et al*. Differential activity of the cytochrome P450 17α-hydroxylase and steroidogenic acute regulatory protein gene promoters in normal and polycystic ovary syndrome theca cells. *J Clin Endocrinol Metab* 2000;85:2304–11

11. Gharani N, Waterworth DM, Batty S, *et al*. Association of the steroid synthesis gene CYP11a with polycystic ovary syndrome and hyperandrogenism. *Hum Mol Genet* 1997;6:397–402

12. Dunaif A, Segal KR, Shelley DR, *et al*. Evidence for distinctive and intrinsic defects in insulin action in polycystic ovary syndrome. *Diabetes* 1992;41:1257–66

13. Dunaif A, Segal KR, Futterweit W, *et al*. Profound peripheral insulin resistance, independent of obesity, in polycystic ovary syndrome. *Diabetes* 1989;38:1165–74

14. Rosenbaum D, Haber RS, Dunaif A. Insulin resistance in polycystic ovary syndrome: decreased expression of GLUT-4 glucose transporters in adipocytes. *Am J Physiol* 1993;264:E197–202

15. Ehrmann DA, Sturis J, Byrne MM, *et al*. Insulin secretory defects in polycystic ovary syndrome. Relationship to insulin sensitivity and family history of non-insulin-dependent diabetes mellitus. *J Clin Invest* 1995;96:520–7

16. Plymate SR, Matej LA, Jones RE, *et al*. Inhibition of sex hormone-binding globulin production in the human hepatoma (Hep G2) cell line by insulin and prolactin. *J Clin Endocrinol Metab* 1988;67:460–4

17. Schena M, Shalon D, Heller R, *et al*. Parallel human genome analysis: microarray-based expression monitoring of 100 genes. *Proc Natl Acad Sci USA* 1996;93:10614–9

18. Liang P, Pardee AB. Differential display of eukaryotic messenger RNA by means of the polymerase chain reaction. *Science* 1992;257:967–71

19. Velculescu VE, Zhang L, Vogelstein B, *et al*. Serial analysis of gene expression. *Science* 1995;270:484–7

20. Diatchenko L, Lau Y-FC, Campbell AP, *et al*. Suppression subtractive hybridization: a method for generating differentially regulated or tissue-specific cDNA probes and libraries. *Proc Natl Acad Sci USA* 1996;93:6025–30

21. Neilson LI, Andalibi A, Kang D, *et al*. Molecular phenotype of the human oocyte by PCR-SAGE. *Genomics* 2000;63:13–24

22. Strauss I, Jerome F, Wood JR, *et al*. Strategies to elucidate the mechanism of excessive theca cell androgen production in PCOS. *Mol Cell Endocrinol* 2001;in press

23. Urbanek M, Legro RS, Driscoll DA, *et al*. Thirty-seven candidate genes for polycystic ovary syndrome: strongest evidence for linkage is with follistatin. *Proc Natl Acad Sci USA* 1999;96:8573–8

24. Urbanek M, Wu X, Vickery KR, *et al*. Allelic variants of the follistatin gene in polycystic ovary syndrome. *J Clin Endocrinol Metab* 2000;85:4455–61

25. de Belle I, Mercola D, Adamson ED. Method for cloning *in vivo* targets of the Egr-1 transcription factor [In Process Citation]. *Biotechniques* 2000;29:162–9

26. Kuo MH, Allis CD. *In vivo* cross-linking and immunoprecipitation for studying dynamic protein : DNA associations in a chromatin environment. *Methods* 1999;19:425–33

27. Spencer VA, Davie JR. Role of covalent modifications of histones in regulating gene expression. *Gene* 1999;240:1–12

Polycystic ovary disease: heritability and heterogeneity

7

P. G. Crosignani

Introduction

The polycystic appearance of the ovary is the essential sign of polycystic ovary syndrome (PCOS), but there is a wide range of associated clinical and biochemical features such as elevated serum concentrations of androgens, insulin, luteinizing hormone (LH) and decreased insulin sensitivity. These conditions are frequently associated with obesity. Since insulin resistance in PCOS patients is predominantly extrasplanchnic[1], the fasting blood sugar is normal.

According to Franks *et al.*[2] ovarian morphology is the essential marker of the syndrome and the wide range of related phenotypes can be explained by the interaction of a small number of key genes with environmental factors.

Since the symptoms of PCOS are found in up to 10% of young women, it is certainly the most frequent endocrine disorder diagnosed in these subjects. Despite the high prevalence of the isolated polycystic ovarian morphology (22%), the syndrome may be accompanied by minimal clinical manifestation, and in particular no uniformly deleterious effect on fertility has been reported[3].

The high prevalence of affected individuals and the wide range of related phenotypes can be explained by the interaction of a small number of key genes with environmental factors. Heritability of PCOS has been inferred from the study of the syndrome in various ethnic groups[4–6], twins[7] and PCOS families[2,8]. These data suggest that the condition is passed down through either sex according to the autosomal dominant model of genetic transmission.

Mechanism of heritability

Ovarian steroidogenesis

Though the secretion of androgens by adrenals may by increased, the main source of androgen excess in PCOS is the ovary[9]. It is well known that there is a primary abnormality in the theca cells of PCOS patients, leading to excessive production of progesterone and androgen[10,11]. Therefore, the abnormal steroidogenesis observed in PCOS is related to an intrinsic abnormality of the theca cells rather than to abnormal gonadotropin stimulation[12]. This finding prompted a study of the cholesterol side-chain cleavage gene (CYP11a) as a possible cause of deranged steroidogenesis. Gharani *et al.*[13] studied the segregation of CYP11a in 20 PCOS families. The most common polymorphism of the gene (indicated as the absence of 216 allele) was significantly associated with PCOS families. A non-parametric linkage analysis using polymorphic markers in that region similarly suggested that the steroid synthesis gene CYP11a is a very important locus for the genetic susceptibility of PCOS hyperandrogenism (non parametric linkage (NPL) score 3.03, $p = 0.003$)[13].

Adrenal and ovarian hyperandrogenism

The increased ovarian and adrenal steroidogenic activity in PCOS can also be caused by enhanced lyase activity, exclusively by the cytochrome P450c17α. Serine phosphorylation of this enzyme system selectively increases its enzymatic activity, leading to hypersecretion of ovarian and adrenal androgen, with no

Table 1 PCOS: pathophysiology for the inheritable susceptibilities

Gene	Molecular lesion	Target	Phenotype
CYP11a locus (gene coding cholesterol side-chain cleavage)	216 genotype	ovarian theca cells	hyperandrogenism
Autosomal dominant gene	point mutation encoding serine hyperphosphorylation	adrenal and ovarian P450c17α lyase activated insulin receptor	hyperandrogensim insulin resistance
11p 15.5 locus (insulin gene)	class III alleles at VNTR	pancreatic β-cells	hyperinsulinemia

VNTR, variable number of tanden repeats

rise in adrenocorticotropic hormone (ACTH) or other steroidogenic activity[14].

Insulin resistance

Insulin resistance is another common feature in women with PCOS. The cause is still unknown. Interestingly, only women with an endocrine syndrome of hyperandrogenism and chronic anovulation appear to be insulin resistant and at high risk of glucose intolerance[15,16]. There appears to be a genetic target cell defect as a cause of the metabolic condition[17].

The same hyperphosphorylation process described for cytochrome P450c17α lyase activity, leading to adrenal and ovarian hyperandrogenism, has been implicated as the cause of a specific post-receptor defect of transduction of the insulin signal in fibroblasts[18]. In affected patients, autophosphorylation of the serine (rather than tyrosine) residue impairs insulin signal transduction and contributes to the 50% insulin resistance observed. Thus a single molecular defect leading to the activation of a serine kinase might explain the two main biochemical disturbances in these patients, i.e. hirsutism and insulin resistance.

Abnormal insulin secretion

Hyperinsulinemia has been reported in patients with PCOS and the syndrome is one of the major risk factors for non-insulin-dependent diabetes mellitus (NIDDM)[19]. The β-cell dysfunction is not obesity-dependent, and in the majority of PCOS women is not associated with glucose intolerance[20].

The direct role of the insulin gene in the etiology of hyperinsulinemia was investigated in three groups of PCOS patients (one of which included 17 families with several affected individuals). All three populations showed an association between class III alleles at the VNTR 5[1] locus to the insulin gene and PCOS[21]. The association was stronger in anovulatory patients, who more frequently have hyperinsulinemia. A non-parametric linkage analysis in the PCOS families showed excess allele sharing at the same locus (NPL score 3.250, $p = 0.002$)[22]. The authors concluded that the VNTR 5[1] region to the insulin gene is a major locus for PCOS-associated hyperinsulinemia. Table 1 summarizes the pathophysiology for the inherited susceptibilities.

Environmental risk factors

Prenatal life

Cresswell et al.[23], from a retrospective study on PCOS patients, suggested the existence of specific prenatal risk factors for the postpubertal expression of the PCOS phenotype. They found two distinct groups of PCOS patients: those who had above-average birthweight and those born to overweight mothers.

The second group comprised women of normal weight who had high plasma LH, but normal testosterone concentrations. These women were born after term (40 weeks' gestation). On the basis of these findings, the authors suggest that the two forms of PCOS have different origins in intrauterine life. Obese, hirsute women with PCOS have higher than normal ovarian secretion of androgens, associated with high birthweight and maternal obesity. Thin women with PCOS have altered hypothalamic control of LH release resulting from prolonged gestation.

Jahnfar et al.[24], on the basis of the high degree of discordance in sonographic ovarian imaging between twins observed in 34 female twin pairs, suggest that the high prevalence of PCOS among twins may be explained by factors acting in prenatal life.

Postnatal risk factors

Chronic anovulation The role of chronic anovulation as an environmental risk factor for PCOS is suggested by several pathophysiological mechanisms where androgen, LH and sex hormone-binding globulin (SHBG)

play key roles. A subgroup of patients with PCOS and hypogonadotropic anovulation has also been described[25].

Obesity Obesity is an independent risk factor for chronic anovulation[26] and body fat distribution (waist to hip ratio) seems more important than weight itself[27]. In obese women, the two main mechanisms leading to anovulation are similar to those in patients with PCOS: (1) excess LH and androgen secretion; and (2) hyperinsulinemia and insulin resistance. In fact, short-term fasting reduces LH secretion in normal weight women[28]. In overweight women, caloric restriction lowers insulin levels and raises SHBG concentrations[29], while in severely obese patients, postgastroplasty recovery of ideal weight restores normal glucose and insulin metabolism[30].

In contrast, in women with PCOS, obesity worsens the syndrome; in these patients, insulin resistance appears to be directly related to body mass index (BMI)[31] while weight reduction in obese PCOS women lowers LH hypersecretion and reverses insulin insensitivity[32,33].

References

1. Dunaif A, Segal KR, Shelley DR, *et al.* Evidence for distinctive and intrinsic defects in insulin action in polycystic ovary syndrome. *Diabetes* 1992;41:1257–66
2. Franks S, Gharani N, Waterworth D, *et al.* The genetic basis of polycystic ovary syndrome. *Hum Reprod* 1997;12:2641–8
3. Kousta E, White DM, Cela E, *et al.* The prevalence of polycystic ovaries in women with infertility. *Hum Reprod* 1999;14:2720–3
4. Carmina E, Koyama T, Chang L, *et al.* Does ethnicity influence the prevalence of adrenal hyperandrogenism and insulin resistance in polycystic ovary syndrome? *Am J Obstet Gynecol* 1992;167:1807–12
5. Norman RJ, Mahabeer S, Masters S. Ethnic differences in insulin and glucose response to glucose between white and Indian women with polycystic ovary syndrome. *Fertil Steril* 1995;63:58–62

6. Legro RS, Kunselman AR, Dodson WX, *et al.* Prevalence and predictors of risk for type 2 diabetes mellitus and impaired glucose tolerance in polycystic ovary syndrome: a prospective, controlled study in 254 affected women. *J Clin Endocrinol Metab* 1999;84:165–8
7. Hutton C, Clark F. Polycystic ovarian syndrome in identical twins. *Postgrad Med J* 1984; 60:64–5
8. Govind A, Obhrai MS, Clayton RN. Polycystic ovaries are inherited as an autosomal dominant trait: analysis of 29 polycystic ovary syndrome and 10 control families. *J Clin Endocrinol Metab* 1999;84:38–43
9. Franks S. Polycystic ovary syndrome: a changing perspective. *Clin Endocrinol* 1989;31: 87–120
10. Gilling-Smith C, Willis DS, Beard RW, *et al.* Hypersecretion of androstenedione by isolated

theca cells from polycystic ovaries. *J Clin Endocrinol Metab* 1994;79:1158–65

11. Gilling-Smith C, Story EH, Rogers V, *et al.* Evidence for a primary abnormality of thecal cell steroidogenesis in the polycystic ovary syndrome. *Clin Endocrinol* 1997;47:93–9

12. Ibañez L, Hall JE, Potau N, *et al.* Ovarian 17-hydroxyprogesterone hyperresponsiveness to gonadotropin-releasing hormone (GnRH) agonist challenge in women with polycystic ovary syndrome is not mediated by luteinizing hormone hypersecretion: evidence from GnRH agonist and human chorionic gonadotropin stimulation testing. *J Clin Endocrinol Metab* 1996;81:4103–7

13. Gharani N, Waterworth DM, Batty S, *et al.* Association of the steroid synthesis gene CYP11a with polycystic ovary syndrome and hyperandrogenism. *Hum Mol Genet* 1997;6:397–402

14. Zhang LH, Rodriguez H, Ohno S, *et al.* Serine phosphorylation of human P450c17 increases 17,20-lyase activity: implications for adrenarche and the polycystic ovary syndrome. *Proc Natl Acad Sci USA* 1995;92:10619–23

15. Robinson S, Kiddy D, Gelding SV, *et al.* The relationship of insulin insensitivity of menstrual pattern in women with hyperandrogenism and polycystic ovaries. *Clin Endocrinol (Oxf)* 1993;39:351–5

16. Dunaif A, Graf M, Mandeli J, *et al.* Characterization of groups of hyperandrogenic women with acanthosis nigricans, impaired glucose tolerance, and/or hyperinsulinemia. *J Clin Endocrinol Metab* 1987;65:499–507

17. Holte J. Disturbance in insulin secretion and sensitivity in women with the polycystic ovary syndrome. *Clin Endocrinol Metab* 1996;10:221–47

18. Dunaif A, Xia J, Book CB, *et al.* Excessive insulin receptor serine phosphorylation in cultured fibroblasts and in skeletal muscle. A potential mechanism for insulin resistance in the polycystic ovary syndrome. *J Clin Invest* 1995;96:801–10

19. Holte J, Bergh T, Berne C, *et al.* Restored sensitivity but persistently increased early insulin secretion after weight loss in obese women with polycystic ovary syndrome. *J Clin Endocrinol Metab* 1995;80:2586–93

20. Dunaif A, Finegood DT. β cell dysfunction independent of obesity in the polycystic ovary syndrome. *J Clin Endocrinol Metab* 1996;81:942–7

21. Bennett ST, Lucassen AM, Gough SCL, *et al.* Susceptibility to human type 1 diabetes at IDDM2 is determined by tandem repeat variation at the insulin gene minisatellite locus. *Nat Genet* 1995;9:284–92

22. Waterworth DM, Bennett ST, Gharani N, *et al.* Linkage and association of insulin gene VNTR regulatory polymorphism with polycystic ovary syndrome. *Lancet* 1997;349:986–90

23. Cresswell JL, Barker DJP, Osmond C, *et al.* Fetal growth, length of gestation, and polycystic ovaries in adult life. *Lancet* 1997;350:1131–5

24. Jahnfar S, Eden JA, Warren P, *et al.* A twin study of polycystic ovary syndrome. *Fertil Steril* 1995;63:478–86

25. Shoham Z, Conway GS, Patel A, *et al.* Polycystic ovaries in patients with hypogonadotropic hypogonadism: similarity of ovarian response to gonadotropin stimulation in patients with polycystic ovarian syndrome. *Fertil Steril* 1992;58:37–45

26. Grodstein F, Goldman MB, Cramer DW. Body mass index and ovulatory infertility. *Epidemiology* 1994;5:247–50

27. Zaadstra BM, Seidell JC, Van Noord PA, *et al.* Fat and female fecundity: prospective study of effect of body fat distribution on conception rates. *Br Med J* 1993;306:484–7

28. Olson BR, Cartledge T, Sebring N, *et al.* Short-term fasting affects luteinizing hormone secretory dynamics but not reproductive function in normal-weight sedentary women. *J Clin Endocrinol Metab* 1995;80:1187–93

29. Kiddy DS, Hamilton-Fairley D, Bush A, *et al.* Improvement in endocrine and ovarian function during dietary treatment of obese women with polycystic ovary syndrome. *Clin Endocrinol (Oxf)* 1992;36:105–11

30. Letiexhe MR, Scheen AJ, Gerard PL, *et al.* Post-gastroplasty recovery of ideal body weight normalizes glucose and insulin metabolism in obese women. *J Clin Endocrinol Metab* 1995;80:364–9

31. Pasquali R, Fabbri R, Venturoli S, *et al.* Effect of weight loss and antiandrogenic therapy on sex hormone blood levels and insulin resistance in obese patients with polycystic ovaries. *Am J Obstet Gynecol* 1986;154:139–44

32. Bützow TL, Lehtovirta MT, Väinämö U, *et al.* The effect of weight reduction on gonadotrophin, insulin and androgen metabolism in

hyperandrogenic overweight infertile women. Presented at the 12th Annual Meeting of the European Society of Human Reproduction and Embryology, Maastricht, The Netherlands, 30 June–3 July 1996. *Hum Reprod* 1996;11 (Suppl. 1):47–8

33. Kiddy DS, Sharp PS, White DM, *et al.* Differences in clinical and endocrine features between obese and non-obese subjects with polycystic ovary syndrome: an analysis of 263 consecutive cases. *Clin Endocrinol (Oxf)* 1990; 32:213–20

Physiopathology of hyperinsulinemia in polycystic ovary syndrome

8

A. Lanzone, M. Ciampelli, F. Cucinelli, M. Guido, P. Villa, G. Muzj,
D. Romualdi, F. Murgia, C. Belosi, R. Apa and A. M. Fulghesu

Introduction

Polycystic ovary syndrome (PCOS) represents one of the most discussed, controversial and explored areas of reproductive medicine, as this syndrome affects up to 10% of women of reproductive age[1]. Within the past decade, it has become apparent that hyperinsulinemia and insulin resistance are prominent features of many women with PCOS, affecting more than 50% of cases. Although about 70% of obese women with PCOS exhibited an exaggerated insulin secretion, this feature is also represented in 20–40% of non-obese subjects[2].

Role of hyperinsulinemia in PCOS

Hyperinsulinemia plays a pivotal role in the disorder by stimulating ovarian androgen production and impeding ovulation, thus leading to the symptomatological features of the syndrome, which are hirsutism and chronic anovulation with menstrual disorders[3]. Insulin is able to stimulate thecal cell production of androgens[4]; this is probably achieved through binding of insulin to the insulin-like growth factor-I (IGF-I) receptor[5]. Alternatively, insulin could act via a hybrid insulin/IGF-I receptor or via the insulin receptor, which may be differentially regulated in the ovary[5]. Willis and co-workers[6] proposed that hyperinsulinemia, by increasing the response of granulosa cells to luteinizing hormone (LH), amplifies the effects of LH levels that may already be elevated in these women. Thus, the effect of LH on the maturing follicle is similar to that which, in the normal cycle, is exerted only at the onset of the

LH surge. This would be expected to lead to terminal differentiation of granulosa cells, resulting in premature arrest of follicular growth and, hence, failure of ovulation. Furthermore, insulin is known to directly inhibit IGF binding-protein I production in the liver, allowing increased local activity of IGF-I to lead to androgen production in the ovary[7].

Rosenfield and co-workers[1,8] have postulated that hyperinsulinemia is a candidate cause for dysregulated hyperactivity of ovarian cytochrome P450 C17α in women with PCOS. The cytochrome P450 C17α is a key enzyme expressed in both adrenals and gonads; it induces the conversion of pregnenolone to dehydroepiandrosterone (DHEA) and, at least in the rat, of progesterone to the corresponding 4-ene 17-ketosteroid androstenedione by a sequence of two steps, namely 17,20 hydroxylation followed by 17,20-lyase activity[9,10]. Both these enzyme activities seem to be upregulated in PCOS[1,8].

Adrenal steroidogenesis

In recent years, the influence of insulin on adrenal steroidogenesis in PCOS has received a great deal of attention. Starting from data suggesting an exaggerated steroidogenic adrenal response to pharmacological doses of adrenocorticotropic hormone (ACTH) in hyperinsulinemic PCOS patients[11], Moghetti and co-workers[12] evaluated the effects of insulin infusion on P450 C17α activity at the adrenal level. The authors showed that hyperinsulinemia, within the high physiological range, did not determine measurable changes in the basal concentrations of any of the evaluated steroid hormones. Nevertheless, insulin infusion was associated with increased ACTH-stimulated levels of 17α-hydroxycorticosteroid intermediates (17OH-pregnenolone and 17OH-progesterone) without significant variations in stimulated cortisol and androstenedione production, thus suggesting a relative impairment of 17,20 lyase activity. Superimposable results were obtained in another study, in which an insulin-lowering drug (metformin) was used to modify circulating insulin levels in PCOS[13]; the treatment was effective in reducing the 17α-hydroxylase and 17,20-lyase activity at the adrenal level.

In a similar study protocol, Nestler and Jakubowicz[14] hypothesized that, by reducing hyperinsulinemia in PCOS subjects, metformin led to a reduction in ovarian cytochrome P450 C17α activity, as shown by a reduced response of 17OH-progesterone to gonadotropin-releasing hormone (GnRH) stimulation. Insulin may also affect the free androgen levels, and thus the biologically active fraction of these hormones, by directly suppressing the hepatic synthesis of sex hormone-binding globulin (SHBG)[15].

Several clinical studies also suggest that the insulin disorders found in PCOS are an effect, and not a cause, of hyperandrogenism; indeed androgens and increased free fatty acids (FFA), as seen in android obesity, inhibit hepatic insulin extraction resulting in hyperinsulinism and insulin resistance[16,17]. However, many studies[2,15,18], although not all[19], showed that pharmacological reduction of androgen levels through GnRH analog administration was not able to modify the hyperinsulinemia of PCOS subjects, thus arguing against this hypothesis.

Diabetes and cardiovascular disease

The insulin alterations as well as the presence of obesity found in PCOS also have profound clinical implications in terms of morbidity due to diabetes mellitus, dyslipidemia, hypertension and cardiovascular disease. The risk of impaired glucose tolerance or frank diabetes mellitus in obese hyperinsulinemic PCOS women aged 20–30 years, estimated to be about 15–20%[15,20] up to 35%[21], is shifted towards that observed in the 45–55 year old normal population[15]. In a risk-factor model (taking into consideration the metabolic variables of waist-to-hip circumference ratio, triglyceride concentration, hypertension and diabetes mellitus), the estimated risk of developing cardiovascular disease in women with PCOS aged 40–49 years was the same as for males of corresponding ages (four times the estimated risk in the normal female population)[22,23]. In women with PCOS aged 50 to 60 years, the same risk was increased eleven-fold[23].

Relationship between insulin resistance and PCOS

In subjects with normal β-cell function, hyperinsulinemia occurs secondary to insulin resistance. An association between insulin resistance and PCOS was initially established by Kahn et al.[24], who reported a lack of insulin receptors, with insulin resistance and hyperinsulinemia, in hyperandrogenic women with polycystic ovaries. However, there is controversy as to whether insulin resistance results from PCOS itself or from the obesity that is frequently associated with the syndrome. Several authors have reported results showing the presence of insulin resistance in obese as well as lean PCOS women[25]; in contrast, recent data failed to find decreased glucose uptake, either using a euglycemic–hyperinsulinemic clamp or intravenous glucose tolerance test (GTT) in lean women with PCOS. Holte and co-workers[26] showed that both women with PCOS and controls were characterized by a linear decline in insulin-mediated glucose disposal, parallel with increasing body mass index (BMI), but this decline was significantly more pronounced in the PCOS group. Indeed, the regression lines (insulin sensitivity versus BMI) for the two groups crossed in the lower part of the normal BMI and diverged linearly with increasing BMI, resulting in similar insulin sensitivity at BMI 21 kg/m², but 50% lower insulin sensitivity in the PCOS group compared with controls at BMI 30 kg/m².

On the other hand, the exaggerated insulin secretion found after an intravenous or oral GTT is not necessarily comparable to data obtained by the clamp technique. In an attempt to better clarify the metabolic features of PCOS, we evaluated the impact of reduced hepatic insulin clearance in determining the hyperinsulinemia of lean and obese PCOS patients[27]. Our results indicate that exaggerated insulin secretion and insulin resistance may coexist in PCOS in a heterogeneous manner partially independent of BMI. Obese patients with hyperinsulinism may have exaggerated pancreatic insulin secretion, reduced hepatic insulin clearance and insulin resistance at the same time. In hyperinsulinemic lean subjects, the contribution to hyperinsulinemia may be due mainly to both increased pancreatic secretion and reduced hepatic clearance. Therefore, it can be speculated that hyperinsulinemia represents a primary feature of PCOS while insulin sensitivity is more influenced by the degree of obesity.

Another factor indicating the dissociation between hyperinsulinemia and insulin resistance in PCOS is the possibility of improving insulin sensitivity in severely insulin-resistant women with the syndrome by weight reduction to levels similar to those of BMI-matched women with normal ovaries, while the exaggerated early insulin response to intravenous GTT remains unchanged[28]. Furthermore naltrexone (an oral opioid antagonist) administration in hyperinsulinemic PCOS women has been shown to be able to reduce the insulin response to a glucose load without influencing the peripheral insulin resistance[29].

Conclusion

While in the past years the attention of many investigators has been focused mainly on the management of two typical features of PCOS, i.e. hirsutism and anovulation, it has recently become evident that the metabolic alterations of the syndrome may have important implications for long-term health.

The importance of the introduction of insulin-lowering drugs as an effective therapeutic strategy in the management of the metabolic disturbances associated with PCOS must be highlighted. These substances could be very helpful, not only in the improvement of menstrual function and in the fall of androgen levels, but also in the prevention of many pathologies, such as diabetes mellitus, hypertension, cardiovascular disease, and endometrial and breast cancer.

We hope that current and future research efforts will not only provide much needed answers about the physiopathology of hyperinsulinemia in PCOS, but they will also lead to short- and long-term tangible benefits for the PCOS population.

References

1. Ehrman DA, Barnes RB, Rosenfield RL. Polycystic ovary syndrome as a form of functional ovarian hyperandrogenism due to dysregulation of androgen secretion. *Endocr Rev* 1995;16:322–53
2. Lanzone A, Fulghesu AM, Andreani CL, *et al.* Insulin secretion in polycystic ovarian disease: effect of ovarian suppression by GnRH agonist. *Hum Reprod* 1990;5:143–9
3. Nestler JE. Obesity, insulin, sex steroids and ovulation. *Int J Obes* 2000;24(Suppl. 2):S71–3
4. Sozen I, Arici A. Hyperinsulinism and its interaction with hyperandrogenism in polycystic ovary syndrome. *Obstet Gynecol Survey* 2000;55:321–8

5. Giudice LG. Insulin-like growth factors and ovarian follicular development. *Endocr Rev* 1992;13:641–69

6. Willis D, Mason H, Gilling-Smith C, *et al*. Modulation by insulin of follicle-stimulating hormone and luteinizing hormone action in human granulosa cells of normal and polycystic ovaries. *J Clin Endocrinol Metab* 1996;81:302–9

7. Conover CA, Lee PDK, Kanaley JA, *et al*. Insulin regulation of insulin-like growth factor binding protein-1 in obese and non obese humans. *J Clin Endocrinol Metab* 1992;74:1355–60

8. Rosenfield RL, Barnes RB, Cara JF, *et al*. Dysregulation of cytochrome P450$17\alpha$ as the cause of polycystic ovarian syndrome. *Fertil Steril* 1990;53:785–91

9. Miller WL. Molecular biology of steroid hormone synthesis. *Endocr Rev* 1988;9:295–318

10. Fevold HR, Lorence MC, McCarthy JL, *et al*. 45017α from testis: characterization of a full length cDNA encoding an unique steroid hydroxylase capable of catalyzing both Δ4- and Δ5-steroid-17,20-lyase reactions. *Mol Endocrinol* 1989;3:968–75

11. Lanzone A, Fulghesu AM, Guido M, *et al*. Differential androgen response to adrenocorticotropic hormone stimulation in polycystic ovary syndrome: relationship with insulin secretion. *Fertil Steril* 1992;58:296–301

12. Moghetti P, Castello R, Negri C, *et al*. Insulin infusion amplifies 17α-hydroxycorticosteroid intermediates response to adrenocorticotropin in hyperandrogenic women: apparent relative impairment of 17,20-lyase activity. *J Clin Endocrinol Metab* 1996;81:881–6

13. LaMarca A, Morgante G, Paglia T. Effects of metformin on adrenal steroidogenesis in women with polycystic ovary syndrome. *Fertil Steril* 1999;72:985–9

14. Nestler JE, Jakubowicz DJ. Decreases in ovarian cytochrome P450$17\alpha$ activity and serum free testosterone after reduction of insulin secretion in polycystic ovary syndrome. *N Engl J Med* 1996;335:617–23

15. Dunaif A, Segal K, Futterweit W, *et al*. Profound peripheral insulin resistance independent of obesity in polycystic ovary syndrome. *Diabetes* 1989;38:1165–74

16. Peiris AN, Mueller RA, Struve MF. Relationship of androgenic activity to splanchnic insulin metabolism and peripheral glucose utilization in premenopausal women. *J Clin Endocrinol Metab* 1987;64:162–7

17. Rebuffe SM, Martin P, Bjorntorp P. Effect of testosterone on abdominal adipose tissue in men. *Int J Obes* 1991;15:791–5

18. Guido M, Pavone V, Ciampelli M, *et al*. Involvement of ovarian steroids in the opioid-mediated reduction of insulin secretion in hyperinsulinemic patients with polycystic ovary syndrome. *J Clin Endocrinol Metab* 1998;83:1742–5

19. Cagnacci A, Paoletti AM, Arangino S, *et al*. Effect of ovarian suppression on glucose metabolism of young lean women with and without ovarian hyperandrogenism. *Hum Reprod* 1999;14:893–7

20. Ciampelli M, Fulghesu AM, Cucinelli F, *et al*. Impact of insulin and body mass index on metabolic and endocrine variables in polycystic ovary syndrome. *Metabolism* 1999;48:167–72

21. Legro RS, Kunselman AR, Dodson WC, *et al*. Prevalence and predictors of risk for type 2 diabetes mellitus and impaired glucose tolerance in polycystic ovary syndrome: a prospective, controlled study in 254 affected women. *J Clin Endocrinol Metab* 1999;84:165–9

22. Dahlgren E, Janson PO, Johansson S, *et al*. Hemostatic and metabolic variables in women with polycystic ovary syndrome. *Fertil Steril* 1994;61:455–60

23. Dahlgren E, Janson PO, Johansson S, *et al*. Polycystic ovary syndrome and risk for myocardial infarction evaluated from a risk factor model based on a prospective population study of women. *Acta Obstet Gynecol Scand* 1992;71:599–604

24. Kahn CR, Flier JS, Bar RS, *et al*. The syndromes of insulin resistance and acanthosis nigricans. Insulin-receptor disorders in man. *N Engl J Med* 1976;294:739–45

25. Ciampelli M, Lanzone A. Insulin and polycystic ovary syndrome: a new look at an old subject. *Gynecol Endocrinol* 1998;12:277–92

26. Holte J, Bergh T, Berne C, *et al*. Enhanced early insulin response to glucose in relation to insulin resistance in women with polycystic ovary syndrome and normal glucose tolerance. *J Clin Endocrinol Metab* 1994;78:1052–8

27. Ciampelli M, Fulghesu AM, Cucinelli F, *et al*. Heterogeneity in β-cell activity, hepatic insulin clearance and peripheral insulin sensitivity in women with polycystic ovary syndrome. *Hum Reprod* 1997;12:1897–1901

28. Holte J, Bergh T, Berne C, *et al*. Restored insulin sensitivity, but persistently increased early insulin secretion after weight-loss in obese women with polycystic ovary syndrome. *J Clin Endocrinol Metab* 1995;80:2586–93

29. Fulghesu AM, Ciampelli M, Guido M, *et al*. Role of the opioid tone in the pathophysiology of hyperinsulinemia and insulin resistance in polycystic ovarian disease. *Metabolism* 1998; 47:1–5

Weight loss and insulin-sensitizers in the treatment of polycystic ovary syndrome

9

A. Gambineri, V. Vicennati, C. Pelusi and R. Pasquali

Introduction

Polycystic ovary syndrome (PCOS) is a disorder of unknown and probably heterogeneous etiology, characterized by chronic anovulation, biochemical and/or clinical evidence of hyperandrogenism, and enlarged polycystic ovaries. PCOS affects 5–10% of women of reproductive age, with the onset of clinical manifestations often occurring at puberty. A consensus definition of PCOS was reached in 1990 under National Institutes of Health (NIH) auspices, requiring the presence of hyperandrogenism of ovarian origin and of oligomenorrhea or amenorrhea for diagnosis, with exclusion of other specific disorders such as steroid 21-hydroxylase deficiency[1]. However, other endocrine abnormalities such as obesity, particularly the abdominal phenotype, peripheral insulin resistance and hyperinsulinemia are frequently described in women with PCOS. In addition, a reduction of high-density lipoproteins and cholesterol, together with an increase in very-low-density lipoproteins and triglyceride blood levels, are common features of PCOS. All these alterations are described as being part of the so-called metabolic syndrome.

Taking into account the promoting role of insulin in the pathogenesis of PCOS, therapeutic approaches aimed at improving the insulin resistance and the concomitant hyperinsulinemia have recently been proposed by different clinical trials in women with PCOS[1–3]. This 'metabolic way' of treatment has been demonstrated to substantially ameliorate some of the pathological features characterizing PCOS, in particular the hyperandrogenism and the infertility frequently associated with the syndrome. This article will review the pathophysiological aspects of hyperinsulinemia-related hyperandrogenism and the clinical evidence of the efficacy of weight loss and insulin-sensitizing agents, particularly metformin, in the treatment of hyperandrogenism and chronic anovulation in women with PCOS and obesity.

The association of obesity and PCOS

Epidemiological studies have shown that in premenopausal women fertility may be negatively affected by excess body weight. The reason for this must be attributed to the hyperandrogenic state frequently described in obese women. A close association between obesity and hyperandrogenism has been proposed to also occur in PCOS, which is the most frequent cause of infertility in young women.

Mechanisms by which obesity interferes with the pathophysiology of PCOS and related infertility are complex and still under debate[1–3]. However, two distinct mechanisms appear to play a major role. First, obesity *per se* affects both androgen secretion and metabolism, thus favoring the increased availability of androgens at the level of peripheral target tissues[4,5]. Second, hyperinsulinemia, which is systematically associated with obesity, particularly when the abdominal phenotype is present, is involved in the regulation of the hypothalamic–pituitary–gonadal axis activity consequently affecting ovarian function and sex steroid metabolism in women with PCOS[1,2,6].

Obesity has been described in nearly half of women with PCOS[7]. This prompted us to consider the presence or the absence of obesity in the characterization of the different phenotypes occurring in PCOS. Moreover, we propose that particular attention should be paid to the analysis of the obesity phenotype[5,6], since it is known that the majority of obese women with PCOS have abdominal body fat distribution. The significance of abdominal obesity may be greater than expected, since this phenotype is often associated with insulin resistance, thus with a condition of 'functional hyperandrogenism'.

The notion that the metabolic syndrome may very often be an integral part of PCOS is an important factor in the evaluation of PCOS throughout life, and indicates that PCOS by itself is not a disorder exclusively related to fertile age women, but may have some health implications even after menopause. Therefore, PCOS should be evaluated according to the age of the woman affected.

Amenorrhea, oligomenorrhea and/or hirsutism are the typical features of PCOS during adolescence, whereas infertility and/or hirsutism are the most frequent symptoms affecting women with PCOS during the reproductive age. In premenopausal or postmenopausal phases, women affected by PCOS may present with diabetes, hypertension, lipid abnormalities and cardiovascular diseases more often than the same age reference population[8,9]. In conclusion, a picture which changes with age should always be kept in mind by physicians, in order to obtain a better understanding of the physiopathological mechanisms which develop this syndrome, and to provide a precise diagnosis and specific and appropriate therapeutic approaches.

Hyperinsulinemia and insulin resistance and their relationship with hyperandrogenism

The concept that hyperinsulinemia is a pathological condition which could promote hyperandrogenism was proposed by an early finding that young women with type A and B Kahn's syndrome, who presented with hyperinsulinemia and insulin-resistance, were often virilized[10]. A few years later, Burghen et al.[11] were the first to describe a close association between hyperinsulinemia and PCOS and a correlation between insulin and androgen levels. Further studies confirmed these preliminary observations[1,2,5,12,13], extending the findings of high level of insulin also to lean women with PCOS[1,2]. These data were substantiated by further reports which have demonstrated a significant positive correlation between fasting and glucose-stimulated insulin levels and plasma testosterone or androstenedione levels in women with PCOS[1,2]. The important role of insulin in the regulation of ovarian steroidogenesis was provided by several *in vitro* findings whose results are summarized in Table 1.

In summary, at the end of nearly thirty years of research, two distinct theories have been proposed to explain the pathophysiological mechanisms leading to the association of hyperandrogenism and hyperinsulinemia. Hyperandrogenism has been proposed as the cause of insulin resistance on the basis of clinical findings which have shown that administration of estrogens and progesterone to women with PCOS resulted in remission of insulin resistance[14]. Further confirmation was obtained by observations that, in women affected by PCOS, androgen administration was able to induce insulin resistance[15] and anti-androgen treatment (e.g. spironolactone) was able to revert this metabolic alteration[16]. It is noteworthy that this effect is completely independent of the type of anti-androgen used, since similar results were obtained after treatment with drugs having different mechanisms of action, such as spironolactone, flutamide, finasteride

Table 1 Direct and indirect insulin effects on ovary function

Direct stimulation of ovarian steroidogenesis acting at level of P450c17α enzyme

Potentiation of LH and FSH effect through an up-regulation of LH ovarian receptors and an amplification of the GnRH effect on gonadotropins at pituitary level

Inhibition of SHBG production at hepatic level

Inhibition of insulin growth factor binding protein-1 production at hepatic and ovarian level

Promotion of the ovarian growth and of the cyst formation acting in synergistic fashion with LH and hCG

Up-regulation of the insulin growth factor type 1 receptors and hybrid insulin/type 1 insulin growth factor receptors

LH, luteinizing hormone; FSH, follicle-stimulating hormone; GnRH, gonadotropin-releasing hormone; SHBG, sex hormone-binding globulin; hCG, human chorionic gonadotropin
Table modified from Poretsky et al.[2]

or gonadotropin-releasing hormone (GnRH)-agonists[17,18]. In order to obtain a full effect from these drugs, a condition of insulin resistance is required in woman with PCOS. It is possible that the favorable effects of anti-androgens reflect the negative effects of androgens (specifically testosterone) on insulin target tissues, such as the muscles. In fact, excessive androgen exposure may reduce muscle insulin sensitivity in both rodents and humans[19].

In contrast to the assumption that hyper-androgenism may cause insulin resistance, hyperinsulinemia has been alternatively proposed as the pathogenetic reason for the hyperandrogenism detected in women with PCOS. This point of view was originated by several in vitro and in vivo findings, which demonstrated that insulin may act as a gonadotropic hormone at ovarian level[1,2,5,6,12,13].

High affinity insulin receptors have been detected in the ovary, and their stimulation by insulin has been shown to induce in vitro androgen synthesis. It is still under debate whether insulin action at ovarian level is also mediated by the cognate insulin-growth factor receptor. This topic was recently carefully

reviewed by Poretsky et al.[2] In vitro data showed that stromal cell cultures or tissue derived from ovaries of women with PCOS are much more responsive to insulin challenge in terms of androgen secretion than those obtained from normal subjects. The same experiments also showed that insulin is not only able to stimulate per se androgen secretion but is also capable of enhancing the effect induced by simultaneous application of luteinizing hormone (LH). Altogether, these data indicate a greater sensitivity to the insulin effects in ovaries of women with PCOS than those of normal women[20].

More conflicting data concerning the putative role of insulin to induce hyperandrogenism are obtained from in vivo studies[1]. Early studies failed to demonstrate an increase in androgen levels following experimentally-induced hyperinsulinemia[2]. Limitations such as the short time of hyperinsulinemia induction and the inappropriately elevated levels of insulin, well above those found in women with PCOS, may explain the inability of these studies to show an insulin effect on androgen secretion.

However, it was recently demonstrated that a significant reduction of androgen concentration and a concomitant increase of sex hormone-binding globulin (SHBG) occurs in obese women and women with PCOS after administration of drugs capable of reducing insulin concentrations, therefore proving the primary role of insulin in the induction of hyperandrogenism.

Ehrmann et al.[21,22] showed that excessive ovarian androgen production may be related to a dysregulation of P450c17α, an ovarian enzyme which is responsible for the transformation of 17 hydroxyprogesterone into androstenedione. The same authors administered nafarelin, a GnRH-analog, to PCOS hyperandrogenic women, after suppressing adrenal androgen production by dexamethasone, and found that androstenedione, 17 hydroxyprogesterone and LH serum levels were significantly higher both before and 24 hours after nafarelin administration in women with PCOS than in normal women. The differences in ovarian steroid response to nafarelin could not be explained by the LH overproduction due to the GnRH analog[21]. Interestingly, similar results in anovulatory women with PCOS were also observed in ovulatory women with PCOS[22]. Altogether, these data support the concept that 17 hydroxylase/17,20 lyase activity is abnormally regulated in the ovary of women with PCOS, thus suggesting that hyperandrogenism in PCOS is due to an intrinsic abnormality of ovarian theca–interstitial cell function[22]. Recent studies using insulin-sensitizer agents have provided direct evidence that hyperinsulinemia may dysregulate ovarian P450c17α function. In particular, Nestler *et al.*[23,24] have studied in detail this issue by administering metformin to obese and non-obese women with PCOS who are affected by insulin resistance, showing that both basal and leuprolide- (another GnRH agonist agent) induced 17α-hydroxyprogesterone levels were significantly reduced after short-term metformin administration. Altogether, these data have clearly proved that chronic hyperinsulinemia may be a key factor in determining P450c17α hyperactivity in women with PCOS. This assumption is further supported by the observation that metformin administration not only favored spontaneous ovulation, but also significantly enhanced low-dose clomiphene-induced ovulation in obese women affected by PCOS and by chronic anovulation[25], the latter usually being resistant even to very high dosages of compounds like clomiphene.

As mentioned above, *in vitro* and *in vivo* studies have shown that insulin may affect both SHBG synthesis and metabolism, therefore indirectly influencing endogenous androgen secretion. Insulin has been shown to inhibit SHBG production in a human hepatoma cell line (Hep G2)[26]. The existence of an inverse correlation between insulin and SHBG concentration has been proved in both pre- and postmenopausal women[27–29]. Moreover, in obese women, particularly in those with abdominal body fat distribution, lower SHBG levels are usually found when compared with normal[30,31]. Decreased basal SHBG

concentrations have been found in women with PCOS[32] and even lower SHBG concentrations have been detected in obese women with PCOS when compared with normal weight women with PCOS[5,32]. Nestler *et al.*[33] found that GnRH agonist administration in obese women with PCOS did not change SHBG concentrations despite a marked reduction in androgen concentrations. However, inhibition of insulin release and a significant increase in SHBG levels were obtained with a concomitant ten days' diazoxide administration. These data clearly indicate that pre-existing hyperinsulinemia may play a more prominent role in suppression of SHBG concentrations than hyperandrogenism. In conclusion, insulin seems to regulate the delivery of androgens in peripheral tissues and appears to be an important factor in determining the clinical expression of the androgenization characterizing PCOS.

The molecular mechanisms underlying the reduction of insulin sensitivity in women with PCOS are not completely elucidated. An excessive serine phosphorylation induced by a serine/threonine kinase has been proposed as the pathogenetic mechanism responsible for the association of PCOS and insulin resistance[1]. Serine phosphorylation appears to modulate the activity of the key regulatory enzyme of androgen biosynthesis, P450c17α[34]. This intriguing fact led to the hypothesis that a single defect may concurrently induce insulin resistance and the hyperandrogenism observed in some women with PCOS.

Glucose tolerance in women with PCOS

Although insulin resistance seems to play a determinant role in the development of PCOS, the presence of insulin resistance does not immediately imply a concomitant alteration of glucose tolerance. Nevertheless, the percentage of women affected by PCOS and obesity, also presenting with glucose intolerance, is rather high, ranging from 20 to 40%[1]. These percentages are substantially above the prevalence rates reported in premenopausal women in population-based studies. Much less frequent is the finding of glucose intolerance in normal-weight or lean women with PCOS. Altogether, this may indicate that obesity *per se* plays an important role in altering the insulin–glucose system in PCOS.

Most obese women with PCOS are characterized by a pre-diabetic state, and may be at increased risk of developing type II diabetes. This has been shown by preliminary studies by Dalhgren et al.[8], who found that middle-aged women, who were histopathologically diagnosed with PCOS 20 to 30 years before the study took place, showed a 15% possibility of developing type II diabetes, in comparison with the 2.3% of the control age-matched group. In addition, the same authors found that these women also had an increased susceptibility to developing arterial hypertension and coronary heart disease. Based on a 10-year follow-up study, we recently found that hyperinsulinemia, insulin resistance and glucose tolerance tended to worsen spontaneously in women with PCOS, without any further worsening of hyperandrogenism. This finding prompted us to suggest that increased susceptibility to type II diabetes may be anticipated by a progressive impairment of insulin sensitivity associated with the development of glucose intolerance[35]. Our observations seem to confirm what has been described in obese women with PCOS by the above-mentioned cross-sectional clinical studies.

Evidence for a defect of insulin secretion in PCOS

Several recent studies have identified insulin secretion defects in obese women with PCOS, suggesting that such impairments could be most severe in those women who have a first-degree familial history of diabetes type II[36,37]. Using a modified frequently-sampled intravenous glucose tolerance test to determine acute insulin response to glucose, Dunaif et al.[37] reported that women with PCOS, particularly obese ones, had significantly decreased insulin

sensitivity when compared with normal-weight controls, and exhibited a first-phase insulin secretion pattern that was inadequate for the insulin-resistant state. Interestingly, these alterations of insulin action and secretion were not associated with glucose intolerance in the majority of women with PCOS investigated. These studies underline the importance of assessing β-cell function in the context of insulin sensitivity. However, longitudinal studies are needed in order to determine whether such defects are predictive of glucose intolerance and type II diabetes in women with PCOS, in particular when affected by abdominal obesity phenotype.

Treatment of women with obesity and PCOS: the effect of weight loss on hyperandrogenism and ovulation

There is long-standing clinical evidence concerning the efficacy of weight loss upon clinical and endocrinological features of obese women presenting with PCOS. However, the effects of weight loss on the clinical course of women with obesity and PCOS have not been as deeply investigated as was the pharmacological management of the syndrome. Weight loss improves menses abnormalities and, most importantly, both ovulation and fertility rate[2,7]. Other beneficial effects include reduction of hirsutism and disappearance of acanthosis nigricans, which is a cutaneous marker of insulin resistance[2,7]. The reduction of testosterone, androstenedione and dehydroepiandrosterone sulfate levels and the increase of SHBG concentrations appear to be responsible for the amelioration of the signs and symptoms reported after weight loss in obese women with PCOS. Moreover, there are indications that weight loss may decrease LH pulse amplitude which, in turn, can be followed by reduced androgen production[38]. The key factor responsible for these effects is the reduction of the insulin level, which is obviously associated with an improvement in the insulin-resistant state.

Table 2 Beneficial effects of weight loss in obese women with PCOS

Final effect	Parameters examined
Reduction	Total and visceral body fat
Improvement	Hirsutism score, menstrual cycle, ovulation and pregnancy rate, acanthosis nigricans
Reduction	Testosterone, androstenedione, insulin
Improvement	Insulin sensitivity
Unchanged/increased	Sex hormone-binding globulin
Unchanged/increased	Luteinizing hormone

A concomitant decrease in testosterone and insulin concentrations (both basal- and glucose-stimulated) has been described regardless of body weight variations[39]. Diet-induced reduction of insulin levels has been demonstrated to decrease P450c17α enzyme activity and consequently ovarian androgen production[40]. In addition, the weight-loss-associated reduction of leptin may lead to a deactivation of the neuroendocrine control of ovarian steroid secretion[41].

To summarize, weight loss in women with obesity and PCOS not only reduces total and visceral fat, but also restores normal menses cycles and improves the fertility rate, reducing androgen and insulin concentrations and improving insulin sensitivity (Table 2). It is important to notice that the effects of dietary-induced weight loss on androgens seem to be specific to obese hyperandrogenic women, since they have not been reported in obese women without PCOS[41].

Agents reducing insulin levels and insulin resistance in the treatment of hyperandrogenism and anovulation in PCOS

As concluded above, diet itself may positively affect hormonal and metabolic parameters in obese women with PCOS. However, insulin suppression obtained after diazoxide administration has been shown to reduce testosterone and to increase SHBG concentrations in obese and hyperandrogenic women with PCOS without affecting body weight. The same treatment has been described to be ineffective in normal-weight controls[33]. Therefore, the reduction of insulin levels has been proposed as the primary goal to be achieved. For this reason, insulin-sensitizing agents have been suggested as one of the therapeutic options for ameliorating hyperandrogenism and anovulation affecting women with PCOS. This therapeutic regimen has been proposed alone or in combination with standard body-weight-reduction procedures such as hypocaloric diet, exercise and behavioral or cognitive approaches. We will briefly summarize the principal characteristics of commercially available insulin-sensitizers and the novel analog drugs currently under investigation.

Metformin

Metformin is a drug belonging to the class of biguanides. This drug has been widely used in Europe and Canada for several decades for the treatment of type II diabetes and it has been recently introduced in the USA. Its mechanism of action includes a reduction of hepatic glucose production and an increased sensitivity of peripheral tissues to insulin (i.e. by increasing insulin-receptor tyrosine kinase activity in vascular smooth muscle), without significant effects on β-cell insulin production[42] (Table 3). Therefore, metformin can reduce peripheral insulin concentrations and improve glucose tolerance and metabolism. Metformin does not appear to display a direct effect on ovarian steroidogenesis and on insulin growth factor binding protein-1 synthesis[2,43]. According to its pharmacokinetic properties, this drug should be administered at dosages ranging from 1500 to 2550 mg/day. The effective maintenance dose may often be 850 mg twice a day, taken with morning and evening meals. Absolute bioavailability is 50 to 60% under fasting conditions. Food intake can slightly decrease and delay absorption, but

Table 3 Mechanisms of the antihyperglycemic effect of metformin

Mechanism	Comment
Suppression of hepatic glucose output	Contributes to postabsorptive and postprandial plasma glucose-lowering effect
Increased insulin-mediated glucose disposal	Demonstrated by glucose-clamp procedures; due at least in part to a reduction in blood glucose concentrations
Increased intestinal glucose use	Shown only in studies in animals
Decreased fatty-acid oxidation	

From Bailey CJ *et al.*[42] *N Engl J Med* 1996;334:574–9. Copyright © Massachusetts Medical Society. All rights reserved

the clinical relevance of this effect is largely unknown. Side-effects are uncommon. Gastrointestinal discomforts may affect around 10% of patients, although these side-effects tend to disappear with time. Rarely, metformin may induce lactic acidosis and, even more rarely, hematological problems.

Thiazolidinediones

Thiazolidinediones are selective ligands for peroxisome proliferation activated receptor (PPAR)γ, a member of the nuclear receptor superfamily of ligand-activated transcription factors[44]. To date, three mammalian PPAR subtypes, PPARα, PPARγ and PPARδ, have been identified, each of them exhibiting distinct tissue-distribution and ligand-binding domain. Natural ligands for these receptors include fatty acids and eicosanoids. PPARγ is expressed mainly in white and brown adipocytes and at lower levels in skeletal muscle and liver. The exact mechanism of action of these compounds is not yet fully elucidated. Lipophilic thiazolidinediones readily enter cells and bind to PPARγ. Genes involved in carbohydrate and lipid metabolism are known to be regulated by PPARγ. Cell culture studies have demonstrated that after activation of PPARγ, thiazolidinediones promote differentiation of pluripotent stem cells and pre-adipocytes into mature

adipocytes[44]. Euglycemic hyperinsulinemic clamp experiments have clearly demonstrated that thiazolidinedione therapy is able to increase insulin-mediated rates of glucose disposal[45]. This effect is associated with a reduction in fasting and post-prandial glucose levels together with a decrease in systemic free fatty acids. One of these compounds, troglitazone, has been shown to suppress basal hepatic glucose production at high doses (600 mg/day), whereas no effect was detectable at lower doses (100–400 mg/day)[46]. It is still unclear whether this suppression is a directly mediated or a secondary effect related to a reduction in circulating free fatty acid levels. The reports of liver damage after troglitazone administration in some patients have provided the rationale for producing analog drugs displaying fewer hepatotoxicity side-effects. For this reason, analogs such as rosiglitazone and pioglitazone have been produced and are now commercially available.

D-Chiro-inositol

Some of the actions of insulin may involve low-molecular-weight inositol phosphoglycan mediators. When insulin binds to its own receptor, members of this class are generated by hydrolysis of glycosyl-phosphatidyl-inositol lipids located in the outer layer of the cell membrane. Released mediators are then internalized, affecting intracellular metabolic processes. Although different species have been identified, an inositol phosphoglycan molecule containing D-chiro-inositol and galactosamine has been described as playing a role in activating key enzymes controlling the oxidative and non-oxidative glucose metabolism[47]. Moreover, there is evidence that inositol glycans may be components of the signal transduction system leading to insulin-triggered testosterone biosynthesis in human thecal cells[48]. D-Chiro-inositol phosphoglycan mediator deficiency has been described as resulting in insulin resistance[49]. Administration of D-chiro-inositol has been shown to improve insulin resistance in both animals and humans[49].

Clinical studies with insulin sensitizers in PCOS

Velasquez et al.[50] first demonstrated that metformin administration in obese women with PCOS was not only able to significantly improve insulin levels, but also to decrease LH and testosterone concentrations, regardless of changes in body weight, while a significant improvement of menstrual abnormalities was also described in most patients. This first report was confirmed by many other studies which proved the beneficial effect of long-term metformin treatment on fertility[51]. As mentioned before, short-term metformin administration (1500 mg/daily for 1 month) has been shown to reduce insulin levels and 17α-hydroxyprogesterone and LH response to leuprolide[23]. Higher plasma insulin and lower serum androstenedione levels associated with less severe menstrual abnormalities seem to be predictive of a beneficial outcome of metformin treatment[52].

An improvement in ovulation rate in obese women with PCOS has also been described after short-term use of metformin. In addition, recent data indicate that administration of this drug may also markedly increase clomiphene-induced ovulation in comparison with placebo, thus suggesting that obese women with PCOS have increased ovarian cytochrome P450c17α activity, resulting in excessive ovarian androgen production, as documented by the increased production of 17α-hydroxyprogesterone after stimulation with GnRH agonist nafarelin[25] (and personal communication by S. Kadkhodayan). As reported above, similar effects have also been observed after dietary-induced weight loss. Recently, we performed a 6-month double-blind controlled study to investigate the effect of a combined metformin administration (850 mg twice daily) and hypocaloric diet on insulin, androgens and fat distribution in a group of abdominally obese women with and without PCOS[41]. Interestingly, a greater reduction of body weight and abdominal fat, particularly the visceral depots, and a

Table 4 Statements for eligibility of PCOS patients when using insulin-sensitizing agents

(1)	The metabolic syndrome as an integral part of the polycystic ovary syndrome in approximately 2/3 of affected women
(2)	Obesity, particularly the abdominal phenotype, affects 40–60% of women with PCOS
(3)	Hyperinsulinemia may play a role in determining hyperandrogenism in PCOS
(4)	Insulin resistance, whatever the cause, may be present not only in obese but also in lean women with PCOS
(5)	Long-term implications of PCOS in adult age and in postmenopause

more consistent decrease of serum insulin, testosterone and leptin concentrations were observed after metformin administration in abdominally obese women with PCOS when compared with placebo. In the patients affected by PCOS these changes were associated with a significant improvement of hirsutism and menstrual abnormalities. These findings led us to conclude that hyperinsulinemia and abdominal obesity may have complementary effects in the pathogenesis of PCOS.

There are few studies on the effects of thiazolidinediones in PCOS. Troglitazone (400 mg daily) has been shown to improve total body insulin sensitivity in obese women with PCOS, resulting in lower circulating insulin levels. A substantial improvement of the PCOS-derived metabolic and hormonal disorders was observed after administration of this drug, as indicated by a decline in testosterone, triglycerides and plasminogen activator inhibitor type I, the last two being well-known risk factors for the development of cardiovascular diseases[53,54]. In addition, short-term troglitazone administration can improve spontaneous ovulation in anovulatory women with PCOS[2]. To our knowledge, there are no clinical studies using the new thiazolidinediones, rosiglitazone and pioglitazone, in women with PCOS.

Among other insulin-sensitizing agents, the potential use of D-chiro-inositol in PCOS treatment is currently under investigation. As mentioned above, inositol glycans have been described as mediating insulin action on thecal steroidogenesis[48]. Taking into consideration these *in vitro* findings, Nestler *et al.*[55] proposed D-chiro-inositol therapy for women with PCOS, demonstrating in a placebo-controlled trial that this drug is able to decrease insulin secretion during the oral glucose tolerance test and to concomitantly increase plasma SHBG. These hormonal changes have been described as being accompained by a significant restoration of spontaneous ovulation.

Altogether these data indicate that insulin sensitizers may constitute an appropriate treatment for women with PCOS. A proposed selection criteria of eligibility of women with PCOS for insulin-lowering agent treatment is illustrated in Table 4.

In conclusion, the data strongly support the hypothesis that in women with obesity and PCOS improvement of hyperinsulinemia can be associated with various clinical benefits. These women exhibit an increased susceptibility of developing diabetes and cardiovascular diseases later in life, particularly when they are postmenopausal. An improvement of insulin sensitivity and hyperinsulinemia in susceptible individuals, as a preventive intervention, may be of great importance as demonstrated by epidemiological and clinical studies[56]. Whether this is the case in the subgroup of insulin-resistant obese women with PCOS is a question that needs to be answered by appropriate long-term intervention studies.

References

1. Dunaif A. Insulin resistance and the polycystic ovary syndrome: metabolism and implication for pathogenesis. *Endocr Rev* 1997;18:774–800
2. Poretsky L, Cataldo NA, Roseuwaks Z, *et al.* The insulin-related ovarian regulatory system in health and disease. *Endocr Rev* 1999;20:545–82
3. Franks S. Polycystic ovary syndrome. *N Engl J Med* 1995;333:853–61
4. Pasquali R. The endocrine impact of obesity in eumenorrheic women. In Azziz R, Nestler JE, Dewailly D, eds. *Androgen Excess Disorders in Women*. Philadelphia, New York: Lippincot-Raven, 1997;455–61
5. Pasquali R, Casimirri F. The impact of obesity on hyperandrogenism and polycystic ovary syndrome in premenopausal women. *Clin Endocrinol* 1993;39:1–16
6. Holte J. Disturbances in insulin secretion and sensitivity in women with the polycystic ovary syndrome. *Baillière's Clin Endocrinol Metab* 1996;10:221–47
7. Pasquali R, Casimirri F, Vicennati V. Weight control and its beneficial effect on fertility in women with obesity and polycystic ovary syndrome. *Hum Reprod* 1997;12(Suppl. 1):82–7
8. Dahlgren E, Johansson S, Lindstedt G, *et al.* Women with polycystic ovary syndrome wedge resected in 1956 to 1965: a long term follow-up focusing on natural history and circulating hormones. *Fertil Steril* 1992;57:505–13
9. Talbott E, Guzick D, Clerici A, *et al.* Coronary heart disease risk factors in women with polycystic ovary syndrome. *Arterioscler Thromb Vasc Biol* 1995;15:821–6
10. Kahn CR, Flier JS, Bar RS, *et al.* The syndromes of insulin resistance and acanthosis nigricans. *N Engl J Med* 1976;294:739–45
11. Burghen GA, Givens JR, Kitabchi AE. Correlation of hyperandrogenism with hyperinsulinism in polycystic ovarian disease. *J Clin Endocrinol Metab* 1980;50:113–16
12. Poretsky L, Kalin MF. The gonadotropic function of insulin. *Endocr Rev* 1987;8:132–41
13. Poretsky L. On the paradox of insulin-induced hyperandrogenism in insulin-resistant states. *Endocr Rev* 1991;12:3–13
14. Cole C, Kitabchi AE. Remission of insulin resistance with Orthonovum® in a patient with polycystic ovarian disease and acanthosis nigricans. *Clin Res* 1978;26:412A
15. Woodward TL, Burghen GA, Kitabki AE, *et al.* Glucose intolerance and insulin resistance in aplastic anemia treated with oxymetholone. *J Clin Endocrinol Metab* 1981;53:905–8

16. Shoupe D, Lobo RA. The influence of androgens on insulin resistance. *Fertil Steril* 1984;4: 385–8

17. Moghetti P, Tosi F, Castello R, *et al*. The insulin resistance in women with hyperandrogenism is partially reversed by antiandrogen therapy: evidence that androgens impair insulin action in women. *J Clin Endocrinol Metab* 1996;81:952–60

18. Diamanti-Kandarakis E, Mitrakou A, Hennes MMI, *et al*. Insulin sensitivity and antiandrogenic therapy in women with polycystic ovary syndrome. *Metabolism* 1995;44:525–31

19. Bjorntorp P. Metabolic implications of body fat distribution. *Diabetes Care* 1991;14:1132–43

20. Barbieri RL, Makris A, Randall RW, *et al*. Insulin stimulates androgen accumulation in incubations of ovarian stroma obtained from women with hyperandrogenism. *J Clin Endocrinol Metab* 1986;62:904–10

21. Ehrmann DA, Rosenfield RL, Barnes RB, *et al*. Detection of functional hyperandrogenism in women with androgen excess. *N Engl J Med* 1992;327:157–62

22. Ehrmann DA, Barnes RB, Rosenfield RL. Polycystic ovary syndrome as a form of functional ovarian hyperandrogenism due to dysregulation of androgen secretion. *Endocr Rev* 1995;16:322–53

23. Nestler JE, Jakubowicz DJ. Decreases in ovarian cytochrome P450c17alpha activity on serum free testosterone and reduction of insulin secretion in polycystic ovary syndrome. *N Engl J Med* 1996;335:617–23

24. Nestler JE, Jakubowicz DJ. Lean women with polycystic ovary syndrome respond to insulin reduction with decreases in ovarian P450c17alpha activity and serum androgens. *J Clin Endocrinol Metab* 1997;82:4075–9

25. Nestler JE, Jakubowicz DJ, Evans WS, *et al*. Effects of metformin on spontaneous and clomiphene-induced ovulation in the polycystic ovary syndrome. *N Engl J Med* 1998;338: 1876–80

26. Plymate SR, Matej LA, Jones RE, *et al*. Inhibition of sex hormone-binding globulin in the human hepatoma (HepG2) cell line by insulin and prolactin. *J Clin Endocrinol Metab* 1988;6:460–4

27. Evans DJ, Hoffmann RG, Kalkhoff RK, *et al*. Relationship of androgenic activity to body fat topography, fat cell morphology and metabolic aberrations in premenopausal women. *J Clin Endocrinol Metab* 1983;57:304–10

28. Plymate SR, Fariss BL, Bassett ML, *et al*. Obesity and its role in polycystic ovary syndrome. *J Clin Endocrinol Metab* 1981;52:1246–9

29. Haffner SM, Katz MS, Stern MP, *et al*. The relation of sex hormones to hyperinsulinemia and hyperglycemia. *Metabolism* 1988;37:683–8

30. Glass AR, Burman KD, Dahms WT, *et al*. Endocrine function in human obesity. *Metabolism* 1981;30:89–104

31. Purifoy FE, Koopmans LH, Tatum RW, *et al*. Serum androgen and sex hormone-binding globulin in obese Pima Indian females. *Am J Physiol* 1981;55:491–6

32. Pasquali R, Casimirri F, Cantobelli S, *et al*. Insulin and androgen relationship with abdominal body fat distribution in women with and without hyperandrogenism. *Horm Res* 1993; 39:179–87

33. Nestler JE, Baralascini CO, Matt DW, *et al*. Suppression of serum insulin by diazoxide reduces serum testosterone levels in obese women with polycystic ovary syndrome. *J Clin Endocrinol Metab* 1989;68:1027–32

34. Zhang LH, Rodriguez H, Ohno S, *et al*. Serine phosphorylation of human P450c17 increases 17,20-lyase activity: implications for adrenarche and polycystic ovary syndrome. *Proc Natl Acad Sci USA* 1995;92:10619–23

35. Pasquali R, Gambineri A, Anconetani B, *et al*. The natural history of the metabolic syndrome in young women with the polycystic ovary syndrome and the effect of long-term estroprogestogen treatment. *Clin Endocrinol* 1999; 50:517–27

36. Ehrmann DA, Sturis J, Byrne MM, *et al*. Insulin secretory defects in polycystic ovary syndrome. Relationship to insulin sensitivity and family history of non-insulin dependent diabetes mellitus. *J Clin Invest* 1995;96:520–7

37. Dunaif A, Finegood DT. β-cell dysfunction independent of obesity and glucose intolerance in the polycystic ovary syndrome. *J Clin Endocrinol Metab* 1996;81:942–7

38. Harlass FE, Plymate SR, Fariss BL, *et al*. Weight loss is associated with correction of gonadotropin and sex steroid abnormalities in the obese anovulatory females. *Fertil Steril* 1984;42:649–52

39. Pasquali R, Antenucci D, Casimirri F, *et al*. Clinical and hormonal characteristics of obese amenorrheic hyperandrogenic women before and after weight loss. *J Clin Endocrinol Metab* 1989;68:173–9

40. Jakubowicz D, Nestler JE. 17α-hydroxyprogesterone responses to leuprolide and serum androgens in obese women with and without polycystic ovary syndrome after dietary weight loss. *J Clin Endocrinol Metab* 1997;82: 556–60

41. Pasquali R, Gambineri A, Biscotti D, *et al.* Effect of long-term treatment with metformin added to hypocaloric diet on body composition, fat distribution, and androgen and insulin levels in abdominally obese women with and without the polycystic ovary syndrome. *J Clin Endocrinol Metab* 2000;85:2767–74

42. Bailey CJ, Turner RC. Metformin. *N Engl J Med* 1996;334:574–9

43. Lacy C. Metformin: drug information. UpToDate® *Drug information Handbook*. Wellesley Hills, MA: UpToDate Inc, 2000:Vol. 8, No. 2

44. Lehmann JM, Moore LB, Smith-Oliver TA, *et al.* An antidiabetic thiazolidinedione is a high affinity ligand for peroxisome proliferation-activated receptor γ (PPARγ). *J Biol Chem* 1995; 270:12953–6

45. Nolan JJ, Ludvik B, Beerdsen P, *et al.* Improvement in glucose tolerance and insulin resistance in obese subjects treated with troglitazone. *N Engl J Med* 1994;331:1188–93

46. Murphy E, Nolan JJ. Insulin sensitizer drugs. *Exp Opin Invest Drugs* 2000;9:1347–61

47. Larner J. Multiple pathways in insulin signalling – fitting the covalent and allosteric puzzle pieces together. *Endocr J* 1994;2:167–71

48. Nestler JE, Jakubowicz DJ, Falcon de Vargas A, *et al.* Insulin stimulates testosterone biosynthesis by human thecal cells from women with polycystic ovary syndrome by activating its own receptor and using inositolglycan mediators as the signal transduction system. *J Clin Endocrinol Metab* 1998;83:2001–5

49. Ortmeyer HK, Huang LC, Zhang L, *et al.* Chiro-inositol deficiency and insulin resistance. II. Acute effects of D-chiro-inositol administration in streptozotocin-diabetic rats, normal rats given a glucose load, and spontaneously insulin-resistant rhesus monkeys. *Endocrinology* 1993;132:646–51

50. Velasquez EM, Mendoza S, Hamer T, *et al.* Metformin therapy in polycystic ovary syndrome reduces hyperinsulinemia, insulin resistance, hyperandrogenemia, and systolic blood pressure, while facilitating normal menses and pregnancy. *Metabolism* 1994;43: 647–54

51. Oberfield SE. Editorial: Metabolic lessons from the study of young adolescents with polycystic ovary syndrome – is insulin, indeed, the culprit? *J Clin Endocrinol Metab* 2000;85:3520–5

52. Moghetti P, Castello R, Negri C, *et al.* Metformin effects on clinical, endocrine and metabolic profiles, and insulin sensitivity in polycystic ovary syndrome: a randomized, double-blind, placebo-controlled 6-month trial, followed by open, long-term clinical evaluation. *J Clin Endocrinol Metab* 2000;85:139–46

53. Dunaif A, Scott D, Finegood D, *et al.* The insulin-sensitizing agent troglitazone improves metabolic and reproductive abnormalities in the polycystic ovary syndrome. *J Clin Endocrinol Metab* 1996;81:3299–306

54. Ehrmann DA, Schneider DJ, Sobel BE, *et al.* Troglitazone improves defects in insulin action, insulin secretion, ovarian steroidogenesis, and fibrinolysis in women with polycystic ovary syndrome. *J Clin Endocrinol Metab* 1997; 82:2108–17

55. Nestler JE, Jakubowicz DJ, Reamer RD, *et al.* Ovulatory and metabolic effects of d-chiro-inositol in the polycystic ovary syndrome. *N Engl J Med* 1999;340:1314–20

56. Ferranini E. Insulin resistance *vs* insulin deficiency in non-insulin dependent diabetes mellitus: problems and prospects. *Endocr Rev* 1998; 19:477–90

New insights into polycystic ovary syndrome by color Doppler, three-dimensional ultrasound and vascular endothelial growth factor

10

S. L. Tan and T. J. Child

Introduction

Polycystic ovary syndrome (PCOS) is a common clinical disorder characterized by chronic anovulation, hyperandrogenism and ovaries of polycystic morphology (Figure 1). Although the syndrome was first described more than 65 years ago, the pathogenesis of this condition has yet to be fully elucidated[1]. In addition, there is a lack of consensus over the clinical and laboratory findings necessary to constitute the syndrome. However, it is recognized that women may have ovaries of polycystic morphology in the absence of all the clinical and laboratory manifestations associated with polycystic ovary syndrome. As such, we distinguish two separate entities. Polycystic ovaries (PCO) describes the ultrasonic appearance of the ovaries. Women with PCO may have regular, ovulatory menstrual cycles with normal serum luteinizing hormone (LH), testosterone and androstenedione levels. PCOS identifies the condition where there are polycystic ovaries seen on ultrasound, together with clinical (amenorrhea, oligomenorrhea, irregular menstrual cycles) and/or endocrine features (raised LH and androgen levels, high LH/follicle-stimulating hormone (FSH) ratio). Recently, three research tools have been applied to the study of PCOS, and they are increasing our insight into this condition. The first of these is high-resolution transvaginal ultrasound combined with color and pulsed Doppler; the second is three-dimensional (3D) ultrasonography; the third is assays for vascular endothelial growth factor (VEGF).

Color and pulsed Doppler ultrasonography

Because of its noninvasive nature, ultrasonography has emerged as an invaluable tool in the diagnosis of the polycystic ovary. The most commonly used ultrasonographic criterion for PCO is the presence of ≥ 10 cysts measuring 2–8 mm in diameter arranged peripherally or scattered throughout a dense, ultrasonically bright ovarian stroma (Figure 1)[2]. With color Doppler ultrasound, it is apparent that the stroma of a polycystic ovary is more densely vascularized than that of a normal ovary. This concurs with histological findings of increased vascularity within the PCO[3]. Color and pulsed Doppler ultrasonography allow the assessment of intraovarian stromal blood flow velocity. In two prospective studies we showed that women with polycystic ovaries had a significantly higher maximum ovarian stromal blood flow velocity during both the spontaneous menstrual cycle[4], and in the *in vitro* fertilization (IVF) treatment cycle[5], compared with women with normal ovaries. We suggested that increased ovarian stromal blood velocity was

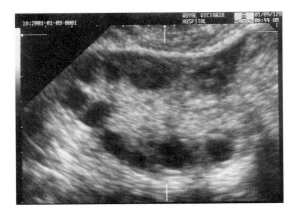

Figure 1 Transvaginal ultrasound picture of a polycystic ovary. Note the multiple small cysts and the enlarged echogenic stroma

an additional parameter for the ultrasound diagnosis of PCO[4]. We also found that during IVF treatment, the maximum ovarian stromal blood flow velocity at the baseline scan[5], and following pituitary down-regulation[6], are correlated with the subsequent follicular response to gonadotropin stimulation. We suggested that the greater degree of vascularization within a polycystic ovary could be the cause of the exuberant response of the PCO to gonadotropin stimulation compared with the normal ovary[4,5,7]. The greater vascularization may result in higher levels of gonadotropins being delivered to the target cells within the ovary. This could also explain the increased risk of developing ovarian hyperstimulation syndrome (OHSS), the main iatrogenic complication of ovarian stimulation in women with polycystic ovaries[5,7]. The maximum ovarian stromal blood velocities are comparable in women with PCO and PCOS, and are significantly higher than in women with normal ovaries[4]. This is a cardinal observation and it supports the notion that all women undergoing induction of ovulation or ovarian stimulation for assisted conception should have a baseline early follicular phase ultrasound scan. If they have polycystic ovaries they are more sensitive to gonadotropin stimulation, irrespective of whether they have the clinical and endocrine features of PCOS. Battaglia

et al.[8] showed that there were differences in ovarian stromal blood flow parameters between polycystic ovaries with a peripheral and general cystic pattern. However, PCOS did not predetermine a single intraovarian blood flow pattern.

Most recently, we have shown that *in vitro* maturation (IVM) of immature oocytes retrieved from women with polycystic ovaries in a natural, unstimulated menstrual cycle is a successful treatment[9,10]. We have found that the pregnancy rates with IVM treatment are higher if more than ten immature oocytes are retrieved. We have also found that the maximum ovarian stromal blood velocity is an independent predictor of both the number of immature oocytes retrieved and the pregnancy rate following *in vitro* maturation of oocyte treatment (unpublished observations).

Color and pulsed Doppler can be used to measure the blood flow velocities within the uterine arteries. The pulsatility index (PI) can be derived from the peak systolic and diastolic velocities [(systolic velocity – diastolic velocity)/average velocity over the cardiac cycle]. An increased PI implies increased resistance to blood flow down-stream from the point of Doppler sampling; consequently, when calculating the PI at the uterine arteries we are indirectly assessing the resistance to blood flow within the uterus. Women with PCOS have a significantly higher uterine artery PI compared with women with normal ovaries, and obese, hyperinsulinemic women with PCOS have a higher uterine artery PI than women with PCOS who are not obese and who have insulin levels in the normal range[11]. The uterine artery PI is also positively correlated with serum androstenedione concentrations and the body mass index in women with PCOS[12,13]. For women with normal ovaries undergoing IVF we have shown a uterine artery PI of between two and three to indicate maximum receptivity of the uterus to embryo implantation[14,15]. Although the average uterine artery PI of women with PCOS is higher than that in women with normal ovaries[11–13,16,17], controlled studies comparing the pregnancy rates between women undergoing IVF with normal ovaries and women with PCO do not suggest any detrimental effect from polycystic ovaries[7,18]. The uterine artery PI of women with PCOS has been reported to significantly reduce following three months of treatment with gonadotropin-releasing hormone agonist and/ or the oral contraceptive pill[13].

Three-dimensional ultrasonography

A two-dimensional (2D) transvaginal probe provides images of the lower pelvis only in the sagittal and coronal planes. Images in the third, transverse, plane can only be provided with use of a 3D transvaginal ultrasound system. 3D ultrasonography entails the acquisition and storage of a volume of images by manual or automatic sweeping of the transducer across a region of interest. The stored data-set can then be digitally manipulated to display a multiplanar view, in which all three planes of the pelvis are displayed simultaneously, centered around the point of interest (Figure 2). As the point of interest is moved through the image volume, all three planes are simultaneously altered. In addition to displaying the transverse plane of the pelvis, 3D ultrasound has the ability to measure volumes with high accuracy and reproducibility[19,20]. Using 3D ultrasound, we measured the follicular, stromal and ovarian volumes of 50 women with normal ovaries and regular menstrual cycles, 24 women with PCO and regular cycles, and 26 women with PCOS[21]. We found that the ovarian volumes of the PCO and PCOS group were significantly greater than in the normal group and that this increase was due to a greater stromal rather than follicular volume. Although polycystic ovaries contain many more follicles than normal ovaries, there was no significant difference in the follicular volume between the two groups of women. There were no differences in ovarian or stromal volume between the PCO and PCOS groups. In addition, we showed that the theca-derived serum concentration of

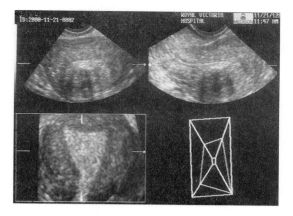

Figure 2 Three-dimensional multiplanar view of a normal uterus. The frontal view of the endometrial cavity can be seen in the lower left image

androstenedione was positively correlated with stromal volume in the PCOS group[21]. No correlation was found between stromal LH, 17-OH-progesterone or testosterone concentrations in any of the three groups[21].

An exciting development in 3D ultrasonography is the ability to combine this technique with power Doppler. Power Doppler allows an estimate of the total blood flow whereas color and pulsed Doppler measure the velocity of flow in selected vessels[22]. If the power Doppler function is activated during 3D volume acquisition, the total amount of blood flow within the volume of interest, such as the ovary, can be quantified[22]. As yet, this technology has not been systematically studied in the polycystic ovary.

Vascular endothelial growth factor

There is increasing interest in the role of VEGF in ovarian physiology and pathophysiology[23]. This glycoprotein growth factor is expressed and secreted in the premenopausal normal ovary in a cyclic manner and it is regulated by gonadotropin secretion during the menstrual cycle. VEGF has a paracrine and/or autocrine function necessary for normal ovarian function, mediating angiogenesis and vascular permeability. VEGF not only mediates angiogenesis but also induces connective tissue stromal growth by increasing microvascular permeability, which leads to extravasation of plasma proteins. The extra-vascular matrix thus formed favors in-growth of new blood vessels and fibroblasts, which in turn organizes the avascular fibrin matrix into a mature, vascularized connective tissue stroma[24,25]. VEGF is therefore critical for normal reproductive function[23].

We investigated the relationship between serum concentrations of VEGF and ovarian morphology in a prospective study[25]. Sixty women were studied in the early follicular phase: 36 had normal ovaries, 14 had regular menstrual cycles and normal hormonal levels with PCO seen on ultrasound scan, while 10 had PCOS[25]. Each woman had pulsed and color Doppler measurements of blood flow within the ovarian stroma and serum VEGF concentrations measured. The mean serum VEGF concentrations were significantly higher in the PCO and PCOS groups compared with women with normal ovaries ($p < 0.001$). The peak systolic blood flow velocities in the ovarian stroma of the PCO and PCOS groups were greater than that found in normal ovaries ($p < 0.001$) confirming our previous findings[5]. We found the serum VEGF concentrations to be positively correlated with stromal blood flow in all three groups of women[25]. We also found, in a study involving patients undergoing IVF treatment, that the follicular concentrations of VEGF were significantly higher in women with PCO than in women with normal ovaries[26]. Higher intraovarian concentrations of VEGF in women with PCO are likely, through angiogenesis, to cause the increased vascularization of the PCO. This may explain the higher risk of OHSS in women with PCO compared with those with normal ovaries[7,26]. We further explored this concept in a prospective study of 107 women undergoing IVF who had serum VEGF concentrations measured before treatment, after pituitary desensitization, and on the days of human chorionic gonadotropin (hCG) administration, oocyte collection, and embryo transfer[27]. Serum VEGF concentrations were higher throughout the treatment cycle in women in whom OHSS developed. Additionally, the

increase in VEGF concentration that occurred between the day of hCG administration and the day of oocyte collection was an important marker of OHSS. A higher VEGF rise predicted all cases of OHSS with a sensitivity of 100% and a specificity of 60%[27].

The question is whether higher serum VEGF concentrations in PCO are a response to the hormonal milieu or are a constitutive feature of PCO, due to inherent increased VEGF expression. *In vitro* studies have been performed on granulosa lutein cells. After cells were stimulated with gonadotropins and hCG, VEGF production was higher in granulosa cells obtained from women with PCO compared with those obtained from women with normal ovaries under similar culture conditions[28]. The expression of VEGF messenger RNA is also increased in the theca cells of PCO compared with normal ovaries, further supporting an inherent difference in terms of VEGF production[24].

Conclusions

Recent results from studies of color, pulsed Doppler and 3D ultrasound, and VEGF are increasing our insight into the pathogenesis of PCOS. It appears that polycystic ovaries secrete higher levels of VEGF than do normal ovaries, regardless of whether there are clinical and endocrine features of PCOS. The hyperthecotic stroma of PCO demonstrates extensive immunohistochemical VEGF staining, and granulosa cells from PCO follicles secrete greater levels of VEGF *in vitro* than do granulosa cells from normal ovarian follicles[24,28]. VEGF is an angiogenic factor, which explains the greater vascularization of the PCO both on histological and color and pulsed Doppler ultrasound examination. During the normal ovulatory cycle, Doppler ultrasound studies show that there is diversion of blood towards the dominant follicle[29], which may contribute to continued growth of the dominant follicle and atresia of the other follicles. It is tempting to speculate that the excessive amount of VEGF and increased vascularity of PCO may result in reduced diversion of blood away from cohort follicles to the leading follicle, thereby permitting uncoordinated or uninhibited growth of other follicles[27,28]. This may explain the multifollicular response to gonadotropin stimulation and increased risk of OHSS. The high levels of VEGF cause increased stromal growth which contribute to the typically increased volume of the PCO compared with the normal ovary. The pivotal involvement of VEGF in neovacularization makes it an attractive candidate for a central role in the pathophysiology of PCO, PCOS and OHSS[28].

References

1. Stein IF, Leventhal ML. Amenorrhea associated with bilateral polycystic ovaries. *Am J Obstet Gynecol* 1935;29:181–91

2. Adams J, Franks S, Polson DW, *et al.* Multifollicular ovaries: clinical and endocrine features and response to pulsatile gonadotrophin releasing hormone. *Lancet* 1985;2(8469–70): 1375–9

3. Hughesdon PE. Morphology and morphogenesis of the Stein-Leventhal ovary and of so-called 'hyperthecosis'. *Obstet Gynecol Surv* 1982;37:59–77

4. Zaidi J, Campbell S, Pittrof R, *et al.* Ovarian stromal blood flow in women with polycystic ovaries – a possible new marker for diagnosis? *Hum Reprod* 1995;10:1992–6

5. Zaidi J, Barber J, Kyei-Mensah A, *et al.* Relationship of ovarian stromal blood flow at baseline ultrasound to subsequent follicular response in an *in vitro* fertilization program. *Obstet Gynecol* 1996;88:779–84

6. Engmann L, Sladkevicius P, Agrawal R, *et al.* The value of ovarian stromal blood flow velocity measurement after pituitary suppression in the prediction of ovarian responsiveness and outcome of *in vitro* fertilization treatment. *Fertil Steril* 1999;71:22–9

7. MacDougall MJ, Tan SL, Balen A, *et al.* A controlled study comparing patients with or without polycystic ovaries undergoing *in vitro* fertilization. *Hum Reprod* 1993;8:233–7

8. Battaglia C, Artini PG, Salvatori M, *et al.* Ultrasonographic patterns of polycystic ovaries: color Doppler and hormonal correlations. *Ultrasound Obstet Gynecol* 1998;11:332–6

9. Chian RC, Gulekli B, Buckett WM, *et al.* Priming with human chorionic gonadotropin before retrieval of immature oocytes in women with infertility due to the polycystic ovary syndrome. *N Engl J Med* 1999;341:1624–6

10. Chian RC, Buckett WM, Tulandi T, *et al.* Prospective randomized study of human chorionic gonadotrophin priming before immature oocyte retrieval from unstimulated women with polycystic ovarian syndrome. *Hum Reprod* 2000;15:165–70

11. Dolz M, Osborne NG, Blanes J, *et al.* Polycystic ovarian syndrome: assessment with color Doppler angiography and three-dimensional ultrasonography. *J Ultrasound Med* 1999;18: 295–302

12. Battaglia C, Artini PG, Genazzani AD, *et al.* Color Doppler analysis in lean and obese women with polycystic ovary syndrome. *Ultrasound Obstet Gynecol* 1996;7:342–46

13. Battaglia C, Genazzani AD, Artini PG, *et al.* Ultrasonographic and color Doppler analysis in the treatment of polycystic ovary syndrome. *Ultrasound Obstet Gynecol* 1998;12:180–7

14. Steer CV, Campbell S, Tan SL, *et al.* The use of transvaginal color flow imaging after *in vitro* fertilization to identify optimum uterine conditions before embryo transfer. *Fertil Steril* 1992;57:372–6

15. Zaidi J, Pittrof R, Shaker A, *et al.* Assessment of uterine artery blood flow on the day of human chorionic gonadotropin administration by transvaginal color Doppler ultrasound in an *in vitro* fertilization program. *Fertil Steril* 1996; 65:377–81

16. Tan SL, Zaidi J, Campbell S, *et al.* Blood flow changes in the ovarian and uterine arteries during the normal menstrual cycle. *Am J Obstet Gynecol* 1996;175:623–31

17. Zaidi J, Jacobs H, Campbell S, *et al.* Blood flow changes in the ovarian and uterine arteries in women with polycystic ovary syndrome who respond to clomiphene citrate: correlation with serum hormone concentrations. *Ultrasound Obstet Gynecol* 1998;12:188–96

18. Engmann L, Maconochie N, Sladkevicius P, *et al.* The outcome of *in vitro* fertilization treatment in women with sonographic evidence of polycystic ovarian morphology. *Hum Reprod* 1999;14:167–71

19. Kyei-Mensah A, Zaidi J, Pittroff R, *et al.* Transvaginal three-dimensional ultrasound: accuracy of follicular measurements. *Fertil Steril* 1996; 65:371–6

20. Kyei-Mensah A, Maconochie N, Zaidi J, *et al.* Transvaginal three-dimensional ultrasound: reproducibility of ovarian and endometrial volume measurements. *Fertil Steril* 1996;65:717–22

21. Kyei-Mensah A, Tan SL, Zaidi J, *et al.* Relationship of ovarian stromal volume to serum androgen concentrations in patients with polycystic ovary syndrome. *Hum Reprod* 1998;13:1437–41

22. Pairleitner H, Steiner H, Hasenoehrl G, *et al.* Three-dimensional power Doppler sonography: imaging and quantifying blood flow and vascularization. *Ultrasound Obstet Gynecol* 1999; 14:139–143

23. Geva E, Jaffe RB. Role of vascular endothelial growth factor in ovarian physiology and pathology. *Fertil Steril* 2000;74:429–38

24. Kamat BR, Brown LF, Manseau EJ, *et al.* Expression of vascular permeability factor/ vascular endothelial growth factor by human granulosa and theca lutein cells. Role in corpus luteum development. *Am J Pathol* 1995; 146:157–65

25. Agrawal R, Sladkevicius P, Engmann L, *et al.* Serum vascular endothelial growth factor concentrations and ovarian stromal blood flow are increased in women with polycystic ovaries. *Hum Reprod* 1998;13:651–5

26. Agrawal R, Conway G, Sladkevicius P, *et al.* Serum vascular endothelial growth factor and Doppler blood flow velocities in *in vitro* fertilization: relevance to ovarian hyperstimulation syndrome and polycystic ovaries. *Fertil Steril* 1998;70:651–8

27. Agrawal R, Tan SL, Wild S, *et al.* Serum vascular endothelial growth factor concentrations in *in vitro* fertilization cycles predict the risk of ovarian hyperstimulation syndrome. *Fertil Steril* 1999;71:287–93

28. Agrawal R. What's new in the pathogenesis and prevention of ovarian hyperstimulation syndrome? *Hum Fertil* 2000;3:112–5

29. Sladkevicius P, Valentin L, Marsal K. Blood flow velocity in the uterine and ovarian arteries during the normal menstrual cycle. *Ultrasound Obstet Gynecol* 1993;3:199–208

Relationship between hyperandrogenism and disorders of glucose metabolism and uterine perfusion

11

G. B. Melis, A. M. Paoletti, S. Guerriero, M. Orrù, S. Campagnoli, R. Bargellini, C. Usala and S. Ajossa

The recent incorporation of color Doppler processing in the transvaginal transducer extends the scope of sonographic imaging from an anatomical to a physiological basis. The ability to assess utero-ovarian blood flow has several applications: detection and differentiation of sonographically complex benign ovarian masses from malignant ones; diagnosis of ovarian torsion; assessment of perfusion in either normotopic or ectopic early pregnancies; and evaluation of women with infertility problems. Following the pioneering work of Goswamy[1], many authors have found a relationship between uterine perfusion and infertility in both spontaneous[2-4] and stimulated[5,6] cycles.

Several studies using transvaginal color Doppler ultrasonography have found higher impedance in the blood flow of the uterine artery[7-10], and some authors have suggested including color Doppler evaluation of the uterine artery in the traditional investigation used for the diagnosis of this disease[7-10]. In contrast, Pinkas *et al.*[11] demonstrated that polycystic ovaries do not disturb blood flow in the uterine artery[11]. This different result may be a reflection of differences in subgroups of women with polycystic ovary syndrome (PCOS) considered in the studies.

In our experience[12,13], the mean pulsatility index (PI) of the uterine artery in women with PCOS is significantly higher than that of the control group, but we demonstrated also that PCOS by itself does not predetermine a single uterine blood flow pattern; in fact, in the group of women affected by this syndrome a very wide range of values of PI of the uterine artery is present[12]. Many authors have studied the influence of reproductive hormones on uterine perfusion. The vasodilatory effect of estradiol (E_2) is well known: estrogen receptors have been found in the wall of human uterine arteries[14]; midcycle elevation of plasma E_2 induces a decrease in vascular resistance[15]; and the administration of a gonadotropin-releasing hormone agonist increases the vascular resistance of uterine arteries[16]. Besides, the marked increase in serum E_2 levels during induction of multiple follicular development for *in vitro* fertilization–embryo transfer determines a significant decrease in PI of the uterine artery[17].

Other hormonal factors are involved in the modulation of uterine perfusion. In our previous study[12] we demonstrated that the administration of cabergoline to patients affected by PCOS determined a significant decrease in the PI in the uterine artery, while E_2 levels remained unchanged and no correlation was found with the PI. In this study, during cabergoline administration, we described a statistically significant reduction in total and free testosterone, androstenedione, dehydroepiandrosterone sulfate (DHEAS) and 17-OH-progesterone (17-OHP), and correlations were found between the PI of the uterine artery and luteinizing hormone (LH), free testosterone, 17-OHP, androstenedione, and DHEAS[12,18,19].

Androgens have been demonstrated to have a direct vasoconstrictive effect on vascular tissues[20], and a fibrotic process has been described, mediated in part by androgen-dependent collagen and elastin deposition in smooth muscle cells[21]. Also, DHEAS seems to have a role in modulation of uterine perfusion. In a study performed in our institute[13], we demonstrated that plasma levels of DHEAS were significantly higher in women with PCOS with PI of uterine artery > 3 than in those with PI < 3, and a significant correlation was found between the two parameters.

Recently, a substantial advance in the field of PCOS has been made, and it has been realized that many women with PCOS are resistant to insulin[22]. The pancreas compensates for insulin resistance in PCOS by increasing insulin release; thus in these women both fasting and oral glucose tolerance test-stimulated levels of insulin and C-peptide are significantly higher[20]. Hyperinsulinemia seems to be a primary cause of hyperandrogenism in women with PCOS, stimulating ovarian testosterone production, decreasing sex hormone-binding globulin concentration and stimulating pituitary LH secretion[22]. On the other hand, it is possible that hyperandrogenism may cause insulin resistance. In fact, exogenous androgens reduce insulin sensitivity, and, in patients with idiopathic hirsutism, treatment with flutamide can completely reverse hyperinsulinism, which suggests that the efficacy of the drug is dependent on peripheral androgen hyperactivity[22]. The same effect was not observed in women with PCOS; this result suggests a more complex pathogenesis of hyperinsulinism in this syndrome[22]. Recently, some authors[23,24] have studied the possible relationship between lower insulin sensitivity and artery hemodynamics; they found that increased thickness of the intima–media complex of the common carotid artery is significantly associated with insulin resistance and with decreased distensibility of the common carotid artery[25]. In addition, Hedblad et al.[24] found that fasting serum insulin covaries with a number of factors and conditions known to influence the development of atherosclerosis[24]. We found no study on the immediate effect of hyperinsulinism on vascular resistance.

The effect of hyperinsulinism on uterine perfusion has not been studied yet, but Battaglia et al.[8] found higher insulin levels, more adverse lipid profile, higher hematocrit values and higher PI of the uterine artery in obese women with PCOS than in lean women with PCOS.

In conclusion, PCOS is not only an endocrinological disease but also has to be considered a metabolic disorder affecting multiple body systems. For this reason it requires comprehensive and long-term evaluation and management. Above all, a gynecologist who sees women with PCOS has to consider not only infertility problems or hyperandrogenism but also the possibility of diabetes mellitus, and would be wise to check blood pressure and serum lipid profile.

References

1. Goswamy RK, Williams G, Steptoe PG. Decreased uterine perfusion – a cause of infertility. *Hum Reprod* 1988;3:955–9
2. Kurjak A, Kupesic-Urek S, Shulman H, et al. Transvaginal color flow Doppler in the assessment of ovarian and uterine blood flow in infertile women. *Fertil Steril* 1991;56:870–3
3. Fujimo Y, Ito F, Matuoka I, et al. Pulsatility index of uterine artery in pregnancy and non-pregnant women. *Hum Reprod* 1993;8:1126–8
4. Steer CV, Tan SL, Mason BA, et al. Midluteal phase vaginal color Doppler assessment of uterine artery impedance in a subfertile population. *Fertil Steril* 1994;61:53–8
5. Cacciatore B, Simberg N, Fusaro P, et al. Transvaginal Doppler study of uterine artery blood flow in *in vitro* fertilization-embryo transfer cycles. *Fertil Steril* 1996;61:130–4
6. Tsai Y-C, Chang J-C, Tai M-J, et al. Relationship of uterine perfusion to outcome of

intrauterine insemination. *J Ultrasound Med* 1996;15:633–6

7. Battaglia C, Artini PG, D'Ambrogio G, *et al*. The role of color Doppler imaging in the diagnosis of polycystic ovary syndrome. *Am J Obstet Gynecol* 1995;72:108–13

8. Battaglia C, Artini PG, Gennazzani AD, *et al*. Color Doppler analysis in lean and obese women with polycystic ovary syndrome. *Ultrasound Obstet Gynecol* 1996;7:342–6

9. Battaglia C, Artini PG, Gennazzani AD, *et al*. Color Doppler analysis in oligo- and amenor-rheic women with polycystic ovary syndrome. *Gynecol Endocrinol* 1997;11:105–10

10. Aalem FA, Predanic M. Transvaginal color Doppler determination of the ovarian and uterine blood flow characteristics in polycystic ovary disease. *Fertil Steril* 1996;65:510–16

11. Pinkas H, Rabinerson D, Avrech OM, *et al*. Doppler parameters of uterine and ovarian stromal blood flow in women with polycystic ovary syndrome and normally ovulating women undergoing controlled ovarian stimulation *Ultrasound Obstet Gynecol* 1998;12:197–200

12. Ajossa S, Paoletti AM, Guerriero S, *et al*. Effect of chronic administration of cabergoline on uterine perfusion in women with polycystic ovary syndrome. *Fertil Steril* 1999;71:314–18

13. Ajossa S, Guerriero S, Paoletti AM, *et al*. Uterine perfusion and hormonal pattern in patients with polycystic ovary syndrome. *J Assis Reprod Genet*;in press

14. Perrot-Applanat M, Groyer-Picard MT, Garcia E, *et al*. Immunocytochemical demonstration of estrogen and progesterone receptors in muscle cells of uterine arteries in rabbits and humans *Endocrinology* 1988;123:1511–14

15. Goswamy R, Steptoe PC. Doppler ultrasound studies of the uterine artery in spontaneous ovarian cycle. *Hum Reprod* 1988;3:721

16. Matta WHM, Stabile I, Show RW, *et al*. Doppler assessment of uterine blood flow changes in patients with fibroids receving the gonadotropin-releasing hormone agonist buserelin. *Fertil Steril* 1988;49:1083

17. Cacciatori B, Tiitnen A. Does ovarian stimulation affect uterine artery impedance? *J Assis Reprod Genet* 1996;13:15–18

18. Paoletti AM, Cagnacci A, Soldani R, *et al*. Evidence that an altered prolactin release is consequent to abnormal ovarian activity in polycystic syndrome. *Fertil Steril* 1995;64: 1094–8

19. Paoletti AM, Cagnacci A, Depau GF, *et al*. The chronic administration of cabergoline normal-izes androgen secretion and improves men-strual cyclicity in women with polycystic ovary syndrome. *Fertil Steril* 1996;66:527–32

20. Horwitz KB, Horwitz LD. Canine vascular tis-sues are targets for androgens, estrogens, progestinics and glucocorticoids. *J Clin Invest* 1982;69:740–8

21. Fisher GM, Swann ML. Effect of sex hormones on blood pressure and vascular connective tis-sue in castrated and non-castrated rats. *Am J Physiol* 1977;232:617–21

22. Paoletti AM, Cagnacci A, Orrù M, *et al*. Treatment with flutamide improves hyperinsu-linemia in women with idiopathic hirsutism. *Fertil Steril* 1999;72:448–53

23. Pergola GD, Ciccone M, Pannacciulli N, *et al*. Lower insulin sensitivity as an independent risk factor for carotid wall thickening in nor-motensive, non-diabetic, non-smoking normal weight and obese premenopausal women. *Int J Obes Relat Metab Disord* 2000;24:825–9

24. Hedblad B, Nilson P, Janson L, *et al*. Relation between insulin resistance and carotid intima-media thickness and stenosis in non-diabetic subjects. Results from a cross-sectional study in Malmo, Sweden. *Diabet Med* 2000;17:299–307

25. van Popele NM, Westendorp IC, Bots ML, *et al*. Variables of the insulin resistance syn-drome are associated with reduced arterial distensibility in healthy non-diabetic middle-aged women. *Diabetologia* 2000;43:665–72

The effect of a herbal treatment (Tian Gui) for polycystic ovary syndrome of the hyperinsulinemic pattern

12

J. Yu

Introduction

Oligomenorrhea and amenorrhea are common in obese women and in women with significant weight loss. Over the last few decades there have been a number of reports describing the adverse effects of obesity on menstruation, but the relevance of these symptoms is unknown, because there is no common pattern in the hormonal parameters of such subjects, and because obesity is a multifactorial problem. Hyperandrogenism and hyperinsulinemia are described in obese women with oligomenorrhea or amenorrhea, especially in polycystic ovary syndrome (PCOS), which sheds light on the endocrine–metabolic mechanism of anovulation. Approximately 50% of women with PCOS are obese, with significant reductions in post-prandial thermogenesis and β_2-adrenoreceptor density on adipocytes, indicating abnormal energy expenditure[1]. Recently, a key regulator of adipogenesia in adipose tissue, the peroxisome proliferator-activated receptor (PPARr), has been identified as being involved in the obesity of PCOS and non-insulin-dependent diabetes mellitus. The regulation of PPARr remains to be studied, though it may be activated by insulin and glucocorticoids[2].

Leptin has been proven to provide a feedback loop between peripheral signals, mainly from fat cells and hypothalamic sites, in the regulation of eating behavior, energy expenditure and reproductive function[3]. Hypothalamic targets for leptin are neurons expressing neuropeptide Y (NPY) via the long form of the leptin receptor (Ob-R_b)[4]. NPY, the most potent stimulator of eating behavior, is one of the steroid-dependent modulators of gonadotropin-releasing hormone (GnRH)[5]. Proopiomelanocortin (POMC), recognized as a basic estrogen-dependent neurosuppressor on GnRH release, also increases food intake. In accounting for adiposity, serum leptin levels are more sensitive than the body mass index (BMI)[3], but the relationship between peripheral leptin levels and central NPY/POMC expressions in PCOS is not clear.

In 1996, a herbal formula known as Tian Gui was reported to be effective for anovulation, infertility and obesity in the treatment of patients with PCOS manifesting hyperinsulinemia/insulin resistance, obesity and clomiphene resistance[6,7]. Herbs in the Tian Gui formula were selected according to the holistic and dialectic views of traditional Chinese medicine, and 15 years of clinical experience by this author. The details of the neuroendocrine–metabolic defects of PCOS in biomedicine were used and developed in examining the mechanism of action of the Tian Gui formula. An animal model was created by modification of Barraclough's androgen-sterilized rat (ASR) model[8], by administering testosterone propionate to female rats at the age of 9 days, which manifested polycystic ovaries, anovulation, infertility, obesity, hyperandrogenism and hyperinsulinemia. This model helped in the investigation of the function of Tian Gui, in addition to the clinical study[9].

Materials and methods

Patients

The study subjects were 54 women aged between 18 and 35 years (mean age 24 years), diagnosed with the hyperinsulinemic pattern of PCOS in the Department of Integrated Traditional Chinese and Western Medicine, Obstetrics and Gynecology Hospital, Shanghai, between 1995 and 1998. All patients manifested amenorrhea or oligomenorrhea with consecutive monophasic basal body temperature, obesity with BMI > 25 kg/m^2 and waist/hip ratio > 0.80, hirsutism, polycystic ovaries on ultrasonography, and failure to ovulate under clomiphene citrate treatment (clomiphene resistance). Significant acanthosis nigricans appeared in 18 cases and infertility was reported in 17 cases. Blood samples were taken on days 3–5 after the first day of the last bleeding episode induced by progesterone, and serum levels of the following were measured: luteinizing hormone (LH), follicle-stimulating hormone (FSH), prolactin (PRL), estradiol, testosterone, dehydroepiandrosterone (DHEA), cortisol, fasting insulin, oral glucose tolerance test (OGTT), 17-hydroxyprogesterone (17-OHP), thyroid-stimulating hormone (TSH), triiodothyronine and thyroxine (T$_4$). The insulin-releasing test was also carried out. Every patient was characterized by high levels of serum testosterone, low estradiol, high fasting and glucose-stimulated insulin, normal or high LH, normal or slightly high 17-OHP, and normal FSH, PRL, DHEA, TSH, triiodothyronine and T$_4$. The traditional Chinese diagnosis was kidney Yin deficiency with phlegm and blood stasis, based on the manifestation of amenorrhea, obesity, thirst, irritability, acne, interior heat, overeating, little vaginal discharge, constipation, dark reddened tongue and fine pulse.

Forty-six patients were administered with the Tian Gui treatment twice a day for 3 months immediately after the diagnosis was made. The treatment contained Chinese foxglove root (*Radix Rehmanniae Glutinosae*), short-horned epimedium herb (*Herba Epiinedii*), Chinese angelica root (*Radix Angelicae Sinensis*), peach seed (*Semen Persicae*) and others. In a control study, 16 patients were allocated randomly into two groups, treated with Tian Gui (8 cases) or metformin (8 cases). The regimen for metformin was 500 mg three times per day for 3 months. The criteria for ovulation were biphasic BBT and elevation of serum progesterone level, and ultrasonic signs of ovulation or pregnancy in infertile women. All patients were re-examined after the 3 months of treatment.

Five normal women with regular menstruation, biphasic BBT and normal body weight, aged 18–30 years, were recruited as controls for hormonal and metabolic measurements on the fifth cycle day.

Animal model

Fifty-five neonatal female Sprague Dawley rats at 9 days of age were injected subcutaneously with testosterone propionate (1.25 mg in neutral tea oil, equivalent to 0.05 ml) or 0.05 ml of neutral tea oil ($n = 15$, control group). All rats were weaned at 21 days of life and housed at 25°C (50% humidity) with 12-h light/dark cycles, with food and water freely available. Vaginal smears were examined daily for 10 consecutive days from 70 days of age, and 40 out of 55 rats with persistent vaginal cornification (72.7%) were used as 9-day androgen-sterilized rat (9d-ASR) models; all rats in the control group showed cyclic estrus changes. A group of 25 9d-ASR rats were administered 1 ml per 100 g body weight of extract from the Tian Gui treatment, and all normal rats and the other 15 9d-ASR rats were administered distilled water, from 80 to 101 days of age.

To prepare the Tian Gui extracts, the Tian Gui treatment was pulverized and refluxed with 95% ethanol three times. The extracts were concentrated under reduced pressure with a rotavapor (Bü CHI Rotavapor R–114, Switzerland) and were evaporated to give 342 mg/ml residue (equivalent to 3 g/ml of crude herbs).

Daily vaginal smears were monitored for 11 days after herbal treatment or distilled water administration was terminated. Rats administered distilled water who did not show cyclic estrus changes were withdrawn from the study.

Food consumption over 24 h was measured from 70 to 100 days of age in all rats. Rats were weighed and perfused transcardially under sodium pentobarbital anesthesia (50 mg/ml, intraperitoneally) at approximately 112 days of age. Normal controls and the 9d-ASR rats administered distilled water were sacrificed in the afternoon of proestrus. Blood was collected from the inferior vena cava before perfusion and stored at −20°C for radioimmunoassays. The retroperitoneal white adipose tissue, pancreas and ovaries of each rat were removed and weighed after fixative perfusion. The brain was removed and coronal sections were cut through the preoptic area and hypothalamus according to a standard method described by Paxions and Watson[10]. The sections were kept at −20°C until further processing.

Single- and double-label immunohistochemistry
Free-floating sections were processed for immunohistochemistry with rabbit antisera directed against estrogen receptor-α (ER$_\alpha$) (diluted to 1 : 400), neuropeptide Y (1 : 8000) and GnRH (1 : 1000). The primary antisera were localized using the avidin–biotin complex system (ABC). The immunoreactive densitometric analyses were performed on a computer-assisted image analysis system. The mean particle density (MPD) provided a semi-quantitative index of average staining intensity within a given region and was used as the unit of analysis.

For the double fluorescence study, the sections were incubated in a mixture of mouse antisera directed against ER$_\alpha$ (diluted to 1 : 400, Santa Cruz) and a rabbit antisera against NPY (1 : 800, Sigma), or in a mixture of a mouse antisera directed against androgen receptor (diluted to 1 : 400, Santa Cruz) and a rabbit antisera against β-endorphin (β-EP) (1 : 8000 Sigma). Then the sections were incubated in a mixture of secondary antibodies: goat anti-mouse immunoglobulin G (IgG) conjugated with rhodamine (diluted to 1 : 20) and swine anti-rabbit IgG conjugated with fluorescein isothiocyanate (FITC, diluted to 1 : 40). The sections were examined with a confocal laser scanning microscope using dual-channel fault scanning (0.9–1 μm thickness) and a powerful three-dimensional rendering and processing module.

Single and dual in situ *hybridization* The specific antisense oligonucleotide hybridization probes of NPY, Ob-R$_b$ and POMC mRNA were terminally labeled with α-^{33}P deoxytriphosphate [α-^{33}P] dATP and terminal transferase. The sections were digested, acetylated, dehydrated, rinsed in saline sodium citrate (SSC), and then reacted in a hybridization solution containing a radiolabeled probe. After posthybridization treatment, the sections were exposed to X-ray film for further autoradiography. Hybridization signal detection (the relative mRNA contents) was evaluated in an image analysis system.

To detect the relationship between Ob-R$_b$ or POMC and NPY mRNA-containing neurons, we used simultaneously digoxigenin- and radiolabeled oligodeoxyribonucleotide probes. The sections were covered with hybridization solution containing the two probes. The digoxigenin-labeled probes were located by alkaline phosphatase-conjugated antibodies against digoxigenin, and the radiolabeled probes by conventional nuclear emulsion autoradiography. A blocking solution (parlodion in acetone) was used to prevent a chemical interaction between the chromagen products and the autoradiographic emulsion. Staining was observed under a dark-field microscope.

Reverse transcription polymerase chain reaction (RT-PCR) The levels of androgen receptor mRNA expression in hypothalamus and

Table 1 Hormonal and metabolic observations during Tian Gui treatment

| | Estradiol (pg/ml) | Testosterone (nmol/l) | Insulin | | Body mass index (kg/m^2) | Waist/hip ratio |
			Fasting (µU/ml)	AUC (µU/dl/h)		
Controls (n = 5)	51.04 ± 1.18	1.43 ± 1.26	5.06 ± 1.73	1869.00 ± 479.89	21.08 ± 3.65	0.70 ± 1.08
Patients (n = 14)						
before Tian Gui	18.40 ± 2.30*	4.53 ± 1.77*	18.35 ± 11.75*	1301.31 ± 751.13*	30.68 ± 3.91*	0.95 ± 0.08*
after Tian Gui	24.56 ± 1.67	1.93 ± 0.89	11.10 ± 5.16	864.56 ± 343.46*	29.81 ± 2.86*	0.91 ± 0.18*

AUC, area under curve; *$p < 0.05$ compared with controls

pancreas were determined by RT-PCR. The total RNA of these tissues was isolated with Trizol agents. The RNA samples were converted to DNA–RNA double-stranded hybrids and then converted into double-stranded cDNA with reverse transcriptase. A standard PCR reaction was then performed on the synthesized cDNA with single-base mutant template control. The electrophoretic bands of digested PCR products were evaluated in an image and analysis system and the optical densities were measured.

Northern blot analysis The total RNA was isolated from hypothalamus and electrophoresed through denaturing gels. The RNA fragments were then transferred to nylon membranes by electroblotting. The nylon membranes were hybridized with a solution containing the digoxin-labeled probe of the POMC gene. The staining was revealed with nitro-blue tetrazolium/5-bromo-4-chloro-3-indolylphosphate.

Hormone assays Serum estradiol, total and free testosterone, DHEA, insulin, C-peptide, FSH, LH and leptin concentrations were measured in duplicate by radioimmunoassay. The intra- and inter-assay coefficients of variation were all less than 10%.

Statistical analyses

Group values were expressed as mean ± SD. Variables not normally distributed were log-transformed before analysis by parametric methods. Data were analyzed with the Student–Newman–Keuls test utilizing one-way analysis of variance (ANOVA). Pearson correlation coefficients (r) were presented on simple and/or multiple linear regression analysis. Analysis of covariance (ANCOVA) and partial correlations were used to investigate the relationship between body weight and serum leptin levels or relative amount of central NPY-IR (immunoreactivity), and the body weight was used as a covariate. Differences were considered significant at $p < 0.05$. Statistical analyses were performed using SAS 6.12 computer software package (statistical analysis system, Cary, NC).

Results

Clinical results

Thirty-two (69.7%) of the 46 patients ovulated after the Tian Gui treatment; of these, 10 patients ovulated in the third cycle (21.7%), 11 ovulated in the second cycle (23.9%) and 11 ovulated in the first cycle (23.9%). Acanthosis nigricans completely disappeared in two cases and was reduced in another 16 cases. Body weight decreased in most cases, and symptoms such as overeating, thirst, irritability and constipation were reduced. Seven of the 17 previously infertile patients became pregnant within 3–9 months of the treatment. Serum testosterone and insulin levels decreased and estradiol levels increased in most of the patients. Complete sets of endocrine and metabolic data were obtained in 14 patients (Table 1).

In the control study, six cases in the group treated with Tian Gui and two cases in the group treated with metformin showed

Table 2 Serum testosterone (T) and estradiol (E$_2$) levels in groups treated with Tian Gui and metformin

	Estradiol (pg/ml)	Testosterone (nmol/l)	log(T/E$_2$)
Tian Gui group			
before treatment	29.55 ± 9.47	3.66 ± 0.54	1.70 ± 0.15
after treatment	50.44 ± 9.81*	3.50 ± 0.78	1.26 ± 0.11*
Metformin group			
before treatment	27.69 ± 6.65	3.22 ± 0.28	1.61 ± 0.14
after treatment	26.37 ± 6.37	2.61 ± 0.50	1.21 ± 0.07

*$p < 0.05$ compared with before treatment

evidence of ovulation. Acanthosis nigricans disappeared in two cases in each group, and apparently decreased in the Tian Gui group but not in the metformin group. Symptoms decreased in the Tian Gui group and were unchanged in the metformin group. The waist/hip ratio decreased in seven cases in the Tian Gui group and in one case in the metformin group. Insulin levels were significantly decreased in the metformin group and slightly decreased in the Tian Gui group, serum testosterone decreased in both groups, and serum estradiol significantly increased in the Tian Gui group, resulting in a decline in the log (testosterone)/estradiol ratio (Table 2).

Animal investigation

Effect of Tian Gui on obesity and anovulation Daily food intake, body weight, retroperitoneal white adipose tissue and serum leptin concentrations of the 9d-ASR rats were significantly higher than that in normal rats and in the 9d-ASR rats administered Tian Gui extract ($p < 0.01$ for both comparisons), as were the levels of fasting and glucose-stimulated insulin.

Two consecutive estrus cycles were observed in all 15 control rats and in 15 of the 25 9d-ASR rats treated with Tian Gui extract (60%) after the age of 101 days, whereas persistently keratinized vaginal cells were exhibited in all of the 15 9d-ASR rats treated with distilled water. All ovaries weighed 30–50% less in 9d-ASR rats than in normal rats (31.24 ± 1.13 vs. 67.54 ± 2.15 mg, $p < 0.01$). Absence of corpora lutea, decreased numbers of granulosa cells (one or two layers) in the cystic follicles and high testosterone secretion

of theca-interstitial cells in 9d-ASR rats were significantly improved by Tian Gui treatment. Levels of LH and FSH were significantly lower, and levels of estradiol, testosterone, free testosterone, androstenedione and DHEA, and the LH/FSH ratio, were significantly higher in 9d-ASR than in normal rats and 9d-ASR rats administered Tian Gui extract ($p < 0.01$, Table 3).

Androgen receptor mRNA expression in the pancreas Pancreatic androgen receptor mRNA expression was significantly higher in the 9d-ASR group than in normal rats and 9d-ASR rats treated with Tian Gui ($p < 0.05$, Table 4). This result was correlated to the secretions of C-peptide and insulin from the pancreas and the serum androgen levels in each group.

Colocalization of androgen receptor, estrogen receptor and leptin receptor (Ob-R$_b$) with neuropeptide-containing neurons In the double immunofluorescence study, the majority of β-endorphin neurons in the hypothalamic arcuate nucleus were decorated with androgen receptor-labelled cells (especially in the cytoplasm), and many NPY-IR neurons in the arcuate nucleus and preoptic area were decorated in the cytoplasm with estrogen receptor-labelled cells. The fibers of NPY neurons were also immunoreactive for estrogen receptor.

In the dual *in situ* hybridization study, signals of Ob-R$_b$ mRNA were coexpressed with NPY mRNA-containing neurons in the arcuate nucleus, and synapses from NPY mRNA-containing neurons were found to

Table 3 Metabolic and endocrine values in normal rats (controls), 9-day androgen-sterilized rats (9d-ASR group) and 9-day androgen-sterilized rats treated with Tian Gui (treatment group). Values are presented as mean ± SD

	Controls (n = 15)	9d-ASR group (n = 15)	Treatment group (n = 15)
Body weight (g)	209.5 ± 12.4	243.9 ± 8.3*	207.4 ± 14.3
Retroperitoneal WAT (g)	9.6 ± 0.7	17.9 ± 1.2*	10.2 ± 1.2
Leptin (ng/ml)	1.19 ± 0.21	2.78 ± 0.16*	0.92 ± 0.28
C-peptide (ng/ml)	0.08 ± 0.01	0.12 ± 0.01*	0.09 ± 0.03
Insulin			
Fasting (µU/ml)	21.41 ± 1.59	29.88 ± 2.58*	25.32 ± 1.47
AUC (µU/dl/h)	56.46 ± 2.21	66.72 ± 2.45*	59.20 ± 2.15
FSH (ng/ml)	1.14 ± 0.13	0.25 ± 0.06*	1.06 ± 0.03
LH (ng/ml)	8.28 ± 0.87	1.17 ± 0.58*	8.05 ± 0.91
Estradiol (pg/ml)	65.57 ± 9.33	141.91 ± 24.97*	67.71 ± 7.13
Total testosterone (ng/dl)	0.12 ± 0.04	0.52 ± 0.15*	0.18 ± 0.05
Free testosterone (pg/ml)	0.06 ± 0.05	0.37 ± 0.15*	0.07 ± 0.04
Log (T/E$_2$)	−2.02 ± 0.58	−1.52 ± 0.61*	−1.87 ± 0.49
Androstenedione (ng/ml)	0.08 ± 0.07	1.78 ± 0.38*	0.13 ± 0.19
DHEA (ng/dl)	0.04 ± 0.01	0.08 ± 0.01*	0.05 ± 0.01
Ovarian total testosterone			
theca–interstitial cells (fmol/10^6 cells)	93.33 ± 5.15	156.00 ± 7.76*	123.60 ± 4.95
total per ovary (pg/ovary)	320.12 ± 42.78	497.34 ± 45.62*	138.07 ± 42.43
Adrenal cell testosterone	25.65 ± 11.45	27.66 ± 10.54*	22.75 ± 6.98
total per adrenal gland (pg/adrenal)	201.79 ± 16.59	284.18 ± 27.76*	155.65 ± 36.13

WAT, white adipose tissue; AUC, area under curve; FSH, follicle-stimulating hormone; LH, luteinizing hormone; T, testosterone; E$_2$, estradiol; DHEA, dehydroepiandrosterone; *$p < 0.01$ compared with controls

contact with synapses from POMC mRNA-containing neurons in the arcuate nucleus.

GnRH in the preoptic area and median eminence Immunolabeling of GnRH neurons in the preoptic area and GnRH fibers in the internal zone throughout the median eminence was significantly less in 9d-ASR rats than in normal rats ($p < 0.01$). Both markedly increased to normal concentrations after treatment with Tian Gui ($p < 0.05$ and $p < 0.01$, respectively, Table 4). These results corresponded to changes in serum LH and FSH levels in each group.

Estrogen receptor in the arcuate nucleus/median eminence and hypothalamic androgen receptor mRNA Hypothalamic expression of androgen receptor mRNA significantly increased in the 9d-ASR group ($p < 0.01$), and after Tian Gui treatment was reduced to levels which were lower than in normal rats ($p < 0.05$). This

result corresponded to the high androgen levels in 9d-ASR rats ($p < 0.01$) and the changes in androgen levels in 9d-ASR rats with Tian Gui treatment (Tables 3 and 4).

Dense populations of estrogen receptor IR cells in the arcuate nucleus/median eminence were significantly fewer in the 9d-ASR group than in normal rats ($p < 0.01$), whereas circulating estradiol levels were higher in the 9d-ASR group ($p < 0.01$). After Tian Gui treatment, 9d-ASR rats had similar densities of estrogen receptor and similar levels of serum estradiol, testosterone and free testosterone to those of the normal group ($p > 0.05$) (Tables 3 and 4).

Changes in other types of mRNA in the arcuate nucleus/median eminence In NPY-immunolabeled sections, numerous NPY-IR perikarya and nerve fibers with varicosities were shown rostrocaudally throughout the arcuate nucleus and the internal zone of the median eminence

Table 4 Values of immunoreactivity and mRNA expression in the hypothalamic arcuate nucleus/median eminence and pancreas in normal rats (controls), 9-day androgen-sterilized rats (9d-ASR group) and 9-day androgen-sterilized rats treated with Tian Gui (treatment group). Values are presented as mean ± SD

	Controls (n = 15)	9d-ASR group (n = 15)	Treatment group (n = 15)
Immunoreactivity (MPD)			
Estrogen receptor-IR+	188.00 ± 12.42	79.07 ± 9.91*	178.93 ± 7.89
Neuropeptide Y-IR+	54.87 ± 15.49	102.93 ± 43.01*	57.53 ± 10.24
GnRH-IR+			
median eminence	98.41 ± 5.63	58.47 ± 9.99*	94.85 ± 5.17
preoptic area	31.44 ± 3.26	7.64 ± 4.04*	28.17 ± 4.37
Hybridization (MPD)			
Androgen receptor mRNA (hypothalamus)	3.71 ± 0.46	4.40 ± 0.33*	1.10 ± 0.18
Neuropeptide Y mRNA	24.12 ± 2.41	52.54 ± 2.54*	27.08 ± 1.62
Ob-R_b mRNA	38.62 ± 2.28	16.34 ± 3.63*	34.72 ± 3.62
POMC mRNA	22.34 ± 3.56	60.08 ± 5.26*	24.76 ± 4.18
Androgen receptor mRNA (pancreas)	0.82 ± 0.18	2.24 ± 0.36*	0.74 ± 0.05

MPD, mean particle density; GnRH, gonadotropin-releasing hormone; *$p < 0.01$ compared with controls

in normal rats. The immunohistochemical staining of NPY in the arcuate nucleus was significantly more concentrated in 9d-ASR rats than in normal rats ($p < 0.01$), while no significant differences were found between 9d-ASR rats treated with Tian Gui and normal rats ($p > 0.05$). Expressions of NPY mRNA and POMC mRNA also showed higher values in 9d-ASR rats than in normal rats and in 9d-ASR rats treated with Tian Gui ($p < 0.01$ for both comparisons, Table 4).

The mean particle density (MPD) of Ob-R_b mRNA highly concentrated in the arcuate nucleus of normal rats was markedly decreased with a 58% reduction in the 9d-ASR group ($p < 0.01$). After Tian Gui treatment, local expression of Ob-R_b mRNA was elevated to levels in the normal range ($p > 0.05$, Table 4).

Correlation analysis In linear regression analysis, serum leptin levels were negatively correlated with serum FSH ($r = -0.7517$) and LH ($r = -0.8444$) levels in the three groups. An inverse correlation was also observed between the relative amount of NPY-IR and estrogen receptor-labeled nuclei ($r = -0.7104$), and between NPY-IR and GnRH-IR fibers in the arcuate nucleus ($r = -0.8802$). With ANCOVA analysis, serum leptin levels and hypothalamic NPY levels were all positively correlated with body weight in the three groups of rats ($r = 0.8977$, $r = 0.8568$, respectively), though no significant association between serum leptin concentrations and NPY expression was detected in these groups of rats after correcting for body weight.

Discussion

Obesity has a huge impact on the human being, and 20% of the world population are reported as being obese. In China the obese population has increased from 9% in 1980 to 15% in the 1990s. Besides the gene factor, the main biomedical changes occurring in obesity are hyperinsulinemia/insulin resistance, leptin resistance and catecholamine resistance[1,3], which are more likely to affect reproductive and metabolic activities, and may induce hypertension, cardiovascular disease, diabetes or cancer in later life[10]. In women, insulin, leptin and catecholamine resistances commonly correlate with low reproductive function, oligomenorrhea, amenorrhea, premature ovarian fading, scanty menorrhea, etc. The majority of cases of both obesity and amenorrhea may appear in PCOS, a heterogeneous disease. Since Stein and Leventhal in 1935 described this symptom complex associated with anovulation, this syndrome has been further studied in the fields of neuroendocrinology and metabolism. Moreover, PCOS is inevitably accelerated and complicated by increasing obesity[11]. Despite this, the authentic symptoms in PCOS are anovulation with oligomenorrhea or amenorrhea, obesity, hirsutism, polycystic ovaries (which involves hyperandrogenemia), accelerated GnRH pulsatile frequency and hyperinsulinemia/insulin resistance, and PCOS can be observed in the peripubertal period, because female puberty is a period of relatively high androgen and insulin resistance[12]. Obesity acts as a modifier of PCOS, but PCOS itself can cause obesity due to hyperandrogenemia, hyperinsulinemia and impairment of catecholamine-induced lipolysis due to a reduction of β_2-adrenoreceptor density on the adipocytes.

In 1961, Barraclough characterized the androgen-sterilized rat, with polycystic ovaries, anovulation and high androgen levels[8]. Since 1981, for the purpose of observing the effects of herbal treatment on anovulation, the study of the ASR model has been extended until hyperinsulinemia, hyperandrogenemia, hypogonadotropic anovulation and obesity were found and proved by testosterone injection in female rats at 9 days of age (9d-ASR) to mimic a period of peripuberty in women[9]. The 9d-ASR model also manifested with hyperphagia, higher storage in abdominal adipose tissue, obesity and hyperleptinemia/leptin resistance, as seen in adolescent girls with PCOS[13]. This 9d-ASR model was selected to be an animal model in the study of PCOS. In PCOS, mutual functions and the relative importances of hyperinsulinemia and hyperandrogenemia have been controversially discussed[14]. Besides the fact that the 9d-ASR model is initiated by testosterone administration, the upregulation of pancreatic androgen receptor mRNA by high androgen resulting in oversecretion of C-peptide and insulin in the 9d-ASR model may explain the fact that the major factor causing hyperinsulinemia in PCOS is hyperandrogenemia.

NPY and POMC gene products are involved in the steroid-dependent regulation of body weight and reproduction. Overexpression of NPY mRNA and an increase in NPY release of the arcuate nucleus/paraventricular nucleus contribute to obesity in Zucker (*fa/fa*) rats or *ob/ob* mice. Central administration of NPY or β-endorphin increases food intake and inhibits GnRH secretion[15,16]. In this study, the colocalization of estrogen receptor and NPY neurons in the hypothalamic arcuate nucleus and preoptic area, and the negative correlations between estrogen receptor and NPY and GnRH, shed light on an estrogen cascade regulation of GnRH. In the 9d-ASR model, high serum estrogen levels metabolized from high serum testosterone levels down-regulate the number of estrogen receptor-oriented NPY-containing neurons in the arcuate nucleus, which enhances local NPY expression, resulting in suppression of GnRH release in the median eminence and hypogonadotropic anovulation[17]. β-Endorphin is the basic estrogen-dependent suppressor of GnRH. The colocalization of androgen receptors in the β-endorphin neurons of the arcuate nucleus in this study may also contribute to steroid-dependent regulation of GnRH. Both upregulation of androgen receptor mRNA due to hyperandrogenemia and down-regulation of estrogen receptor due to high serum estradiol levels push the release of β-endorphin and expression of POMC mRNA to high levels resulting in supression of GnRH levels in the 9d-ASR model. In addition, the close axonal contact between NPY- and POMC-containing neurons further strengthens this relation, which makes the reproductive function worse and more complicated.

In metabolic terms, the high central NPY and POMC levels in the 9d-ASR rats stimulate food intake, which induces obesity and high serum leptin levels. It has been reported that the ratio of leptin levels in cerebrospinal fluid/serum is decreased in obese women (leptin resistance), and the obesity is also hypothesized to be due to leptin resistance[3]. In 9d-ASR rats, a decrease in expression of Ob-R$_b$

mRNA leading to a high NPY concentration in the arcuate nucleus stimulates higher food intake – a vicious circle leading to obesity.

It is suggested that in the 9d-ASR model, high levels of testosterone in the female subjects influence central NPY and POMC via a steroid–receptor cascade, resulting in more food intake and in anovulation. Moreover, high peripheral leptin levels may also influence central NPY and POMC via the leptin system to affect reproduction and obesity. This feedback mechanism may further worsen the neuro-endocrine–metabolic network in the 9d-ASR model.

Leptin receptor has been found in ovary, liver and other tissues, and a recent report on leptin-promoting aggregation of human platelets via Ob-R$_b$[18] may suggest one of the causes of development of cardiovascular disease in people with obesity or PCOS.

In the literature relating to traditional Chinese medicine, reproduction is recorded to be mainly controlled by the kidney (one of the five organs in traditional Chinese medicine). According to the view of Dan-xi Zhu (1281–1359), amenorrhea and infertility are commonly caused by 'obstruction of fat', and are manifested by symptoms of deficiency in kidney Yin. In 1740, Chi-yuan Shu wrote 'amenorrhea and fatty abdomen usually happen when kidney Yang is insufficient to stem the Yin fluid, which might flow down to the womb system (including the ovary), forming phlegm masses'. Thus amenorrhea with obesity may be manifested with deficiency of kidney Yin or deficiency of kidney Yang. The different pattern diagnoses in traditional Chinese medicine are often related to different lifestyles and environments.

In terms of integrated traditional Chinese and Western medicine, patients with menstrual disorders and normal or high serum FSH levels usually have thirst, irritability, constipation, lack of vaginal discharge and dark reddened tongues, and are usually diagnosed with deficiency of kidney Yin and blood stasis. Patients with low FSH levels who manifest with intolerance of cold, back pain, less vaginal discharge and plump tongues are diagnosed with deficiency of kidney Yang and phlegm. Based on these disease diagnoses, treatment with different herbs or acupuncture, or combining these with hormones, is planned for each individual patient. In patients with PCOS and deficiency of kidney Yang, usually showing an LH/FSH ratio > 2.5, the ovulatory rate was 82.7% with a herbal treatment, and 36.9% with acupuncture treatment[19–21]. During the herbal treatment, serum FSH levels were elevated at first, followed by a rise in serum estradiol, a surge of LH and FSH, and ovulation. Hypothalamic β-endorphin release was depleted by the acupuncture and the frequency of FSH pulsatile secretion increased, resulting in growth of an ovarian follicle and ovulation[22,23]. However, these treatments did not work in patients with PCOS manifesting with obesity and hyperinsulinemia, who had symptoms of deficiency in kidney Yin, with high food intake and clomiphene resistance. Another herbal formula (Tian Gui) was developed after a long period of clinical and laboratory observations. Of all the cases reported, 69.7% ovulated in one cycle, and 45.8% in two or three cycles during the 3 months of treatment. This result correlated with decreases in serum testosterone and insulin, elevation of serum estradiol, relief of symptoms including acanthosis nigricans, and improvement of the waist/hip ratio. In comparison, metformin improved testosterone and insulin levels, but did not improve the level of estradiol or relieve symptoms, and resulted in fewer cases of ovulation[6,9]. The longer the Tian Gui was used, the higher the ovulatory rate appeared, and no side-effects were observed. Those patients who failed to ovulate with Tian Gui treatment showed positive results with clomiphene citrate, to which they had previously been resistant. Clomiphene citrate treatment is only used one cycle at a time, to help women achieve pregnancy, but does not help to establish regular cycles.

The decreases in pancreatic androgen receptor mRNA and secretion of C-peptide and insulin in 9d-ASR rats administered Tian Gui treatment may suggest the original factor that causes hyperinsulinemia in 9d-ASR rats is the high androgen levels, rather than insulin levels, and interaction is possible between the two. This idea may be more realistic and close to the 'exaggerated adrenache' hypothesis[11]. In addition, this may be one of the peripheral actions of Tian Gui, as decreased testosterone and insulin levels may directly effect obesity, ovarian follicular growth, and a decrease in blood viscosity by decreasing platelet aggregation caused by leptin from the fat tissues.

For central regulation of obesity and amenorrhea in patients with PCOS, and in 9d-ASR rats, the Tian Gui treatment decreases peripheral androgen and causes a relative decrease of estradiol, and may mainly attenuate the endocrine and metabolic cascades in 9d-ASR rats via their receptors. Reduction of central NPY and POMC levels decreases gluttony for food, decreases body weight and decreases leptin levels. The normalized leptin levels control central NPY via the leptin receptors, and this may be the metabolic aspect of the Tian Gui function. Normalized NPY and POMC levels establish the central GnRH to normal levels leading to an elevation of FSH and LH, and resulting in ovulation in obese patients with PCOS of the hyperinsulinemic pattern, as well as in 9d-ASR rats.

The present study may not only explain the effectiveness and main mechanism of action of the Tian Gui formula, but may also be an example of a holistic view of PCOS. We diagnosed PCOS with a high serum testosterone level, polycystic ovaries, hirsutism, amenorrhea, oligomenorrhea or dysfunctional uterine bleeding, and obesity, Moreover, we divided PCOS into two patterns: typical PCOS with deficiency of kidney Yang and phlegm, LH/FSH > 2.5 and positive challenge to clomiphene; and PCOS with obesity, deficiency of kidney Yin and blood stasis, significant hyperinsulinemia and negative challenge to clomiphene. Both patterns may occur during the pathological process. There is still a lot to be studied, and it seems that herbal administration is not only a treatment for PCOS but may also aid in the prevention of cardiovascular disease and diabetes.

Acknowledgements

The authors would like to thank Dr Y. L. Wang and Mrs C. D. Da, the State Key Laboratory of Neurobiology, and Shanghai Medical University for their kind help with image analysis, Dr A. F. Parlow from the Hormone Distribution Program of NIDDK (National Institute of Diabetes, Digestion and Kidney) for the kind supply of radioimmunoassay reagent, and Professor L. Z. Zhuang from the State Key Laboratory of Reproductive Biology, Academy of Science, Beijing, for the kind supply of rabbit polyclonal GnRH antibody. We also thank Dr X. M. Guan and Dr Alan Naidoff from Rabway, the Merck Laboratory, USA, for the kind supply of probes, and Dr Steiner from the University of Washington, Seattle, USA, for the kind supply of POMC plasmid.

References

1. Ek I, Arner P, Bergqvist A, et al. Impaired adipocyte lipolysis in non-obese women with the polycystic ovarian syndrome: a possible link to insulin resistance? *J Clin Endocrinol Metab* 1997;82:1147–53

2. Shalev A, Siegrist-kaiser CA, Yen PM, et al. The peroxisome proliferator-activated receptor is a phosphoprotein: regulation by insulin. *Endocrinology* 1996;137:4499–502

3. Laughlin GA, Morles AJ, Yen SSC. Serum leptin levels in women with polycystic ovarian syndrome: the role of insulin resistance/hyperinsulinemia. *J Clin Endocrinol Metab* 1997; 82:1692–6

4. Mercer JG, Hoggard N, Williams LM, et al. Coexpression of leptin receptors and preproneuropeptide Y mRNA in arcuate nucleus of mouse hypothalamus. *J Neuroendocrinol* 1996;8:733–6

5. Kalra SP, Sahu A, Kalra PS, *et al*. Hypothalamic neuropeptide Y: a circuit in the regulation of gonadotropin secretion and feeding behavior. *Ann NY Acad Sci* 1990;611:273–83

6. Zhou LR, Yu J. Clinical observation on treatment of hyperinsulinism and hyperandrogenism in anovulatory patients with replenishing kidney yin herbs. *Chin J Integr Med* (English) 1997;3:2

7. Hou JW, Yu J, Wei MJ. Study on treatment of hyperandrogenism and hyperinsulinism in polycystic ovary syndrome with the Chinese herbal formula 'Tiangui fang'. *Chinese J Integr Traditional Western Med* (Chinese) 2000;20:589–92

8. Barraclough CA. Production of anovulatory sterile rats by injection of testosterone propionate. *Endocrinology* 1961;68:62–7

9. Yu J, Yang SP, Zhang YP, *et al*. An androgen-induced hyperinsulinemic and hyperandrogenemic anovulatory rat model. *J Reprod Med* 1995;4(Suppl.):45–50

10. Dahlgren E, Johansson S, Lindstedt G. Women with polycystic ovarian syndrome wedge-resected in 1956 to 1965: a long-term follow-up focusing on natural history and circulating hormones. *Fertil Steril* 1992;57:505–13

11. Yen SSC. Polycystic ovarian syndrome. In Yen SSC, Jaffe RB, Barbiesi RL, eds. *Reproductive Endocrinology*, 4th edn. Philadelphia: Saunders 1999:436–78

12. Dramusic V. Hyperandrogenism (polycystic ovarian syndrome, hirsutism, acne, obesity). In Dramusic V, Ratnam SS, eds. *Clinical Approach to Paediatric and Adolescent Gynaecology*. Singapore: Oxford University Press, 1998:157–87

13. Sun F, Yu J. The effect of a special herbal tea on obesity and anovulation in androgen-sterilized rats. *Proc Soc Exp Biol Med* 2000;223:295–301

14. Dunaif A. Insulin resistance and the polycystic ovarian syndrome: mechanism and implications for pathogenesia. *Endocr Rev* 1997;18:774–800

15. White BD, Martin RJ. Evidence for a central mechanism of obesity in the Zucker rat: role of neuropeptide Y and leptin. *Proc Soc Exp Biol Med* 1997;214:222–32

16. Erickson JC, Hollopeter G, Palmiter RD. Attenuation of the obesity syndrome of ob/ob mice by the loss of neuropeptide Y. *Science* 1996;274:1704–7

17. Sun F, Yu J. The effect of TGR on serum leptin and pituitary LH and FSH levels. *J Integr Med* 2000;10(2):65–6

18. Nakata M, Yada T, Soejima N, *et al*. Leptin promotes aggregation of human platelets via the long form of its receptor. *Diabetes* 1999;48:426–9

19. Yu J, Li CJ. Regulation of the hypothalamic–pituitary–ovarian axis in the treatment of polycystic ovarian disease with herbs for tonifying the kidney and resolving phlegm. *Chinese J Integr Traditional Western Med* (Chinese) 1986;6:218–21

20. Yang QY, Yu J. Central opioid and dopamine activities in polycystic ovary syndrome in induction of ovulation with electroacupuncture. *J Reprod Med* 1992;1:16–19

21. Yu J. Polycystic ovary syndrome (PCOS). In Chris H, ed. *Handbook of Obstetrics and Gynecology in Chinese Medicine: An Integrated Approach*. Seattle: Eastland Press, 1998:59–62

22. Yang SP, Yu J, He LF. Release of GnRH from the MBH induced by electroacupuncture in conscious female rabbits. *Acupunct Electrother Res* 1994;19:9–27

23. Yu J, Zheng HM, Bing SM. Changes of serum follicular stimulation hormone, luteinizing hormone and follicular sizes during electroacupuncture for induction of ovulations. *Chinese J Integr Med* 1995;1:13–16

Ovulation induction in polycystic ovary syndrome patients

13

B. C. Tarlatzis and H. N. Bili

Introduction

Polycystic ovary syndrome (PCOS) is one of the most common causes of anovulation and infertility[1]. Although the etiology of PCOS remains unknown, recent data indicate that a small group of abnormally functioning genes are the possible underlying cause in some cases[2,3]. Treatment is currently symptomatic, aiming either to normalize the menstrual cycle or to induce ovulation in those women desiring pregnancy. Various compounds and treatment regimens have been used for ovulation induction in PCOS but none of them has been universally accepted.

The reported conception rates with the different protocols are lower than the ovulation rates, and are associated with a high incidence of miscarriage, which has been attributed to the high basal luteinizing hormone (LH) levels[4,5]. Furthermore, the incidence of multiple gestations and ovarian hyperstimulation syndrome (OHSS) is increased. Thus, the current goal is to improve the achievement of pregnancy but with fewer complications.

Clomiphene citrate

Clomiphene citrate has been used extensively for ovulation induction in PCOS. Clomiphene administration increases follicle-stimulating hormone (FSH) concentrations, and this broadens the window of endogenous FSH increase, enhancing follicular recruitment and selection[6]. Clomiphene is usually given at any time between cycle days 2 and 5 following menstruation, for 5 days. Although there

has been no difference in results observed between the onset on days 2 or 5[7], day 2 may have an advantage over day 5 in that ovulation occurs earlier and this may be closer to the normal profile of FSH increase for follicle recruitment and selection. The daily dose of clomiphene that is recommended for the first treatment attempt is 50 mg, which can be increased up to a total daily dose of 150 mg, although a total daily dose of 250 mg has also been used[8].

The results with clomiphene vary considerably among different studies. Ovulation rates range between 40 and 80%[9] but with consistently lower pregnancy rates. In properly selected patients with no other causes of infertility apart from anovulation, cumulative pregnancy rates as high as 60–75% after 6 months of treatment have been reported[10]. Recently, it has been observed that body weight, free androgen index, ovarian volume and serum leptin levels are the predominant predictors of ovulation after clomiphene treatment[9,11]. On the other hand, age and cycle history (especially amenorrhea) can predict the achievement of pregnancy in clomiphene-induced ovulatory women[12]. When clomiphene fails to induce ovulation or conception after treatment for a period of 6 months, the situation is considered to be clomiphene resistance or failure, and other treatment alternatives should be explored.

Combinations of clomiphene with gonadotropins have also been used, more often in the past than nowadays. Moreover, tamoxifen (another antiestrogenic compound) has been tried instead of clomiphene for inducing ovulation but has gained only limited popularity.

Human gonadotropins

Human gonadotropins used for ovulation induction are either derived from the urine of menopausal women (human menopausal gonadotropin (hMG), purified FSH) or are synthesized by recombinant DNA technology. In the conventional protocol, the usual starting dose of gonadotropin is two ampoules (150 IU) per day and, depending on ovarian response, the dose is increased in a stepwise manner[13]. However, PCOS patients are more prone to hyper-respond when treated with gonadotropins, and this may lead to a high rate of multiple pregnancies and OHSS.

For this reason, during the last few years, the treatment of PCOS patients with gonadotropins has changed, involving low-dose regimens (step-up and step-down protocols). In the low-dose step-up protocol, the starting dose is 75 IU FSH per day, which in some cases can be even lower, i.e. 37.5 IU. The initial dose is kept constant for 7–14 days and is increased by 37.5 IU per day every 7 days, up to a maximum of 225 IU (three ampoules) per day[14]. Once a leading follicle of 12–14 mm is seen by ultrasound, the dose of FSH is maintained constant up to the day of human chorionic gonadotropin (hCG) administration. Alternatively, a step-down mode of administration has also been used successfully[15]. According to this protocol, a dose of two (150 IU) to three ampoules (225 IU) of gonadotropins is used for 1–2 days which is then decreased by half an ampoule once a leading follicle starts to emerge, and this dose is maintained constant up to the day of hCG administration.

The main advantage of these protocols over conventional ones is that monofollicular development is achieved in approximately 75% of cycles together with a reasonable pregnancy rate and a significantly lower risk of multiple pregnancies and OHSS[16].

GnRH agonists with gonadotropins

Gonadotropin releasing hormone (GnRH) agonists are used in PCOS patients in the long desensitization protocol aiming to reduce the high basal LH levels and to improve the outcome of treatment with gonadotropins. It has been found that GnRH agonists prevent premature luteinization in gonadotropin-treated cycles, with pregnancy rates similar or even higher than the conventional regimens[17]. Furthermore, some studies indicate that the miscarriage rate may be reduced[17,18]. On the other hand, an increased risk of OHSS (~25%) and multiple gestation has been observed in PCOS patients pre-treated with a GnRH agonist[19].

GnRH antagonists

GnRH antagonists could be useful in ovulation induction in patients with PCOS in order to enable minimal ovarian stimulation protocols[20]. However, the optimal dose and protocol of the antagonist administration as well as the need for luteal support need to be explored further.

Conclusions

In conclusion, conventional ovulation induction protocols, with clomiphene citrate or gonadotropins, seem to be effective in women with PCOS. In those who failed to conceive, the use of GnRH-agonists in the long desensitization protocol may improve pregnancy rates, probably due to suppression of high endogenous LH and premature LH surges. There is no great experience yet with the use of GnRH antagonists for ovulation induction in PCOS, but it appears to be a promising approach allowing minimal ovarian stimulation.

References

1. van Santbrink EJ, Hop WC, Fauser BC. Classification of normogonadotropic infertility: polycystic ovaries diagnosed by ultrasound vs endocrine characteristics of PCOS. *Fertil Steril* 1997;67:452–8

2. Simpson JL. Elucidating the genetics of polycystic ovary syndrome. In Dunaif A, Givens JR, Haseltine FP, *et al.*, eds. *Polycystic Ovary Syndrome* Boston, MA: Blackwell Scientific 1992:59–69

3. Carey AH, Chan KL, Short F, *et al.* Evidence for a single gene effect causing polycystic ovaries and male pattern baldness. *Clin Endocrinol* 1993;38:653–8

4. Homburg R, Armar AN, Eshel A, *et al.* The influence of serum luteinizing hormone concentrations on ovulation, conception and early pregnancy loss in patients with polycystic ovary syndrome. *Br Med J* 1998;297:1024–6

5. Tarlatzis BC, Grimbizis G, Pournaropoulos F, *et al.* The prognostic value of basal luteinizing hormone: follicle-stimulating hormone ratio in the treatment of patients with polycystic ovarian syndrome by assisted reproduction techniques. *Hum Reprod* 1995;10:2545–9

6. Messinis IE, Koutsoyiannis D, Milingos S, *et al.* Changes in pituitary response to GnRH during the luteal-follicular transition of the human menstrual cycle. *Clin Endocrinol* 1993;38:159–63

7. Wu CH, Winkel CA. The effect of therapy initiation day on clomiphene citrate therapy. *Fertil Steril* 1989;52:564–8

8. Gorlitsky GA, Kase NG, Speroff L. Ovulation and pregnancy rates with clomiphene citrate. *Obstet Gynecol* 1978;51:265–9

9. Imani B, Eijkemans MJC, te Velde ER, *et al.* Predictors of patients remaining anovulatory during clomiphene citrate induction of ovulation in normogonadotropic oligoamenorrheic infertility. *J Clin Endocrinol Metab* 1998;83:2361–5

10. Kelly AC, Jewelewicz R. Alternate regimens for ovulation induction in polycystic ovarian disease. *Fertil Steril* 1990;54:195–202

11. Imani B, Eijkemans MJC, de Jong FH *et al.* Free androgen index and leptin are the most prominent endocrine predictors of ovarian response during clomiphene citrate induction of ovulation in normogonadotropic oligoamenorrheic infertility. *J Clin Endocrinol Metab* 2000;85:122–8

12. Imani B, Eijkemans MJC, te Velde ER, *et al.* Predictors of chances to conceive in ovulatory patients during clomiphene citrate induction of ovulation in normogonadotropic oligoamenorrheic infertility. *J Clin Endocrinol Metab* 1999;84:1617–22

13. Brown JB. Pituitary control of ovarian function – concepts derived from gonadotrophin therapy. *Aust NZ J Obstet Gynaecol* 1978;18:47–54

14. Franks S, Adams J, Mason H, *et al.* Ovulatory disorders in women with polycystic ovary syndrome. *Clin Obstet Gynaecol* 1985;12:605–32

15. Fauser BCJM, Donderwinkel P, Schoot DC. The step-down principle in gonadotrophin treatment and the role of GnRH analogues. *Bailliere's Clin Obstet Gynaecol* 1993;7:309–30

16. Meldrum DR. Low dose follicle-stimulating hormone therapy for polycystic ovarian disease. *Fertil Steril* 1991;55:1039–40

17. Dodson WC, Hughes CL, Yancy SE, *et al.* Clinical characteristics of ovulation induction with human menopausal gonadotropins with and without leuprolide acetate in polycystic ovary syndrome. *Fertil Steril* 1989;52:915–8

18. Homburg R, Eshel A, Kilbom J, *et al.* Combined luteinizing hormone releasing hormone analogue and exogenous gonadotrophins for the treatment of infertility associated with polycystic ovaries. *Hum Reprod* 1990;5:32–5

19. Smitz J, Ron-El R, Tarlatzis BC. The use of gonadotrophin releasing hormone agonists for *in vitro* fertilization and other assisted procreation techniques: Experience from three centers. *Hum Reprod* 1992;7(Suppl. 1):49–66

20. Macklon NS, Fauser BCJM. Regulation of follicle development and novel approaches to ovarian stimulation for IVF. *Hum Reprod Update* 2000;6:307–12

Transdermal estrogens for the treatment of premenstrual syndrome

14

J. Studd and W. Cronje

Introduction

Severe premenstrual syndrome (PMS) is a poorly understood collection of cyclical symptoms, which cause considerable psychological and physical distress. The psychological symptoms of depression, loss of energy, irritability, loss of libido and abnormal behavior as well as the physical symptoms of headaches, breast discomfort and abdominal bloating may occur for up to 14 days each month. There may also be associated menstrual problems, pelvic pain and menstrual headaches, and the woman may only enjoy as few as 7 symptom-free days per month. It is obvious that the symptoms mentioned can have a significant impact on the day-to-day functioning of affected women. It is estimated that up to 95% of women have some form of PMS, but about 5% of women of reproductive age will be affected severely, with disruption of their daily activities[1]. Considering these figures, it is disturbing that many of the consultations at our specialist PMS clinics start with women saying that for many years they have been told by everyone, including the family physician, that there are no treatments available and that they should simply 'live with it'. In addition, many commonly used treatments only make the symptoms worse.

The exact cause of PMS is uncertain, but fundamentally it is due to hormonal or biochemical changes, and the resulting complex interaction between ovarian steroids and neuroendocrinological factors that occur with ovulation. This produces varied symptoms in women who are somehow vulnerable to changes in their normal hormone levels. The cyclical chemical changes, probably attributable to progesterone or one of its metabolites, produce the cyclical symptoms of PMS.

History

This condition was mentioned in the fourth century BC by Hippocrates, but became a medical epidemic in the nineteenth century. Victorian physicians were aware of menstrual madness, hysteria, chlorosis, ovarian mania, as well as the commonplace neurasthenia. In the 1870s Maudsley[2], the most distinguished psychiatrist of the time, wrote '... the monthly activity of the ovaries which marks the advent of puberty in women has a notable effect upon the mind and body; wherefore it may become an important cause of mental and physical derangement ...' This was somehow recognized, rightly or wrongly, to be attributable to the ovaries, and bilateral oophorecotomy – Battey's operation[3] – was performed in tens of thousands of women in North America and Britain. Longo[4], in his brilliant essay on the decline of Battey's operation, posed the question of whether it worked. Of course there was no knowledge of osteoporosis and the devastation of long-term estrogen deficiency; therefore, on balance the operation was not helpful long-term but probably did, as was claimed, cure the 'menstrual/ovarian madness'. The essential logic of this operation was to remove cyclical ovarian function but happily this can now effectively be achieved by simpler medical therapy. Only in 1931 was the phrase 'premenstrual tension' introduced by Frank[5], who described 15 women with the typical symptoms of PMS as we know it. Greene and Dalton extended the definition to 'premenstrual syndrome' in 1953[6], recognizing the wider range of symptoms.

Treatment strategies

PMS does not occur if there is no ovarian function[7]. Obviously, it does not occur before puberty, after the menopause or after oophorectomy. It also does not occur during pregnancy. However, it is important to realize that hysterectomy with conservation of the ovaries does not often cure PMS[8] as patients are left with the usual cyclical symptoms and cyclical headaches. This condition, best called 'the ovarian cycle syndrome'[9] is usually not recognized to be hormonal in etiology, as there is no reference point of menstruation.

Inhibition of gonadotropins

A medical 'Battey's operation' can be achieved by the use of gonadotropin-releasing hormone (GnRH) analogs, and Leather et al.[10] have demonstrated that 3 months of goserelin (Zoladex®, Astra Zeneca) therapy cures all the symptom groups of PMS. The women do, of course, have hot flashes and sweats, but these are usually far preferable to the cyclical depression, irritability and headaches. The long-term risk of goserelin therapy is bone demineralization, but Leather et al.[11] showed that add-back with a product containing 2 mg estradiol valerate and cyclical levonorgestrel (Nuvelle®; Schering Health) maintains the bone density at both the spine and the hip. Most of the PMS symptoms remain improved with this 'add-back' therapy but bloating, tension and irritability recur – probably due to the cyclical progestogen. In a Scandinavian study, Sundstrom and colleagues[12] used low-dose GnRH analogs (100 µg buserelin) with good results on the symptoms of PMS, but the treatment still caused anovulation in as many as 56% of patients.

Danazol is another method of treating PMS by inhibiting pituitary gonadotropins, but its side-effects include androgenic and virilizing effects. When used in the luteal phase only[13] it only relieved mastalgia and not the general symptoms of PMS, although side-effects were minimal.

Estrogen therapy

Greenblatt et al.[14] showed the effects of an ovulatory dose of estrogen implants for the use of contraception and the first study for its use in PMS was by Magos et al.[15] using 100 mg estradiol implants, which was a dose shown to inhibit ovulation by previous ultrasound and day 21 progesterone studies. The study showed a huge improvement with placebo implants, but the improvements of every symptom cluster was greater in the active estradiol group (Figure 1). In addition, the placebo effect waned after a few months with continued response to estradiol. These patients, of course, were also given 7–13 days of oral progestogen per month to prevent endometrial hyperplasia and irregular bleeding[16]. Subsequently, a placebo-controlled trial of cyclical norethisterone in hysterectomized women reproduced the typical symptoms of PMS[17]. We believe that cyclical oral progestogen in the estrogen-primed woman is the correct model for PMS. It is also significant that progestogen intolerance is one of the principal reasons why older, postmenopausal women stop taking HRT[18]. It is common for progestogens to cause PMS-like symptoms (Figure 2)[19], in the same way that endogenous cyclical progesterone is the probable cause of PMS.

Our group still uses estradiol implants, often with the addition of testosterone for loss of energy and loss of libido, in our PMS clinics, but we use a dose of estradiol lower than 100 mg, inserting pellets of estradiol 50 mg or 75 mg, together with 100 mg testosterone. Endometrial protection is conferred through the oral addition of a progestogen or a Mirena® (Schering Healthcare) levonorgestrel-releasing intrauterine system (IUS). These women with PMS respond well to estrogens but are often intolerant of progestogens, and it is therefore commonplace for us to reduce the orthodox 13-day course of progestogen to

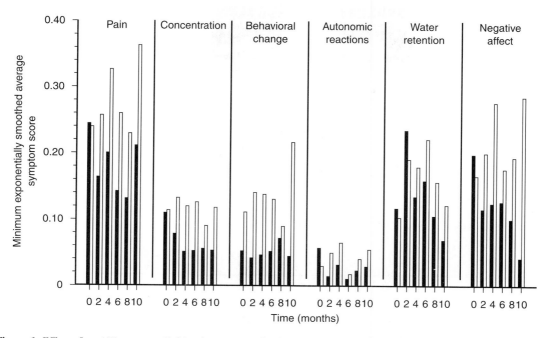

Figure 1 Effect of ■, 100 mg estradiol implant; or □, placebo implant on minimum exponentially smoothed average symptom scores over 10 months of treatment. Figure reproduced with permission of the BMJ Publishing Group from Magos *et al.* BMJ 1986;292:1629–33

10 or 7 days starting, for convenience, on the first day of every calendar month. Thus, the menstrual cycle is reset. The Mirena IUS could also play a vital role in preventing PMS-like symptoms as it performs its role of protecting the endometrium without systemic absorption. In a recent study[20] we have shown a 50% decrease in hysterectomies carried out in our practice (Figure 3) since the introduction of the Mirena IUS in 1995. With its profound effect on menorrhagia and the possibility of fewer progestogenic side-effects, Mirena looks a very promising component of PMS treatment in the future.

Hormone implants are not licensed in all countries and are unsuitable for women who may wish to discontinue treatment easily in order to become pregnant. Estradiol patches are an alternative and our original double-blind crossover study used a 200 μg estradiol patch twice weekly[21]. This produced plasma estradiol levels of 800 pmol/l and suppressed luteal phase progesterone and ovulation.

Once again this treatment was better than placebo in every symptom cluster of PMS. Figure 4 shows the initial response to placebo and active treatment, as well as the respective effects after 3-month crossover. When active treatment was substituted by placebo there was a deterioration in response, whereas there was continued improvement when placebo was replaced by active treatment. Subsequently, an uncontrolled observational study from our PMS clinic indicated that PMS sufferers could have the same response to 100 μg patches with fewer symptoms of breast discomfort and bloating and with less anxiety about high-dose estrogen therapy[22].

The original studies outlined in this paper are all scientifically valid placebo-controlled trials showing a considerable improvement in PMS symptoms with estrogen therapy. Although this treatment is used by most gynecologists in the UK, its value has not been exploited by psychiatrists anywhere in the world. We believe that the benefit of this

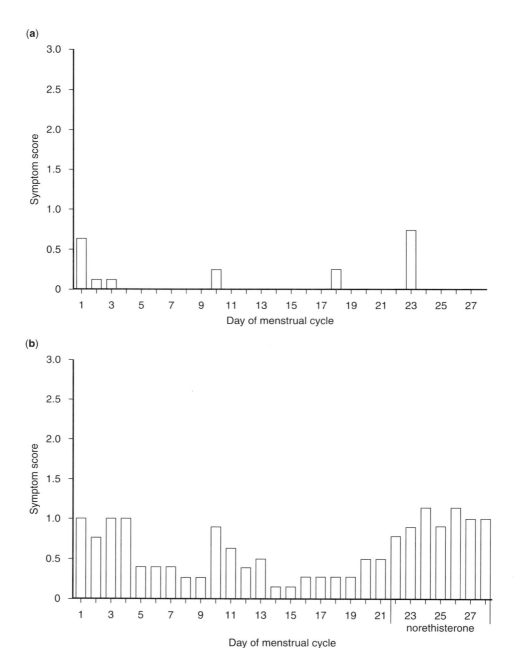

Figure 2 Symptoms scores (a) following suppressing ovulation with 200 μg estradiol; and (b) after the addition of norethisterone (5 mg). Figure reproduced with permission of the RCOG press from Studd *et al.* *Disorders of the Menstrual Cycle*[20]

therapy in severe PMS is due to inhibition of ovulation, but there is probably also a central 'mental tonic' effect. Klaiber *et al.*[23] using very high doses of Premarin® (conjugated estrogens) showed this, and our other psycho-endocrine studies of climacteric depression and postnatal depression have shown the benefit of high-dose transdermal estrogens[24].

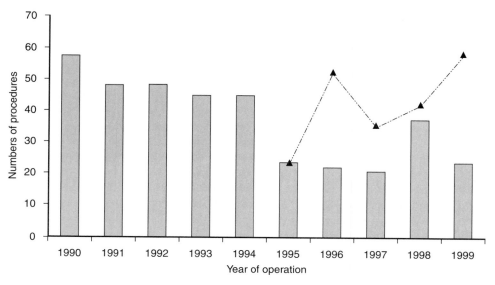

Figure 3 Number of hysterectomies performed (□) and Mirena levonorgestrel intrauterine systems inserted (--▲--), before and after the introduction of Mirena in June 1995[20]

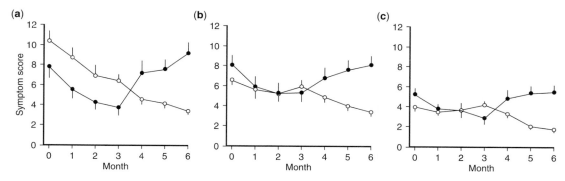

Figure 4 Double-blind 3-month crossover study using a 200 μg estradiol patch twice weekly, showing the effect on symptom clusters of premenstrual syndrome: (a) negative affect; (b) pain; and (c) water retention. Mean (SE) exponentially smoothed average maximum symptom scores, ●—●, active treatment for 3 months and placebo treatment for 3 months; ○—○, placebo treatment for 3 months and active treatment for 3 months. Figure reproduced with permission from Watson NR *et al*. Treatment of severe pre-menstrual syndrome with oestradiol patches and cyclical oral norethisterone. *Lancet* 1989;2:730–4

In general terms, more women suffer from depression than men, and this depression often occurs at times of hormonal flux beginning with puberty[25]. It characteristically occurs as postnatal depression, premenstrual depression or climacteric depression – the triad of hormone-responsive mood disorders[26]. Premenstrual depression is the most common of these disorders, and when severe can be treated effectively by transdermal estrogens together with the appropriate endometrial protection with oral or intrauterine progestogen[16,26].

Ultimately, there are some women who, after treatment with estrogens and the Mirena coils, will prefer to have a hysterectomy in order to prevent cycles with a virtual guarantee of improvement in symptoms. This should not be seen as a failure or even a last resort, as it does carry many other advantages[20].

It is important that women who have had a hysterectomy and bilateral salpingo-oophorectomy have effective replacement therapy, ideally with replacement of the ovarian androgens. Implants of estradiol 50 mg and testosterone 100 mg are an ideal combination for long-term therapy post-hysterectomy, with a continuation rate of 90% at 10 years[20].

Conclusions

Suppression of ovulation is the most sucessful and most logical treatment for severe premenstrual syndrome. This can easily be performed by transdermal estrogens either by patches using 100 to 200 µg patches twice weekly or by hormone implants of 50 to 75 µg of estradiol every 6 months. GnRH analogs are also effective.

Patients having transdermal estrogens require cyclical progestogen to prevent endometrial hyperplasia and irregular bleeding, but PMS symptoms can return with oral progestogen therapy. If this progestogen intolerance occurs, it is more common in patients with PMS, further treatment may consist of insertion of a progestogen releasing Mirena IUS or even hysterectomy and bilateral salpingo-oophorectomy with long-term estrogen therapy.

References

1. O'Brien PMS. Helping women with premenstrual syndrome. *Br Med J* 1993;307:1471–5
2. Maudsley H. Sex in mind and education. *Fortnightly Rev*, 1874
3. Battey R. Battey's operation – its matured results. *Transactions Georgia Med Assoc*, 1873
4. Longo LD. The rise and fall of Battey's operation: a fashion in surgery. *Bull Hist Med* 1979; 53:244–67
5. Frank RT. The hormonal basis of premenstrual tension. *Arch Neurol Psychiat* 1931;26:1053–7
6. Greene R, Dalton K. The premenstrual syndrome. *Br Med J* 1953;I:1007–14
7. Studd JWW. Premenstrual tension syndrome. *Br Med J* 1979;I:410
8. Backstrom T, Boyle H, Baird DT. Persistence of symptoms of premenstrual tension in hysterectomized women. *Br J Obstet Gynaecol* 1981; 88:530–6
9. Studd JWW. Prophylactic oophorectomy at hysterectomy. *Br J Obstet Gynaecol* 1989;96: 506–9
10. Leather AT, Studd JWW, Watson NR, *et al*. The treatment of severe premenstrual syndrome with goserelin with and without 'add-back' estrogen therapy: a placebo-controlled study. *Gynecol Endocrinol* 1999;13:48–55
11. Holland EF, Leather AT, Studd JW, *et al*. The effect of a new sequential oestradiol valerate and levonorgestrel preparation on the bone mineral density of postmenopausal women. *Br J Obstet Gynaecol* 1993;100:966–7
12. Sundstrom I, Nyberg S, Bixo M, *et al*. Treatment of premenstrual syndrome with gonadotropin-releasing hormone agonist in a low dose regimen. *Acta Obstet Gynecol Scand* 1999;78:891–9
13. O'Brien PM, Abukhalil IE. Randomized controlled trial of the management of premenstrual syndrome and premenstrual mastalgia using luteal phase-only danazol. *Am J Obstet Gynecol* 1999;180:18–23
14. Greenblatt RB, Asch RH, Mahesh VB, *et al*. Implantation of pure crystalline pellets of estradiol for conception control. *Am J Obstet Gynecol* 1977;127:520–7
15. Magos AL, Brincat M, Studd JWW. Treatment of the premenstrual syndrome by subcutaneous oestradiol implants and cyclical oral norethisterone: placebo controlled study. *Br Med J* 1986;292:1629–33
16. Studd JWW, Thom MH. Oestrogens and endometrial cancer. In Studd JWW, ed. *Progress in Obstetrics and Gynaecology*, Vol. 1. Edinburgh: Churchill Livingstone, 1981:182–98
17. Magos AL, Brewster E, Singh R, *et al*. The effects of norethisterone in postmenopausal women on oestrogen replacement therapy: a model for the premenstrual syndrome. *Br J Obstet Gynaecol* 1986;93:1290–6

18. Bjorn I, Backstrom T. Drug related negative side-effects is a common reason for poor compliance in hormone replacement therapy. *Maturitas* 1999;32:77–86

19. Watson NR, Studd JWW. Use of oestrogen in treatment of the premenstrual syndrome: a comparison of the routes of administration. *Contemp Rev Obstet Gynaecol* 1990;2:117–23

20. Studd JWW, Domoney C, Khastgir G. The place of hysterectomy in the treatment of menstrual disorders. In *Disorders of the Menstrual Cycle*. London: RCOG Press, 2000;29:313–23

21. Watson NR, Studd JWW, Savvas M, *et al.* Treatment of severe pre-menstrual syndrome with oestradiol patches and cyclical oral norethisterone. *Lancet* 1989;2:730–4

22. Smith RNJ, Studd JWW, Zamblera D, *et al.* A randomised comparison over 8 months of 100 mcgs and 200 mcgs twice weekly doses of transdermal oestradiol in the treatment of severe premenstrual syndrome. *Br J Obstet Gynaecol* 1995;102:475–84

23. Klaiber EL, Broverman DM, Vogel W, *et al.* Estrogen therapy for severe persistent depressions in women. *Arch Gen Psychiatry* 1979;36:550–9

24. Gregoire AJP, Kumar R, Everitt B, *et al.* Transdermal oestrogen for treatment of severe postnatal depression. *Lancet* 1996;347:930–3

25. Montgomery JC, Brincat M, Tapp A, *et al.* Effect of oestrogen and testosterone implants on psychological disorders in the climacteric. *Lancet* 1987;1:297–9

26. Panay N, Studd JWW. The psychotherapeutic effect of oestrogens. *Gynecol Endocrinol* 1998;12:353–63

27. Paterson ME, Wade-Evans T, Sturdee DW, *et al.* Endometrial disease after treatment with oestrogens and progestogens in the climacteric. *Br Med J* 1980;280:822–4

Epidemiology and psychosocial aspects of premenstrual syndrome in Italy

15

F. Facchinetti, G. Sances, M. Tarabusi, N. Ghiotto, A. Tirelli, R. D'Amico and G. Nappi

Introduction

Premenstrual syndrome (PMS) is a progressively worsening group of symptoms that occurs during the luteal phase of the menstrual cycle, interferes with family and social activities, and usually resolves after the onset of menses. The essential features of PMS are a markedly depressed mood, anxiety and emotional instability, accompanied by diminished interest in usual activities. The cluster of physical symptoms may include breast tenderness, bloating, headache, water retention, joint or muscle pain and other discomforts[1]. Owing to the lack of objective clinical signs and typical biological markers, it is difficult to establish operational diagnostic criteria for PMS. Moreover, the exact prevalence of the syndrome and its underlying etiopathogenetic mechanisms are still unknown.

Several studies have shown that PMS symptoms can be severe enough to affect a subject's quality of life and work (causing absenteeism and impaired performance)[2-5]. In this paper we report the results of a small epidemiological study focusing on an Italian population, and also evaluate personality features.

Methods

One hundred women of childbearing age (range 22–51 years) were randomly selected from among the staff of a large university hospital in Pavia, Italy. The women were stratified by job (doctors/nurses/office staff/students). To be included in the study, subjects had to be Italian-born, and to have experienced regular menstrual cycles (lasting 24–32 days) throughout the previous six months. Eight women refused to participate.

A structured clinical interview was carried out in order to gather personal data, and to establish obstetric, gynecological and psychiatric histories. The participants were then requested to fill in daily, for two consecutive cycles, the validated Italian version of the 'Calendar of Premenstrual Experiences' (COPE)[6]. Furthermore, in a subpopulation of 18 PMS and 17 control participants, a marital communication questionnaire[7] was also administered.

Results and discussion

For the actual evaluation, only women completing every questionnaire were taken into consideration. Thus, the data analysis was carried out on 73 out of 92 participants.

In accordance with the criteria established when the Italian version of COPE was validated[6], every women giving both a total score > 35 in the luteal phase and an increase > 80% in the luteal *vs* follicular score, for two consecutive cycles, was diagnosed as having PMS. On the basis of these very restrictive criteria, 18 women were found to be PMS-positive in two cycles (24.7%) while a further 14 met the criteria for only one cycle (19.2%). These latter participants were excluded from the analysis. The remaining 41 women (56.2%) were PMS-negative in both cycles and were treated as the control group. None of the PMS participants had previously consulted a doctor about her complaint, while only two (8.3%) had undergone psycho-pharmacological and/or psychological treatment.

The age of the PMS participants (33.8 ± 6.5 years) and controls (33.2 ± 7.5 years) was similar. In comparison with the control group, the PMS women had experienced an earlier menarche I (< 11 years : 18.1 *vs* 2.9%; $p = 0.02$). All the PMS group had had at least eight years of education while this was true of only 16.4% of the controls ($p = 0.01$). Surprisingly, the distribution of jobs was similar in the two groups. Furthermore, 66.7% PMS sufferers compared with 48.8% controls were married. No differences in obstetric and gynecological history emerged between controls and PMS sufferers, with the exception of a lower rate of contraceptive use in the latter group (83.3% *vs* 58.5%).

The general level of communication underwent a reduction from 160 ± 41 in the follicular phase to 145 ± 33 ($p < 0.05$) in the luteal phase in PMS women. Neither in the control women, nor in the husbands of the PMS women, were there differences dependent on the cycle. In PMS women, the level of communication was reduced premenstrually in every category, particularly those concerning children.

These data demonstrate that PMS is a relatively common disorder, affecting 25% of a northern Italian, urban, employed population. Moreover, in addition to those meeting these strict diagnostic criteria, a further 19% of women reported premenstrual discomfort in one out of the two menstrual cycles studied.

These PMS sufferers were not characterized by any peculiar clinical or demographic feature, although they were found to be more educated than the rest of the sample. This finding could be explained by the fact that women who are more educated exhibit a greater awareness of their psychosocial functioning, and are thus more likely to perceive premenstrual discomfort as a disturbing phenomenon. In addition, PMS participants experienced an earlier menarche, a finding recently reported also in a North American population of PMS sufferers[8]. The authors of this latter study argue in favor of a different (stronger) hormonal milieu in these women. The impact of PMS within the family seems to be considerable. Indeed, our findings indicate that sufferers reduced their level of verbal communication with their partners and the phenomenon is even more marked in relationships of longer standing. This issue has been addressed by several authors who have tended to report, in older partnerships, more conflicts, less intimacy and fewer shared recreational pursuits than normal[9].

It could be that the damage to the family that is mentioned above stems from a lack of overt communication, and interventions should thus be aimed at promoting a family approach[10]. In terms of the impact of PMS, the family seems to constitute a crucial area: in a recent survey of western women, the disorder was claimed to have a greater effect on the family than on work or social spheres[11].

In conclusion, despite PMS being present in a quarter of these Italian women, none of them had previously consulted a doctor for solving the problem. However, the premenstrual distress significantly interferes with marital communication. Although Italian women appear to cope well with premenstrual discomfort the damage to family relationships needs to be addressed.

Acknowledgement

This research was supported by a grant from the Ministry of Public Health ICS 030.91 RF.96.369.

References

1. Moos RH. The development of menstrual distress questionnaire. *Psychosom Med* 1968;30: 853–67

2. Reid RL, Yen SSC. Premenstrual Syndrome. *Am J Obstet Gynecol* 1981;39:85–104

3. Fioroni L, Sances G, Scaccabarozzi S, *et al.* Epidemiological aspects of premenstrual syndrome in Italy. In Nappi G, *et al.*, eds. *Headache and Depression: Serotonin Pathways as a Common Clue.* New York: Raven Press, 1991:305–10

4. Adersch B, Wenderstan C, Maham L, *et al.* Premenstrual complaints. Prevalence of premenstrual symptoms in a Swedish urban population. *J Psychosom Obstet Gynaecol* 1986;5:39–45

5. Johnson SR. The epidemiology and social impact of premenstrual symptoms. *Clin Obstet Gynaecol* 1987;30:367–76

6. Tarabusi M, Sances G, Ghiotto N, *et al.* Diagnostic ability of the Italian version of the Calendar of Premenstrual Experiences. *It J Obstet Gynecol* 1998;3:102–6

7. Martinez Millàn ML, Marvàn ML. Comunicacion Marital y Sìntomas Premestruales. *Acta Psiquiàt Psicol Am Lat* 1995;41:24–8

8. Deuster PA, Tilahun A, South-Paul J. Biological, social, and behavioural factors associated with premenstrual syndrome. *Arch Fam Med* 1999;8:122–8

9. Kuczmierczyk AR, Labrum AH, Johnson CC. Perception of family and work environments in women with premenstrual syndrome. *J Psychosom Res* 1992;8:787–95

10. Watson WL, Nanchoff-Glatt M. A family systems nursing approach to premenstrual syndrome. *Clin Nurse Spec* 1990;4:3–9

11. Hylan TR, Sundell K, Judge R. The impact of premenstrual symptomatology on functioning and treatment-seeking behaviour: experience from the United States, United Kingdom, and France. *J Womens Health Gend Based Med* 1999; 8:1043–52

Hormonal methods of emergency contraception 16

P. C. Ho

Introduction

Emergency contraception is contraception provided to a woman after unprotected intercourse, to prevent pregnancy. The need for emergency contraception may arise because the woman is not using any method of contraception, or when there is failure of the barrier methods such as breakage or slipping of condoms, or in the case of rape. The use of emergency contraception may play an important role in preventing unplanned pregnancies and abortions. It was estimated that the widespread use of emergency contraception in the USA could prevent over 1 million abortions and 2 million unintended pregnancies that end in childbirth[1]. There are hormonal and non-hormonal methods of emergency contraception. The insertion of a copper intrauterine contraceptive device (a non-hormonal method) is a highly effective method of emergency contraception[2], but it may be associated with the complications of bleeding, pain and pelvic inflammatory disease. Therefore, it is not suitable for women who have high risk factors for development of pelvic inflammatory disease. In this article, only hormonal methods of emergency contraception are discussed.

High-dose estrogens

One of the earliest methods of emergency contraception was the use of high-dose estrogens (ethinylestradiol, conjugated estrogens or diethylstilbestrol) for 5 days[3,4]. These regimens are highly effective in the prevention of pregnancy but the incidence of side-effects is very high (nausea, 54–70%; vomiting, 24–33%). The pregnancy rates reported in the literature are mostly less than 1%[5]. A randomized trial showed that the pregnancy rate after use of ethinylestradiol was comparable to that of the Yuzpe regimen[6]. The high incidence of sideeffects and the need for a 5-day treatment regimen made these regimens unpopular and they are now seldom used.

Combined estrogen and progestogen regimen

The Yuzpe regimen consists of administration of two doses of combined pills at a 12-h interval within 72 h of intercourse, each dose containing 100 µg of ethinylestradiol and 1 mg of norgestrel[7]. The main side-effects of this regimen are nausea (54%) and vomiting (16%)[6]. Recently, a randomized trial showed that the incidence of nausea and vomiting was significantly decreased when meclizine was taken 1 h before the first dose of the Yuzpe regimen[8]. The next menstruation usually occurred around the expected time or earlier. Only 11.5% of the women had a delay of more than 3 days[9].

The failure rate of the Yuzpe regimen varied between 0.2 and 7.4%. Trussell and colleagues[10] recently pooled the data from eight studies and estimated that the Yuzpe regimen probably prevented over 74% of pregnancies. A recent large-scale multicenter study conducted by the World Health Organization (WHO) showed that the efficacy of the Yuzpe regimen decreased with increase in the intercourse–treatment interval[11]. The pregnancy rate rose from 2% when treatment was given within 12 h of intercourse to 4.7% when given between 61 and 72 h of intercourse. No serious adverse effects have been reported in the literature. The contraindications for the Yuzpe regimen are different from those of combined oral contraceptive pills for ongoing contraception. According to the WHO, confirmed pregnancy is the only condition in which the Yuzpe regimen is not to be used[12]. This is because the drugs are no longer necessary. While there is no study on the possible teratogenic effect of the Yuzpe regimen, numerous studies on the teratogenic risk of combined oral contraceptive pills did not find any evidence of increased risk[13].

To elucidate the mechanism of action of the Yuzpe regimen, Swahn and co-workers[14] administered the drugs to eight volunteers on day 12 of their cycle and found that the luteinizing hormone (LH) surge was not detectable in three women and was postponed in another three. The mean area under the curve of LH and the pregnanediol glucuronide secretion in the treatment cycles were also significantly lower than those in the control cycles. When the drugs were given 2 days after the LH surge, the morphometric dating did not differ enough from the chronological dating to characterize the endometrium as out of phase. Therefore, it appears that the Yuzpe regimen may act mainly by postponing or suppressing ovulation, although the effect was not consistent.

Levonorgestrel

Ho and Kwan[9] reported the first study comparing levonorgestrel (two doses of 0.75 mg at a 12-h interval) with the Yuzpe regimen for emergency contraception. They showed that the failure rate of levonorgestrel was slightly but not significantly lower than that of the Yuzpe regimen. The incidence of side-effects (nausea, vomiting and fatigue) was significantly lower than in the Yuzpe regimen. The time of return of the next menstruation was similar to that with the Yuzpe regimen. In a recent WHO multicenter randomized study[11], the pregnancy rate of levonorgestrel (1.1%)

was significantly lower than that of the Yuzpe regimen (3.2%). It was estimated that levonorgestrel within 72 h of unprotected intercourse could prevent about 85% of the expected pregnancies. The incidence of side-effects was also significantly lower than in the Yuzpe regimen. As with the Yuzpe regimen, the pregnancy rate increased with increase in the intercourse–treatment interval: 0.4% when given within 24 h and 2.7% when given between 49 and 72 h. Further analysis of the combined data from both the levonorgestrel and Yuzpe regimens showed that a consistent and significant linear relationship existed between the pregnancy rate and the intercourse–treatment interval[15]. Therefore, it is important for women to obtain the drugs early after unprotected intercourse to achieve better results. When the data from the two studies were combined, the pregnancy rate for levonorgestrel was still significantly lower. Therefore, when available, levonorgestrel should be the drug of choice.

The exact mechanism of action of levonorgestrel in emergency contraception is still unknown. Kesseru and associates[16] reported that 0.4 mg of levonorgestrel given 3–10 h after intercourse led to a significant reduction of the number of spermatozoa in the uterine cavity, pronounced alkalinization of intrauterine fluid and increased viscosity of cervical mucus. Landgren and colleagues[17] found that repeated doses of 0.75 mg of levonorgestrel over a few days led to varying effects on ovulation and the endometrium. However, the doses and regimens used in these two studies were different from that used in emergency contraception. Further studies are required to elucidate the mechanism of action of levonorgestrel.

Mifepristone

Mifepristone is a progesterone antagonist at the receptor level and it is highly effective for emergency contraception. In the first two studies undertaken[18,19], 585 women were given 600 mg mifepristone within 72 h of unprotected intercourse and none of them conceived. The difference in pregnancy rates between mifepristone and the Yuzpe regimen was statistically significant[18]. The incidence of side-effects, especially nausea and vomiting, was significantly lower in the mifepristone group. However, in 42% of women, there was a delay of more than 3 days in the onset of the next period[19]. This delay may lead to anxiety for the women.

In a recent multicenter randomized study conducted by the WHO[20], the efficacy and side-effects of three doses of mifepristone (10 mg, 50 mg and 600 mg) in emergency contraception were compared. The pregnancy rates in the 10 mg, 50 mg and 600 mg groups were 1.2%, 1.1% and 1.3%, respectively. Using the estimates of expected recognizable pregnancies, they estimated these regimens to have prevented 84–86% of pregnancies. The incidence of delay in onset of the next menses and bleeding within 5 days of drug administration was significantly lower in the lower-dose group. The results also showed that the efficacy of mifepristone did not decrease with increase in the intercourse–treatment interval up to 120 h after intercourse, an advantage over the Yuzpe regimen and levonorgestrel. Mifepristone is well known as a drug for abortion. This may hinder its acceptance as a method for emergency contraception. The reduction of the dose to 10 mg without loss of efficacy may make this regimen more acceptable, as this dose is much lower than that required for abortion.

Danazol

Danazol is a semi-synthetic steroid derived from 17α-ethinyltestosterone. Rowlands and co-workers[21] first reported the use of danazol for emergency contraception. The pregnancy rate was 6% but the incidence of sideeffects such as nausea and vomiting was much lower than with the Yuzpe regimen. Zuliani and associates[22] reported that the pregnancy rates of danazol in emergency contraception were 1.7% and 0.8% for doses of 800 mg and

1200 mg, respectively. The results of a more recent study were disappointing[18]. The pregnancy rate was 4.7%, which was lower than those of the Yuzpe regimen and mifepristone. In fact, the number of observed pregnancies was not significantly different from that of expected pregnancies. Because of the unfavorable results, danazol is seldom used for emergency contraception.

Self-administration of emergency contraception

Since the pregnancy rates after emergency contraception with either the Yuzpe regimen or levonorgestrel increase with the intercourse–treatment interval, it may be better if women could keep a supply of emergency contraceptive pills at home. In a recent study from Scotland[23], women were assigned to two groups: one group were given a replaceable supply of emergency contraception pills (Yuzpe regimen) to take home, while the other group had to obtain the emergency contraception pills by visiting a doctor. Significantly more women in the treatment group (47%) had used emergency contraception than in the control group (27%), but they were not more likely to use it repeatedly. The use of other methods of contraception was similar in the two groups of women. There were no serious adverse effects. The number of unintended pregnancies was higher (though not statistically significant) in the control group. These data show that, even if women are given a supply of emergency contraceptive pills to keep at home, they are unlikely to stop regular contraception and use emergency contraceptive repeatedly.

Conclusions

Effective and safe methods of emergency contraception are now available. There is evidence that mifepristone and levonorgestrel are more effective than the Yuzpe regimen and they are associated with a lower incidence of side-effects. Both can prevent around 85%

of pregnancies. However, the Yuzpe regimen is still the most widely available method and it can probably prevent over 74% of pregnancies. It is likely that when levonorgestrel is more widely available it may become the drug of choice.

References

1. Trussell J, Stewart F. The effectiveness of the Yuzpe regimen of emergency contraception. *Fam Plann Perspect* 1996;28:58–64

2. Trussell J, Ellertson C. Efficacy of emergency contraception. *Fertil Contracept Rev* 1995;4: 8–11

3. Dixon GW, Schlesselman JJ, Ory HW, *et al.* Ethinylestradiol and conjugated estrogens as postcoital contraceptives. *J Am Med Assoc* 1980; 244:1336–9

4. Haspels AA. Interception: post-coital estrogens in 3016 women. *Contraception* 1976;14:375–81

5. Silvestre L, Bouali Y, Ulmann A. Postcoital contraception: myth or reality? *Lancet* 1991;338: 39–41

6. Van Santen MR, Haspels AA. A comparison of high-dose estrogens versus low-dose ethinylestradiol and norgestrel combination in postcoital interception: a study in 493 women. *Fertil Steril* 1985;43:206–13

7. Yuzpe AA, Lancee WJ. Ethinylestradiol and DL-norgestrel as a postcoital contraceptive. *Fertil Steril* 1977;28:932–6

8. Raymond EC, Crenin MD, Barnhart KT, *et al.* Meclizine for prevention of nausea associated with use of emergency contraceptive pills: a randomized trial. *Obstet Gynecol* 2000;95: 271–7

9. Ho PC, Kwan MSW. A prospective randomized comparison of levonorgestrel with the Yuzpe regimen in post-coital contraception. *Hum Reprod* 1993;8:389–92

10. Trussell J, Rodriguez G, Ellertson C. Updated estimates of the effectiveness of the Yuzpe regimen of emergency contraception. *Contraception* 1999;59:147–51

11. World Health Organization Task Force on Postovulatory Methods of Fertility Regulation. Randomised controlled trial of levonorgestrel versus the Yuzpe regimen of combined oral contraceptives for emergency contraception. *Lancet* 1998;352:428–33

12. World Health Organization. *Improving Access to Quality Care in Family Planning: Medical Eligibility Criteria for Contraceptive Use.* (WHO/FRH/FPP/96.9). Geneva, Switzerland 1996:31–3

13. Bracken MB. Oral contraception and congenital malformations in offspring: a review and meta-analysis of the prospective studies. *Obstet Gynecol* 1990;76:552–7

14. Swahn ML, Westlund P, Johannisson E, *et al.* Effect of post-coital contraceptive methods on the endometrium and the menstrual cycle. *Acta Obstet Gynecol Scand* 1996;75:738–44

15. Piaggio G, Von Hertzen H, Grimes DA, Van Look PFA, on behalf of the World Health Organization Task Force on Postovulatory Methods of Fertility Regulation. Timing of emergency contraception with levonorgestrel or the Yuzpe regimen. *Lancet* 1999; 353:721

16. Kesseru E, Garmendia F, Westphal N, *et al.* The hormonal and peripheral effects of de-norgestrel in postcoital contraception. *Contraception* 1974;10:410–24

17. Landgren BM, Johannisson E, Aedo AR, *et al.* The effect of levonorgestrel administered in large doses at different stages of the cycle on ovarian function and endometrial morphology. *Contraception* 1989;39:275–89

18. Webb AMC, Russell J, Elstein M. Comparison of Yuzpe regimen, danazol, and mifepristone (RU486) in oral postcoital contraception. *Br Med J* 1992;305:927–31

19. Glasier A, Thong KJ, Dewar M, *et al.* Mifepristone (RU486) compared with high-dose estrogen and progestogen for emergency postcoital contraception. *N Engl J Med* 1992;327:1041–4

20. Task Force on Postovulatory Methods of Fertility Regulation. Comparison of three single doses of mifepristone as emergency contraception: a randomised trial. *Lancet* 1999; 353:697–702

21. Rowlands S, Guillebaud J, Bounds W, Booth M. Side effects of danazol compared with an ethinyloestradiol/norgestrel combination when used for postcoital contraception. *Contraception* 1983;27:39–49

22. Zuliani G, Colombo UF, Molla R. Hormonal postcoital contraception with an ethinylestradiol–norgestrel combination and two danazol regimens. *Eur J Obstet Gynecol Reprod Biol* 1990; 37:253–60

23. Glasier A, Baird D. The effects of self-administering emergency contraception. *N Engl J Med* 1998;339:1–4

Benefits of injectable contraception to women's health

17

P. G. Spinola

Introduction

Injectable contraceptives can be classified into progestin-only injectables, depot medroxy-progesterone acetate (DMPA) and norethisterone enanthate (NET-EN). Table 1 shows the brand name, formulations and schedule of the progestin-only injectables. Table 2 shows the brand name, formulations and schedule of the combined estrogen–progestin monthly injectables.

With all injectables, the injection should be given intramuscularly because absorption may be too slow if the provider injects into fat. In contrast, massaging the injection site accelerates absorption and should therefore be avoided.

Injectable contraceptives are chemical derivatives of the natural hormones progesterone, testosterone and estradiol and fulfill many of the features of an ideal contraceptive. They are highly effective, long-acting, simple to use, non-invasive, reversible, unrelated to coitus, need minimal motivation and are relatively inexpensive. It is estimated that about 16 million women worldwide use injectable contraceptives to regulate their fertility. The most widely used injectable is DMPA, which is used by more than 13 million women. The other progestin-only injectable contraceptive currently available is NET-EN, an ester of a 19-nortestosterone derivative, used by approximately one million women. Monthly injectable contraceptives are widely used in Latin America and China by an estimated two million women[1].

The development of injectable contraceptives started with the first publication in the medical literature by Siegel in 1963[2]. He tested the formulation 17α-hydroxyprogesterone caproate 500 mg and estradiol valerate 10 mg. The half-dose of this formulation has been extensively used in China as Chinese Injectable No. 1 or Gravibinon. Subsequently another formulation of 150 mg of dihydroxyprogesterone acetophenide (DHPA) with 10 mg estradiol enanthate (E2-EN) was tested in the 1960s[3–6]. DMPA was first used in humans in 1960 for the prevention of premature labor, given in doses as high as 1–4 g per injection. It was soon recognized that many women who were treated during pregnancy remained infertile for many months afterwards[7]. This led to the recognition of DMPA's contraceptive properties and clinical contraceptive trials were started in 1963. The first reports appeared in 1966, indicating a very high effectiveness in preventing pregnancy, and the product has since become popular as a contraceptive[8]. The combination of progestin and estrogen that became Cyclofem was originally developed in Brazil in 1968[9], and the combination that became Mesigyna was first tested in 1974[10]. When the clinical assessment of Cyclofem and Mesigyna was satisfactorily completed, the World Health Organization initiated a systematic program to introduce Cyclofem into the national family planning programs of several countries.

Progestin-only injectables

DMPA is a remarkable drug with a wide range of applications in gynecology and general

Table 1 Progestin-only injectables: brand name, formulation and injectable schedule

Brand name	Formulation	Injectable schedule
Depo-provera Megestron Tricilon	Depot medroxyprogesterone acetate 150 mg	Every 3 months
Noristerat Doryxus	Norethisterone enanthate 200 mg	Every 2 months

Table 2 Combined estrogen–progestin monthly injectables: brand name, formulation and injectable schedule

Brand name	Formulation	Injectable schedule
Perlutan Uniciclo Ciclovular Perlutal Topasel Agurin	Dihydroxyprogesterone acetophenide 250 mg + estradiol enanthate 10 mg	Monthly between the 7th and 10th day of each menstrual cycle
Anafertin Yectames	Dihydroxyprogesterone acetophenide 75 mg + estradiol enanthate 5 mg	As above
Cyclofem Cyclofemina Cycloprovera Cyclogeston Lunelle	Depot medroxy progesterone acetate 25 mg + estradiol cypionate 5 mg	Monthly: first injection 1st–5th day of the menstrual cycle, subsequently every 30 ± 3 days
Mesigyna Norigynon	Norethisterone enanthate 50 mg + estradiol valerate 5 mg	As above
Gravibinon Chinese Injectable No. 1	17-hydroxyprogesterone caproate 250 mg + estradiol valerate 5 mg	Monthly: two injections in first month, subsequently at 28-day intervals

medicine. A widely studied drug, its efficacy and short-term safety have been repeatedly demonstrated. The advantages of DMPA include the following[11,12]:

(1) very effective (99.7%);

(2) safe;

(3) reversible;

(4) discreet;

(5) long-term pregnancy prevention;

(6) does not interfere with sex;

(7) increased sexual enjoyment;

(8) no daily pill-taking;

(9) flexibility in return visits;

(10) can be used by women of any age;

(11) suitable for lactating women;

(12) no estrogenic side-effects; and

(13) efficacy not reduced by diarrhea or vomiting.

The disadvantages of DMPA are shown below. The discontinuation of the contraceptive method by clients because of these disadvantages can be avoided by adequate counseling prior to initiation[11,12].

(1) changes in menstrual bleeding;

(2) may cause weight gain;

(3) delayed return of fertility;

(4) may cause headaches, nausea, breast tenderness, moodiness and depression; and

(5) does not protect against STDs/AIDS.

One of the principal advantages of DMPA is that it can be used by most women, including[11,12]:

(1) during breast-feeding;

(2) smokers;

(3) nulliparous women;

(4) adolescents;

(5) women with benign breast disease;

(6) women who suffer from mild headaches;

(7) women with high blood pressure;

(8) women with iron deficiency anemia;

(9) women with varicose veins;

(10) women with valvular heart disease;

(11) women with irregular menstrual periods;

(12) women with malaria;

(13) women with schistosomiases;

(14) women with sickle cell disease;

(15) women with thyroid disease;

(16) women with uterine fibroids;

(17) women with epilepsy; and

(18) women with tuberculosis.

In addition to the advantages of DMPA previously mentioned, there are several non-contraceptive benefits of DMPA to women's health, as listed below[11,12]:

(1) amenorrhea;

(2) preventing iron-deficiency anemia;

(3) preventing ectopic pregnancy;

(4) preventing endometrial cancer;

(5) treatment of endometrial carcinoma;

(6) treatment of endometriosis;

(7) treatment of uterine fibroids;

(8) preventing premenstrual syndrome (PMS);

(9) preventing dysmenorrhea;

(10) making epileptic seizures less frequent;

(11) making sickle cell crises less frequent and less painful;

(12) preventing vaginal candidiasis;

(13) preventing pelvic inflammatory disease (PID);

(14) preventing ovarian cysts; and

(15) may help prevent ovarian cancer.

A comparison between DMPA and NET-EN is made in Table 3.

Controversial issues

We should be aware of some of the controversial issues related to progestin-only contraceptives, such as loss of bone mass, depression, delay in return of fertility and HIV transmission.

Combined estrogen-progestin monthly injectables

Combined estrogen–progestin monthly injectables, when properly used, are among the most effective methods of contraception available today and should therefore be considered for inclusion among the family planning methods available at any clinic or other health facility offering an integrated family planning service. The addition of a short- or medium-acting estrogen ester to long-acting progestins to produce combined injectable formulations was a successful strategy to overcome the endometrial bleeding problems associated with progestin-only injectables. The advantages and disadvantages of combined estrogen–progestin monthly injectables compared to progestin-only formulations are shown in Table 4. The main indications for the contraceptive use of combined estrogen–progestin monthly injectables include women who do not tolerate or are unwilling or unable to use oral contraceptive pills, intrauterine devices or barrier methods. Also those who

Table 3 Comparison of the characteristics of depot medroxyprogesterone acetate (DMPA) and norethisterone enanthate (NET-EN)

Characteristic	DMPA	NET-EN
Effectiveness	99.7%	99.6%
Bleeding	More amenorrhea	More irregular
Reinjection window	2–4 weeks early or late	1–2 weeks early or late
Duration	3 months	2 months
Return of fertility	Average delay: 4 months longer than for other contraceptives	Probably less delay
Cost	Less expensive	More expensive

Table 4 Relative advantages and disadvantages of combined estrogen–progestin: monthly injectables compared with long-acting progestin-only formulations

Advantages	Disadvantages
Better cycle control	Not suitable for lactating women
Less endometrial suppression	Shorter-acting and more injections
More rapid return to fertility	Not for women with contraindications
More contact with health personnel	to use of estrogens
Shorter inconvenience if side-effects occur	Presence of estrogenic side-effects
Much lower progestin dose	
Similar or higher contraceptive efficacy and acceptability	

prefer a long-acting method and who accept some menstrual irregularities are among possible candidates for the use of these injections. Contraindications are the same as those of combined oral contraceptives.

Current research on injectable contraceptives

Injectable contraceptives are an extremely effective form of contraception and are gaining over other methods in family planning programs. Due to the changing needs of women as they advance through their reproductive years, it is very important to offer contraceptive choices which will have a more favorable effect on the metabolism than currently available hormone contraceptives.

Despite the good acceptability of the combi- nation of DHPA 150 mg plus E2-EN 10 mg in Latin America, some investigators believe that the doses of both components could be reduced without loss of efficacy[13]. Recently, a clinical trial with this combination was carried out in nine family planning centers in Brazil[14]. The study was a comparative, double-blind, clinical trial in which a combination containing DHPA 90 mg plus E2-EN 6 mg was compared with the regular combination DHPA 150 mg plus E2-EN 10 mg. The study showed that intramuscular injection of the low dose, given at approximately 24-day intervals, is as effective in preventing conception in women as the DHPA 150 mg plus E2-EN 10 mg and the study also showed that the continuation rate with the use of either one of the two combinations was approximately the same. One of the important aspects of this trial is the fact that the women in the study had constant access to other methods of contraception. During their monthly visits to the family planning clinics, they met with women using other methods of contraception such as IUDs and other long-acting methods such as subdermal implants or sterilization. As these methods were also available to patients enrolled in this trial on demand, this may have tempted some of them to switch to another method being praised by the other women. Nevertheless, 60% of the women did not discontinue the study, indicating that at least half of those who used one of the two dosages were genuinely pleased with the method.

The present finding that the combination of a natural estrogen with the simplest progesterone derivative available is as effective and acceptable as its previously available, high-dosage combination will certainly come as good news to users of this product[15].

Many other approaches are being tested in the development of injectable contraceptives. Among them, a compound under study, levonorgestrel butanoate, is a three-monthly injectable contraceptive for women. Clinical trials have already shown it to be an effective method of contraception, providing contraceptive protection at a low dose of 5 to 10 mg every 3 months. Such a preparation would have advantages over DMPA, and may result in less ovarian suppression, less amenorrhea and a more rapid return of fertility. Levonorgestrel has a long safety record as an oral contraceptive and as the active ingredient in Norplant® devices. It has been previously tested successfully as a monthly injectable in combination with estradiol hexabenzoate but was never marketed[16].

New strategies appear to have a promising future in the development of injectable contraceptives such as steroid delivery systems through biodegradable polymers and monolithic microspheres of natural steroids.

Injectable contraceptives in the late premenopause

The late premenopause begins at 35–40 years of age and ends with the menopause. In most parts of the world, childbearing by women in this age group is not desirable. Research has shown that half of all women in their early forties are still fertile. Contraception protects women against pregnancies in this age group. Progestin-only injectable contraceptives can usually be prescribed for these women. Although monthly injectable contraceptives using a combination of the natural hormones, progesterone and estradiol, are suitable for healthy, non-smoking women over the age of 35, there have been no reports in the literature of studies in this age group. I believe that not only can this combination be used as a very safe contraceptive but it can also protect women from menopausal symptoms and reduce the incidence of cardiovascular diseases and osteoporosis, as well as providing other benefits of hormone replacement therapy.

Conclusions

Injectable contraceptives have several advantages and few disadvantages. The accumulated knowledge on injectable contraception must be matched by an equal advance in counseling by family planning providers and clinical management of injectable contraceptives so that this method can be optimally used by family planning programs and their clients.

References

1. D'Arcangues C, Snow R. Injectable contraceptives. In Rabe T, Runnebaum B, eds. *Fertility Control Update and Trends*. Berlin, Heidelberg: Springer-Verlag, 1999;121–49
2. Siegel I. Conception control by long-acting progestogens: preliminary report. *Obstet Gynecol* 1963;21:666–8
3. Taymor ML, Plank S, Yahia C. Ovulation inhibition with a long-acting parenteral progestogen–estrogen combination. *Fertil Steril* 1964;15:653–60
4. Rutherford RN, Banks AL, Coburn WA. Deladroxate for the prevention of ovulation. *Fertil Steril* 1964;15:648–52
5. Reifenstein EC, Pratt TE, Hartzell KA, *et al.* Artificial menstrual cycles induced in ovulating women by monthly injection of progestogen–estrogen. *Fertil Steril* 1965;16:652–64
6. Felton HT, Hoelscher EW, Swartz DP. Evaluation of use of an injectable progestogen–estrogen for contraception. *Fertil Steril* 1965;16:665–76

7. World Health Organization. *Injectable Contraceptives: Their Role in Family Planning Care*. WHO Booklet, Geneva, Switzerland, 1990;1:111

8. Coutinho EM, de Souza JC, Csapo AI. Reversible sterility induced by medroxyprogesterone injections. *Fertil Steril* 1966;17:261

9. Coutinho EM, de Souza JC. Conception control by monthly injections of medroxyprogesterone suspension and a long-acting oestrogen. *J Reprod Fertil* 1968;15:209–14

10. Newton, JR, Darcangues C, Hall PE. Once-a-month combined injectable contraceptives. *J Obstet Gynaecol* 1994;14(Suppl. 1):S1–S34

11. New era for injectables. *Injectables and Implants*. Population Reports: Population Information Program, The Johns Hopkins School of Hygiene and Public Health, Baltimore, USA. Series K, Number 5, August 1995

12. Johns Hopkins Population Information Program. DMPA Injectable Contraceptive. In *The Essentials of Contraceptive Technology*. Baltimore, USA: The Johns Hopkins University School of Public Health, 1997:7-2–7-21

13. Moore LL, Valuck R, McDougall C, *et al.* A comparative study of one-year weight gain among users of medroxyprogesterone acetate, levonorgestrel implants, oral contraceptives. *Contraception* 1995;52:215–20

14. Coutinho EM, Spinola P, Barbosa I, *et al.* Multicenter, double-blind, comparative, clinical study on the efficacy and acceptability of a monthly injectable contraceptive combination of 150 mg dihydroxyprogesterone acetophenide and 10 mg estradiol enanthate compared to a monthly injectable comparative combination of 90 mg dihydroxyprogesterone acetophenide and 6 mg estradiol enanthate. *Contraception* 1997;55:175–81

15. Coutinho EM, Spinola P, Tomaz G, *et al.* Efficacy, acceptability and clinical effects of a monthly injectable contraceptive combination of 90 mg of dihydroxy-progesterone acetophenide and 6 mg of estradiol enanthate. *Contraception* 2000;61:277–80.

16. De Souza JC, Coutinho EM. Control of fertility by monthly injections of a mixture of norgestrel and a long-acting estrogen. *Contraception* 1972; 5:395

Immunobiology of endometriosis: molecular aspects and local cytokines

18

M. Busacca, E. Somigliana, S. Cozzolino, P. Filardo,
P. Viganò and M. Vignali

Introduction

Endometriosis is characterized by the presence of endometrial glands and stroma within the pelvic peritoneum and other extrauterine sites, and is estimated to affect 2–10% of women of reproductive age. Recently, the development of animal models of the disease and data from molecular biology techniques have led to the proposal of novel therapeutic strategies that do not constitute a medically-induced menopause. Specifically, the demonstration of an aberrant expression of the enzyme aromatase in endometriotic tissue, which favors accumulation of estradiol, has led to the possibility of using aromatase inhibitors to treat endometriosis[1]. Moreover, since the angiogenic factor vascular endothelial growth factor (VEGF) has been reported to be essential for endometriotic angiogenesis, a novel therapeutic strategy to treat this disease would be to block the growth of these vessels[2]. These novel therapeutic targets have evolved from the identification of specific changes in endometrial cells that enable them to implant in ectopic locations. The characteristics critical to ectopic implantation include:

(1) The microscopic and molecular structure of refluxed endometrial fragments, such as the expression of specific adhesion molecules[3,4];

(2) The number of regurgitated endometrial cells;

(3) Their ability to proliferate[1];

(4) Their ability to secrete angiogenetic factors[5];

(5) Their ability to disrupt the peritoneal surface by producing metalloproteinases[6].

However, there is also good evidence to indicate that endometriosis is characterized by specific immune changes[7,8]. Indeed, the genetic alterations in endometrial cells in themselves do not guarantee that endometriosis will develop. In other words, the expression of the disease is likely to be associated with the capacity of endometrial cells to counteract an ongoing immunological response.

The aims of this review are:

(1) To show evidence that endometriosis immunology resembles some features characteristic of cells capable of evading immunosurveillance; and

(2) To present findings demonstrating that the subversion of this condition by the use of an immune-stimulating agent is able to control the immunological response *in vitro* and the expression of the disease *in vivo*.

There are, of course, other situations in nature that arise or benefit from the cellular ability to escape immunosurveillance. There are a few strategies through which both malignant and non-malignant cells can counteract the immune system, including:

(1) Modification of surface antigens critical to immune recognition[9–10];

(2) Production of circulating antigens which compete with surface antigens critical to immune recognition[11];

(3) Direct or indirect secretion of inhibitory factors and cytokines, of which the most consistently stipulated to have a role in tumor-mediated immunosuppression are interleukin-10 (IL-10), transforming growth factor-β (TGFβ) and prostaglandin E_2 (PGE_2)[11,12].

Recent evidence indicates that these strategies can also be employed by endometrial cells.

The MHC class I system in the endometrium

Essentially, all nucleated cells of the body carry major histocompatibility complex (MHC) class I molecules. This allows them to present foreign antigens to the T cell system and simultaneously makes them resistant to a particular population of lymphoid cells called natural killer (NK) cells, which lyse specifically cells that lack or have very low levels of class I molecules because they engage inhibitory receptors (KIR) with these molecules. The establishment of the interaction KIR–MHC class I molecules implies a signal to the lymphoid cells of no lysis[13,14]. According to a very interesting study by Komatsu and coworkers[15], the endometrium represents an unusual exception to nucleated cells since normal endometrial cells start to express consistent levels of class I molecules only during the secretory phase and decidualization. Therefore, during retrograde menstruation, these cells could become a potential target of conventional NK cells that are located in peritoneum. In contrast, in endometriosis, as shown in the study by Semino et al.[16], the up-regulation of class I molecules could make ectopic cells able to evade the NK cell-mediated immune response.

The soluble ICAM-1 molecule and endometriosis

NK cell-mediated recognition of deleterious cells also requires the engagement of activatory molecules that are not only necessary but also sufficient to induce lysis[13,14]. Among these costimulatory pathways, one of the most studied for its extensive role in direct cell–cell interaction is the lymphocyte function-associated antigen-1 (LFA-1) intercellular adhesion molecule (ICAM)-1 pathway. LFA-1 is expressed on most lymphoid cells and ICAM-1 is expressed on endometrial cells of women either with or without endometriosis[17]. This pathway has a regulatory physiologic antagonist, which is represented by the soluble form of ICAM-1[18]. The shedding form is still able to bind to LFA-1, and thus competes with the cell-bound molecule for binding to the same receptor on immune cells. As a consequence, high levels of soluble ICAM-1 can disturb the attack of immune cells against their targets and the effective immunological reaction is prevented. This is one of the mechanisms through which eutopic endometrial cells from patients with endometriosis can evade immunesurveillance, as they release significantly higher levels of soluble ICAM-1 when compared to endometrial cells of women without the disease[18]. Consistent with this hypothesis, in a recent study we correlated levels of soluble ICAM-1 released by eutopic endometrial cells with various parameters documenting the severity of the disease, and found a significant correlation between levels of soluble ICAM-1 and the number of peritoneal endometriotic implants ($r = 0.64$, $p < 0.005$)[19].

Immunosuppressive factors in endometriosis

Endometrial cells have been shown to secrete or induce the secretion of several factors able to serve immunosuppressive roles such as TGFβ, PGE_2, placental protein 14 (PP14), and the Th2 cytokines interleukin (IL)-4 and IL-10, all of which have been demonstrated to be increased in the peritoneal cavity and/or endometriotic tissue of patients with endometriosis[6,8,20,21]. An environment rich in these factors implies a suppression of cell-mediated immunity[22], and in keeping with this observation, NK cell activity has been reported to be defective in endometriosis[23–26]. Therefore, endometrial cells may indeed use typical mechanisms to evade immunosurveillance:

(1) They can modify class I antigenic pattern[16];

(2) They produce a soluble protein sICAM-1 that competes with a surface antigen critical to immune recognition[18]; and

(3) They can generate an environment rich in certain immunosuppressive factors which are exactly the same as those used by most cellular systems for the same purpose[22].

However, the most convincing evidence that endometriosis is associated with a defective response at immune level would be the demonstration that the disease may be amenable to control through immune manipulation. Thus, our group has tried to identify a substance that may induce a reversal of this immunesuppression, and in particular focused attention on the major factor involved in the stimulation of NK cell cytotoxic activity, the cytokine IL-12 or formerly termed natural killer cell stimulatory factor[27].

IL-12 and endometriosis

IL-12 is a heterodimeric molecule produced by monocyte–macrophages and dendritic cells. The IL-12 heterodimer is composed of two disulfide-linked chains, p35 and p40, encoded by separate genes. Simultaneous expression of the two genes is required for production of the biologically active IL-12 heterodimer, but all the cell types producing the biologically active heterodimer also produce a large excess of the free p40 chain. The physiological significance of this overproduction still needs to be elucidated; some evidence would indicate that natural p40 may act as a physiological antagonist of IL-12[28].

In vitro experiments

Given the variety of effects exerted by IL-12 on NK cells, we reasoned that IL-12 may play a role in the phenomenon of elimination of refluxed endometrial cells in the peritoneal cavity. Thus, in our studies, we measured concentrations of IL-12 and the free p40 subunit in the peritoneal fluid of 33 patients with endometriosis and 40 women without laparoscopic evidence of the disease. The ratio between p40 and IL-12 was significantly higher in patients with endometriosis (59.1 ± 8.7 pg/ml) compared to women without the disease (32.9 ± 5.4 pg/ml, $p < 0.02$), and was associated with severity, as it tended to increase with the stage of the disease. Thus, a large excess of free p40, which is the natural antagonist of IL-12, is present in peritoneal fluid of patients with endometriosis[28]. We subsequently evaluated the effect of IL-12 and its free p40 subunit on NK cell cytotoxic activity against endometrial cells. We treated NK cells with IL-12 and/or its free p40 subunit and evaluated the ability of these NK cells to lyse specifically endometrial targets[28]. The addition of IL-12 to NK cells caused a strong enhancement of cytotoxicity, while the free p40 subunit was able to completely abolish the increase in cytotoxicity induced by IL-12. This effect cannot be attributed to any toxic action of p40 as treatment of NK cells with the free p40 subunit alone did not alter the basal cytotoxicity[28].

In vivo experiments

Our next step was to evaluate the ability of IL-12 to control the disease in vivo. Thus, we set up a model of endometriosis that could satisfy two specific criteria. First, we needed to work on mice since only mouse and human forms of IL-12 have been cloned and purified. Second, it should be a procedure that models a massive retrograde menses, since the surgical transplantation of endometrium on the peritoneal wall is non-conforming with the pathogenic mechanism for the disease. Briefly, we used syngenic mice and we divided them into donors and challenged animals. Both groups were initially subjected to ovariectomy and estrogen supplementation in order to eliminate differences related to the stage of the estrous cycle. After 7 days, one donor mouse was killed for every two mice to be challenged with endometrium. Both uterine horns of the donor were gently peeled in order to detach the uterine muscle from the endometrium, then chopped and inoculated into the peritoneal cavity of challenged mice. Mice challenged with endometrium were then subjected to estrogen supplementation once a week. After three weeks of endometrial challenge, mice were sacrificed and endometriotic lesions were carefully excised from the surrounding tissue in order to assess their weight and surface area. Lesions appeared as tan multicystic areas bulging under the serosal coat of the abdominal wall. New vessels indicating a process of neovascularization were present on their surface. Microscopic examination confirmed that all the gross lesions analyzed were endometriotic in character. Mice challenged with endometrium were then either treated with IL-12 or vehicle control. IL-12 was administered intraperitoneally by daily injections of 0.15 μg for 5 days, from two days before to two days after the inoculation of endometrium. Control mice received only the vehicle, following the same procedure. Intraperitoneal administration of IL-12 during endometrial challenge in the C57BL/6 strain was able to induce a significant prevention of endometriosis establishment. Indeed, weight and surface area of the lesions as evaluated 3 weeks after inoculation of endometrium was significantly lower in IL-12-treated animals (0.60 ± 0.17 mg and 9.91 ± 1.40 mm^2) than in non-treated mice (2.66 ± 0.45 mg; $p < 0.005$; 25.64 ± 2.87 mm^2; $p < 0.001$)[29].

Conclusions

Therefore, the results of this study support the following observations:

(1) Endometrial cells utilize well-known mechanisms to evade immunesurveillance. The unbalanced regulation of the IL-12 system resulting in the secretion of a substantial excess of the free p40 subunit may indeed represent one of these mechanisms;

(2) IL-12 is able to stimulate the cytolytic arm of the initial immune response *in vitro* and prevent endometriosis establishment *in vivo*. Therefore, this finding supports targeting of the immune system as a novel management approach to the disease.

IL-12 is the single most potent cytokine in animal tumor models. Microgram doses of this drug can cause regression of well-established tumors. Clinical trials with IL-12 are now in progress especially for the treatment of specific tumors such as melanoma and renal cell carcinoma, as well as for asthma and hepatitis C[27]. Side-effects are limited, although these still need to be reduced. We realize that IL-12, with its immunogenic properties, does not represent an ideal candidate for endometriosis treatment. Nevertheless, it is clear that the field of immunotherapy, both in terms of biological therapy or gene therapy, has become more active in the last few years, and that much effort is now directed toward the identification of other less immunogenic compounds that might stimulate the production of IL-12.

References

1. Bulum SE, Zeitoun KM, Takayama K, *et al*. Aromatase as a therapeutic target in endometriosis. *Trends Endo Met* 2000;11:22–7
2. Charnock-Jones DS, Bruner-Tran KL, Chamberlain PD, *et al*. The role of sflt in antagonising growth of endometriotic lesions *in vivo*. *Presented at Endometriosis 2000, 7th Biennal World Congress*, London, May 2000
3. Busacca M, Viganò P, Magri B, *et al*. The adhesion molecules of human endometrial stromal cells. Immunological implications. *Annal N Y Acad Sci* 1994;734:43–6
4. Viganò P, Gaffuri B, Somigliana E, *et al*. Expression of intracellular adhesion molecule (ICAM)-1 mRNA and protein is enhanced in endometriosis versus endometrial stromal cells in culture. *Mol Hum Reprod* 1998;4:1150–6
5. McLaren J. Vascular endothelial growth factor and endometriotic angiogenesis. *Hum Reprod Update* 2000;6:45–55

6. Osteen K. Progesterone and transforming growth factor-α co-mediate matrix metalloproteinase expression in a model of endometriosis. In Minaguchi H, Sugimoto O, eds. *Endometriosis Today: Advances in Research and Practice*. London: Parthenon Publishing, 1997:200–9

7. Braun DP, Dmowski WP. Endometriosis: abnormal endometrium and dysfunctional immune response. *Obstet Gynecol* 1998;10:365–9

8. Ho HN, Wu MY, Yang YS. Peritoneal cellular immunity and endometriosis. *Am J Reprod Immunol* 1997;38:400–12

9. Carosella ED, Dausset J, Rouas-Freiss N. Immunotolerant functions of HLA-G. *Cell Mol Life Sci* 1999;55:327–33

10. Cabestre FA, Lefebvre S, Moreau P, et al. HLA-G expression: immune privilege for tumour cells? *Semin Cancer Biol* 1999;9:27–36

11. Geertsen R, Hofbauer G, Kamarashev J, et al. Immune escape mechanisms in malignant melanoma. *Int J Mol Med* 1999;3:49–57

12. Salazar-Onfray F. Interleukin-10: a cytokine used by tumors to escape immunosurveillance. *Med Oncol* 1999;16:86–94

13. Lanier LL. Natural killer cells: form no receptors to too many. *Immunity* 1997;6:371–8

14. Lanier LL. Follow the leader: NK cell receptors for classical and nonclassical MHC class I. *Cell* 1998;92:705–7

15. Komatsu T, Komishi I, Mandai M, et al. Expression of class I human leukocyte antigen (HLA) and α2-microglobulin is associated with decidualization of human endometrial stromal cells. *Hum Reprod* 1998;13:2246–51

16. Semino C, Semino A, Pietra G, et al. Role of major histocompatibility complex class I expression and natural killer-like T cells in the genetic control of endometriosis. *Fertil Steril* 1995;64:909–16

17. Viganò P, Pardi R, Magri B, et al. Expression of intercellular adhesion molecule-1 (ICAM-1) on cultured human endometrial stromal cells and its role in the interaction with natural killers. *Am J Reprod Immunol* 1994;32:139–145

18. Somigliana E, Viganò P, Gaffuri B, et al. Endometrial stromal cells as a source of intercellular adhesion molecule (ICAM)-1 molecule. *Hum Reprod* 1996;11:1190–4

19. Viganò P, Somigliana E, Gaffuri B, et al. Endometrial release of soluble intercellular adhesion molecule 1 and endometriosis: relationship to the extent of the disease. *Obstet Gynecol* 2000;95:115–18

20. Cornillie FJ, Lauweryns JM, Seppala M, et al. Expression of endometrial PP14 in pelvic and ovarian endometriotic implants. *Hum Reprod* 1991;6:1411–15

21. Koninckx PR, Riittinen L, Seppala M, et al. CA-125 and placental protein 14 concentrations in plasma and peritoneal fluid of women with deeply infiltrating pelvic endometriosis. *Fertil Steril* 1992;57:523–50

22. Somigliana E, Viganò P, Gaffuri B, et al. Modulation of NK cell lytic function by endometrial secretory factors: potential role in endometriosis. *Am J Reprod Immunol* 1996;36:296–300

23. Oosterlynck DJ, Cornillie FJ, Waer M, et al. Women with endometriosis show a defect in natural killer activity resulting in a decreased cytotoxicity to autologous endometrium. *Fertil Steril* 1991;56:45–51

24. Oosterlynck DJ, Meuleman C, Waer M, et al. The natural killer cell activity of peritoneal fluid is decreased in women with endometriosis. *Fertil Steril* 1992;58:290–5

25. Somigliana E, Viganò P, Vignali M. Endometriosis and unexplained recurrent spontaneous abortion: pathological states resulting from aberrant modulation of natural killer cell function? *Hum Reprod Update* 1999;5:40–51

26. Viganò P, Vercellini P, Di Blasio AM, et al. Deficient antiendometrium lymphocyte-mediated cytotoxicity in patients with endometriosis. *Fertil Steril* 1991;56:894–9

27. Smyth MJ, Taniguchi M, Street SEA. The anti-tumor activity of IL-12: mechanisms of innate immunity that model and dose dependent. *J Immunol* 2000;165:2665–70

28. Mazzeo D, Viganò P, Di Blasio AM, et al. Interleukin-12 and its free p40 subunit regulate immune recognition of endometrial cells: potential role in endometriosis. *J Clin Endocrinol Metab* 1998;83:911–16

29. Somigliana E, Viganò P, Rossi G, et al. Endometrial ability to implant in ectopic sites can be prevented by interleukin-12 in a murine model of endometriosis. *Hum Reprod* 1999;14:2944–50

Peritoneal endometriosis, ovarian endometriosis and adenomyotic nodules of the rectovaginal septum: three different entities which require a specific therapy

19

J. Donnez and M. Nisolle

Introduction

It is generally believed that endometriosis is caused by the implantation of retrograde menstrual endometrial cells, or by metaplasia. In the pelvis, we have clearly shown that three different forms of endometriosis must be considered: peritoneal endometriosis; ovarian endometriosis; and endometriosis of the rectovaginal septum[1,2].

Histogenesis of peritoneal endometriosis

Since 1987, many studies have confirmed the numerous subtle appearances of peritoneal endometriosis and a significant increase in the diagnosis of endometriosis at laparoscopy has been noted[3–12]. Our data on stromal vascularization were the first histological evidence providing support for the distinction of three different types of peritoneal endometriotic lesions: black, red and white[13–15]. The presence of a lower mitotic activity and the poor stromal vascularization (Table 1) in white lesions (white opacification) suggests that this type of lesion is a latent form of the disease; meanwhile red lesions, (red vesicles, polypoid lesions, flame-like lesions) are more active forms of the disease. Vascularization of endometriotic implants is the most important factor in growth and invasion of endometrial glands in other tissue. Indeed, an extensive vascular network was observed in red flame-like lesions, revealing the importance of angiogenesis in the early stages of development after implantation[16]. The implantation is due to the adhesion of stromal cells to the mesothelium and degradation of the extracellular matrix by matrix metalloproteinases[17]. The high stromal vascularization suggests an angiogenesis induced by recent implantation via growth factors or cytokine secreted in the stroma[18]. Hypervascularization permits further implantation in the subperitoneal fatty tissue[19].

According to our morphological data and the morphometric evaluation of the stromal vascularization, there is an obvious similarity between eutopic endometrium and red peritoneal lesions[16]. Morphologically, red peritoneal lesions are characterized by numerous proliferative glands with a columnar or pseudostratified epithelium, as can be observed in proliferative eutopic endometrium. The glandular proliferative status of red lesions is similar to that observed in eutopic endometrium, revealing a similar degree of activity. Moreover, the similar stromal vascularization observed in both tissues allows us to confirm our hypothesis that eutopic endometrium and red peritoneal lesions are similar tissues, suggesting that red lesions are recently implanted

Table 1 Morphological and morphometric study of typical and subtle peritoneal lesions

	Black lesions (n = 135)	Red lesions (n = 36)	White lesions (n = 50)	After GnRHa (n = 36)
Typical glandular epithelium and stroma	100%	100%	70%	100%
Tubal metaplasia	70%	70%	44%	44%
Hyperplasia areas	0%	12%	0%	0%
Epithelial height (μm)[b]	15.3 ± 3.6*	22.8 ± 6.3	13.1 ± 3.6[†]	14.3 ± 5.3*
Mitotic index (%)[b]	0.6 ± 1.0*	1.4 ± 2.0	0.2 ± 0.4[†]	0.3 ± 0.6*
Vascularization				
No capillaries per mm² stroma[a]	246*	149	201[†]	225*
Capillary mean surface area (μm²)[b]	117 ± 84*	501 ± 697	76 ± 36[†]	73 ± 43[†]
Capillaries/stroma relative surface area (%)[a]	2.29*	3.99	1.52[†]	1.40[†]

[a]values are medians; [b]values are means ± SD; *significantly different from red lesions; [†]significantly different from black and red lesions; GnRHa, gonadotropin-releasing hormone agonist

regurgitated endometrial cells. These data constitute an argument in favor of the transplantation theory for peritoneal endometriosis.

Thereafter, detachment of glands from viable red endometrial implants, explained by the presence of matrix metalloproteinases, could initiate their implantation in other peritoneal sites, as in a 'metastatic' process[20]. Partial shedding from red lesions throughout the menstrual cycle also explains why the red lesion always has a proliferative aspect. After this partial shedding, the remaining red lesion regrows constantly until the next shedding, but, on the other hand, menstrual shedding finally induces an inflammatory reaction, provoking a scarification process which encloses the implant. The enclosed implant becomes a 'black' lesion because of the presence of intraluminal debris. This scarification process is probably responsible for the reduction in vascularization, as proved by the significant decrease in the capillaries/ stroma relative surface area. In some cases, the inflammatory process and subsequent fibrosis totally devascularize the endometriotic foci, and white plaques of old collagen are all that remain of the ectopic implant. White opacification and yellow-brown lesions are latent stages of endometriosis. They are probably non-active lesions which could be quiescent for a long time.

In agreement with Brosens[11,12], we regard red lesions as early endometriosis, and black lesions as advanced endometriosis[8,13]. White lesions are believed to be healed endometriosis or quiescent or latent lesions. This hypothesis corroborates the clinical findings of Redwine[21] and Goldstein et al.[22] that red lesions precede the others, and that with time their presence decreases, being replaced by black, and ultimately white, lesions.

The ectopic foci are more or less autonomous, not governed by the normal control mechanisms governing the uterine endometrial glands and stroma. The exact reason why a number of implants or cells do not respond to hormonal therapy is not known, but at least four hypotheses have been proposed[23,24]: (1) the drug does not gain access to the endometriotic foci because fibrosis surrounding the foci prevents access locally; (2) endometriotic cells may have their own genetic programming, while endocrine influence appears to be only secondary and dependent on the degree of differentiation of the individual cell; (3) fewer estrogen receptors are present in peritoneal ectopic endometrium[23] when compared with eutopic

Table 2 Morphological and morphometric study of ovarian endometriomas

	Ovarian endometriomas (n = 93)	After GnRHa (n = 40)
Typical glandular epithelium and stroma	100%	97%
Tubal metaplasia	30%	51%
Hyperplasia areas	0%	0%
Epithelium height (μm)	18.5 ± 4.1	17.2 ± 4.8
Mitotic index (%)	0.7 ± 1.9	0.06 ± 1.10
Vascularization	(n = 32)	(n = 8)
No. of capillaries per mm² stroma[a]	105	132
Capillary mean surface area (μm²)[b]	316 ± 161	366 ± 221
Capillaries/stroma relative surface area (%)[a]	3.08	4.18

[a]values are medians; [b]values are means ± SD; GnRHa, gonadotropin-releasing hormone agonist

endometrium[25]; and (4) the different regulatory mechanisms of endometriotic steroid receptors may result in deficient endocrine dependency[23] because the receptors, although present, are biologically inactive[26]. In peritoneal endometriosis, a low rate of mitosis and a poor stromal vascularization after gonadotropin-releasing hormone (GnRH) agonist administration were demonstrated (Table 1). Our hypothesis is that under GnRH agonist, the lesions are in latent stages. They are probably non-active lesions which could be quiescent as long as estrogen secretion is suppressed. But the fact that residual areas of active endometriosis are present in 78% of cases explains the rapid recurrence observed after cessation of therapy[8].

Histogenesis of ovarian endometriosis

Although recent papers and debates[11,27,28] have tried to classify endometriomas, considerable uncertainty still exists. According to our laparoscopic and histological findings, a classification of ovarian endometriosis into two different types was suggested[29]: (1) superficial hemorrhagic lesions, (2) hemorrhagic cysts (endometriomas). In some areas, deep-infiltrating ovarian endometriosis, characterized by active foci deeply infiltrating the ovarian cortex, led us to suggest that different

pathogeneses must be considered for such development from epithelial inclusions in the ovary.

No significant decrease was noted in glandular activity after hormonal therapy (Table 2), and endometriomas did not demonstrate the characteristic changes of the secretory phase[16], suggesting autonomous or relatively hormone-independent proliferation[30]. The high and hormonally-independent stromal vascularization also suggests that the stroma plays a role in the development and maintenance of endometrial cysts. This highly vascularized endometriotic stroma could be responsible for the maintenance and continued growth of endometriomas; numerous hemosiderin-laden macrophages were seen in the stroma and, particularly, just underneath the epithelium lining the cyst. Large vessels were still present after GnRH agonist therapy; that is why in the management of the cyst wall, vaporization instead of cystectomy after three months of GnRH agonist therapy is the procedure of choice[31].

The pathogenesis of typical ovarian endometrioma is a source of controversy. The original paper by Sampson[32] on this condition reported that perforation of the so-called chocolate cyst led to spillage of adhesions and the spread of peritoneal endometriosis. Hughesdon[33] suggested that adhesions are not the consequence but the cause of endometriomas and thus contradicted

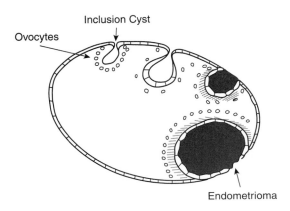

Figure 1 Hypothesis of the histogenesis of ovarian endometriomas

Sampson's hypothesis. The site of perforation, as described by Sampson, could represent the stigma of invagination of the cortex following the accumulation of menstrual debris from bleeding of endometrial implants[33]. This hypothesis corroborates observations based on ovarioscopy and *in situ* biopsies[11,34,35]. Other authors have suggested that large endometriomas may develop as a result of the secondary involvement of functional ovarian cysts in the process of endometriosis[36]. We have proposed a different hypothesis of the development of ovarian endometriosis based on coelomic metaplasia of invaginated epithelial inclusions[19,37]. This hypothesis, based on the metaplastic potential of the pelvic mesothelium, is a widely accepted theory of the pathogenesis of common epithelial ovarian tumors[38].

The fact that primordial follicles were found surrounding the endometriotic cyst is also in agreement with our hypothesis. When the mesothelium invaginates deep in the ovary, the follicles located at the invagination site are pushed concomitantly with the mesothelium (Figure 1).

The endometrioma must be considered as an invagination, but not as the result of the bleeding of a superficial implant. Indeed, metaplasia of the coelomic epithelium invaginated into the ovarian cortex was proved in our study and explains the endometrioma formation. The classification published in 1993[31] has thus to be reconsidered. There would be only two types of ovarian endometriosis: (1) superficial implants, which must be considered as peritoneal implants, resulting from the implantation of regurgitated endometrial cells; (2) intraovarian endometriosis or endometriomas, which are the consequence of metaplasia of invaginated mesothelial inclusions, and whose cyst wall epithelium and stroma are capable of secondary invagination, creating extracystic endometriotic lesions, previously called deep-infiltrating endometriosis. These active extracystic lesions are responsible for recurrence after surgical therapy[31,39].

Histogenesis of adenomyotic nodule

Sampson, in 1922[40], defined cul-de-sac obliteration as 'extensive adhesions in the cul-de-sac, obliterating its lower portion and uniting the cervix or the lower portion of the uterus to the rectum; with adenoma of the endometrial type invading the cervical and the uterine tissue and probably also (but to a lesser degree) the anterior wall of the rectum'.

The endometriotic nodule of the rectovaginal septum was considered by Koninck and Martin[41] to be the consequence of deep-infiltrating endometriosis. On the other hand, some authors[11,42,43] have suggested that it was an adenomyotic nodule, whose histopathogenesis was probably not related to the implantation of regurgitated endometrial cells, but to the metaplasia of Müllerian remnants[19]. Rectovaginal nodular endometriosis or adenomyosis is defined as a large and deep nodule (> 2 cm in size) whose largest area is under the peritoneal surface[44]. The lesion originates from the rectovaginal septum tissue and consists essentially of smooth muscle hyperplasia with active glandular epithelium and scanty stroma[19,44]. In the uterus, adenomyosis is a common condition characterized pathologically by the presence of endometrial

Table 3 Morphological and morphometric study of rectovaginal adenomyomas

	Rectovaginal adenomyomas (n = 68)	After GnRHa (n = 39)
Typical glandular epithelium and stroma	100%	100%
Tubal metaplasia	68%	21%
Hyperplasia areas	1.3%	0%
Epithelium height (μm)[b]	16.8 ± 5.0	12.9 ± 3.3
Mitotic index (%)[b]	0.4 ± 0.7	0.02 ± 0.05*
Vascularization		
No. of capillaries per mm² stroma[a]	142	208
Capillary mean surface area (μm²)[b]	143 ± 99	120 ± 60
Capillaries/stroma relative surface area (%)[a]	1.8	2.2

[a]values are medians; [b]values are means ± SD; *significantly different from control group; GnRHa, gonadotropin-releasing hormone agonist

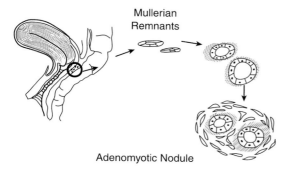

Mullerian Remnants

Adenomyotic Nodule

Figure 2 Hypothesis of the histogenesis of rectovaginal adenomyosis

glands and stroma within the myometrium[42]. In the nodule, endometriotic glands and stroma were often observed by serial sections up to the vaginal mucosa[24]; the invasion process of the smooth muscle by glandular epithelium did not require the presence of stroma[16,24].

As already described for peritoneal and ovarian endometriosis, even if a significant decrease of the mitotic index is observed after GnRH agonist therapy (Table 3), the persistence of mitoses confirmed by the glandular proliferative index[16] suggests the relative hormonal independence of the rectovaginal adenomyotic nodule.

The stromal vascularization did not show any significant cyclic variation, and after GnRH agonist therapy the number of capillaries per mm² of stroma, their mean surface area, and the ratio of capillaries to stroma surface area were found to be similar to the values observed in the non-treated group. The different responses of peritoneal endometriosis and rectovaginal adenomyosis throughout the menstrual cycle and to GnRH agonist provide another argument supporting the hypothesis that these two lesions are two different diseases and have a different physiopathology.

Adenomyosis exhibits a varied functional response to ovarian hormones and secretory changes are absent or incomplete during the second half of the cycle[45]. Histological observations similar to those of uterine adenomyosis can be made at the level of the adenomyotic rectovaginal nodule[24,44]. These similarities lead us to suggest that the so-called endometriotic nodule of the rectovaginal septum is, in fact, just like an adenomyoma or an adenomyotic nodule which can develop from Müllerian rests and consists essentially of smooth muscle with active glandular epithelium and scanty stroma. Because of the poor differentiation and the hormonal independence of these lesions, their growth in the rectovaginal septum tissue is probably not regulated by circulating steroid[46]. The low mitotic activity observed in this pathology can account for the relatively slow evolution of the adenomyoma.

The nodule is an extraperitoneal lesion and is not influenced by peritoneal fluid as is peritoneal endometriosis.

The clinical diagnosis of the nodular lesion is made only when smooth muscle proliferation is sufficient to be felt by vaginal examination. The endometriotic foci involving smooth muscle are typically associated with striking proliferation of the smooth muscle, creating an adenomyomatous appearance similar to that of adenomyosis in the endometrium[47]. When endometriotic glands, whose histogenesis is probably metaplasia, affect the rectovaginal septum which contains smooth muscle, smooth muscle proliferation can take place and the nodule thus develops (Figure 2). Moreover, nodular adenomyotic lesions can be found in other organs, such as the bowel, the bladder and the ureter. Histologically, they are systematically characterized by markedly hyperplastic smooth muscle[48]. In cases of rectovaginal nodules, hyperplasia of the smooth muscle present in the septum provokes perivisceritis at radiography, which is the consequence of serosal retraction due to the inflammatory process and fibrosis on the anterior wall of the rectum.

The absence of evolution of the 'rectal lesion' after removal of the nodule supports our hypothesis concerning its rectovaginal septum origin, and strongly suggests that it is not necessary to excise the anterior wall of the rectum in such circumstances[19,24].

Conclusion

Peritoneal endometriosis is probably caused by the implantation of regurgitated menstrual cells. The ovarian endometrioma is the consequence of non-hormone-regulated bleeding from intraovarian epithelial inclusions after they have undergone metaplasia into endometrial-like tissue. Rectovaginal endometriosis is, in fact, an adenomyotic lesion and develops from Müllerian rests. In conclusion, peritoneal endometriosis, ovarian endometriosis and rectovaginal adenomyotic nodules must be considered as three separate entities with different pathogeneses.

References

1. Nisolle M, Donnez J. Peritoneal endometriosis, ovarian endometriosis and adenomyotic nodules of the rectovaginal septum are three different entities. *Fertil Steril* 1997;68:585–96
2. Nisolle M, Casanas-Roux F, Donnez J. Peritoneal endometriosis, ovarian endometriosis and adenomyotic nodules of the rectovaginal septum: a different histopathogenesis? *Gynaecol Endoscopy* 1997;6:203–9
3. Redwine DB. The distribution of endometriosis in the pelvis by age groups and fertility. *Fertil Steril* 1987;47:173–5
4. Stripling MC, Martin DC, Chatman DL, *et al.* Subtle appearances of pelvic endometriosis. *Fertil Steril* 1988;49:427–31
5. Martin DC, Hubert GD, Vander Zwaag R, *et al.* Laparoscopic appearances of peritoneal endometriosis. *Fertil Steril* 1989;51:63–7
6. Nisolle M, Paindaveine B, Bourdon A, *et al.* Peritoneal endometriosis: typical aspect and subtle appearance. In Donnez J, ed. *Laser Operative Laparoscopy and Hysteroscopy*, Leuven, Belgium: Nauwelaerts Printing, 1989:25–41
7. Donnez J, Nisolle M, Casanas-Roux F, *et al.* Endometriosis: pathogenesis and pathophysiology. In Shaw RW, ed. *Endometriosis.* Carnforth, UK: Parthenon Publishing, 1990:11–29
8. Donnez J, Casanas-Roux F, Nisolle M. Peritoneal endometriosis: new histological aspects. In Brosens J, Donnez J, eds. *Current Status of Endometriosis. Research and Management.* Carnforth, UK: Parthenon Publishing, 1993: 75–87
9. Donnez J, Nisolle M, Casanas-Roux F. Peritoneal endometriosis: two-dimensional and three-dimensional evaluation of typical subtle lesions. *Ann N Y Acad Sci* 1994;734:342–51
10. Brosens I, Puttemans P, Deprest J. Appearances of endometriosis. *Baillière's Clin Obstet Gynaecol* 1993;7:741–57

11. Brosens IA. Is mild endometriosis a disease? Is mild endometriosis a progressive disease? *Hum Reprod* 1994;9:2209–11

12. Brosens IA. New principles in the management of endometriosis. *Acta Obstetrica Gynaecol* 1994;159:18–21

13. Nisolle M, Casanas-Roux F, Anaf V, *et al*. Morphometric study of the stromal vascularization in peritoneal endometriosis. *Fertil Steril* 1993;59:681–4

14. Nisolle M, Casanas-Roux F, Donnez J. Peritoneal endometriosis: new aspects in two-dimensional and three-dimensional evaluation. In Sutton C, Diamond M, eds. *Endoscopic Surgery for Gynaecologists*. Oxford, UK: Saunders, 1993:207–14

15. Nisolle M, Casanas-Roux F, Donnez J. Histogenesis of peritoneal endometriosis. In Nezhat CR, Berger GS, Nezhat FR, eds. *Endometriosis. Advanced Management and Surgical Techniques*. New York: Springer-Verlag, 1995:19–25

16. Nisolle M. Peritoneal, ovarian and rectovaginal endometriosis are three distinct entities. *Thèse d'Agrégation de l'Enseignement Supérieur, Université Catholique de Louvain* 1996

17. Singer C, Marbaix E, Kokorine I, *et al*. Paracrine stimulation of interstitial collagenase (MMP-1) in the human endometrium by interleukin-1 alpha and its dual block by ovarian steroids. *Proc Natl Acad Sci USA* 1997;94:10341–5

18. Smith SK. Angiogenesis and endometriosis. Presented at the *III World Congress on Endometriosis*, Brussels, 1992;Abstr. 18

19. Donnez J, Nisolle M. L'endométriose péritonéale, le kyste endométriotique ovarien et le nodule de la lame rectovaginale sont trois pathologies différentes. Editorial. *Références en Gynécologie et Obstétrique* 1995;3:121–3

20. Marbaix E, Kokorine I, Donnez J, *et al*. Regulation and restricted expression of interstitial collagenase suggest a pivotal role in the initiation of menstruation. *Hum Reprod* 1996;11:134–43

21. Redwine DB. Age-related evolution in color appearance of endometriosis. *Fertil Steril* 1987;48:1062–3

22. Goldstein MP, de Cholnoky C, Emans SJ, *et al*. Laparoscopy in the diagnosis and management of pelvic pain in adolescents. *J Reprod Med* 1980;44:251–8

23. Nisolle M, Casanas-Roux F, Wyns CH, *et al*. Immunohistochemical analysis of estrogen and progesterone receptors in endometrium and peritoneal endometriosis: a new quantitative method. *Fertil Steril* 1994;62:751–9

24. Donnez J, Nisolle M, Casanas-Roux F, *et al*. Stereometric evaluation of peritoneal endometriosis and endometriotic nodules of the rectovaginal septum. *Hum Reprod* 1995;11:224–8

25. Bouchard P, Marraoui J, Massai MR, *et al*. Immunocytochemical localization of oestradiol and progesterone receptors in human endometrium: a tool to assess endometrial maturation. *Baillières' Clin Obstet Gynaecol* 1991;5:107–15

26. Metzger DA. Cyclic changes in endometriosis implants. In Brosens I, Donnez J, eds. *The Current Status of Endometriosis. Research and Management*. Carnforth, UK: Parthenon Publishing, 1993:89–108

27. Nezhat F, Nezhat C, Nezhat C, *et al*. A fresh look at ovarian endometriomas. *Contemporary Ob/gyn* 1994:81–94

28. Nezhat C, Nezhat F, Nezhat C, *et al*. Classification of endometriosis. Improving the classification of endometriotic ovarian cysts. *Hum Reprod* 1994;9:2212–3

29. Brosens IA, Donnez J, Benagiano G. Improving the classification of endometriosis. *Hum Reprod* 1993;8:1792–5

30. Nisolle M, Casanas-Roux F, Donnez J. Histological study of ovarian endometriosis after hormonal therapy. *Fertil Steril* 1988;49:423–6

31. Donnez J, Nisolle M, Casanas-Roux F, *et al*. Endometriosis: rationale for surgery. In Brosens I, Donnez J, eds. *Current Status of Endometriosis. Research and Management*. Carnforth, UK: Parthenon Publishing, 1993: 385–95

32. Sampson JA. Heterotopic or misplaced endometrial tissue. *Am J Obstet Gynecol* 1925;10:649–64

33. Hughesdon PE. The structure of endometrial cysts of the ovary. *J Obstet Gynaecol of the Br Emp* 1957;44:69–84

34. Brosens IA. Classification of endometriosis. Endoscopic exploration and classification of the chocolate cysts. *Hum Reprod* 1994;9:2213–4

35. Brosens IA. Ovarian endometriosis. In Shaw RW, ed. *Endometriosis – Current Understanding and Management*. London: Blackwell Science, 1995:97–111

36. Nezhat F, Nezhat C, Allan CJ, *et al*. A clinical and histological classification of endometriomas: implications for a mechanism of pathogenesis. *J Reprod Med* 1992;37:771–6

37. Donnez J, Nisolle M, Gillet N, *et al*. Large ovarian endometriomas. *Hum Reprod* 1996; 11:641–6

38. Serov SF, Scully RE, Sobin LH. Histological typing of ovarian tumors. In *International Histological Classification of Tumors. No 9*, Geneva: World Health Organization, 1973:17–21

39. Canis M, Wattiez A, Pouly JL, *et al*. Laparoscopic treatment of endometriosis. In Brosens I, Donnez J, eds. *The Current Status of Endometriosis Research and Management*. Carnforth, UK: Parthenon Publishing, 1993:407–17

40. Sampson JA. Intestinal adenomas of endometrial type. *Arch Surg* 1922;5:21

41. Koninck PR, Martin D. Deep endometriosis: a consequence of infiltration or retraction or possible adenomyosis externa? *Fertil Steril* 1992;58:924–8

42. Donnez J, Nisolle M, Casanas-Roux F, *et al*. Laparoscopic treatment of rectovaginal septum endometriosis. In Donnez J, Nisolle M, eds. *An Atlas of Laser Operative Laparoscopy and Hysteroscopy*. Carnforth, UK: Parthenon Publishing, 1994:75–85

43. Donnez J, Nisolle M. Advanced laparoscopic surgery for the removal of rectovaginal septum endometriotic or adenomyotic nodules. *Baillière's Clin Obstet Gynaecol* 1995;9:769–74

44. Donnez J, Nisolle M, Casanas-Roux F, *et al*. Rectovaginal septum, endometriosis or adenomyosis: laparoscopic management in a series of 231 patients. *Hum Reprod* 1995;2:630–5

45. Zaloudek C, Norris HJ. Mesenchymal tumors of the uterus. In Kurman R, ed. *Blaustein's Pathology of the Female Genital Tract*. New York: Springer-Verlag, 1987:373

46. Donnez J, Nisolle M, Casanas-Roux F, *et al*. Peritoneal endometriosis and 'endometriotic' nodules of the rectovaginal septum are two different entities. *Fertil Steril* 1996;66:362–8

47. Scully RE, Richardson GS, Barlow JF. The development of malignancy in endometriosis. *Clin Obstet Gynecol* 1966;9:384–411

48. Clement PB. Endometriosis, lesions of the secondary Müllerian system, and pelvic mesothelial proliferations. In Kurman RJ, ed. *Blaustein's Pathology of the Female Genital Tract*. New York: Springer-Verlag, 1987:516–59

Angiogenesis and endometriosis 20

G. D'Ambrogio, A. Fasciani, F. Cristello, M. Monti,
A. R. Genazzani and P. G. Artini

Introduction

Endometriosis is a very common disease characterized by an ectopic localization of endometrial glands and stromal cells outside the uterine cavity. It affects about 10% of fertile women, reaching a prevalence of 50% in women with infertility problems[1]. In 40–60% of cases the ovary is involved in the disease, representing the most common site of localization[2].

The ectopic endometrium, in advanced endometriosis, has a characteristic appearance, represented by small dark red or blue–black nodules with scar tissue all around. The lesions also display increased vascularization. The fibrotic reaction frequently produces adhesion to near pelvic structures, or the formation of cysts, called endometriomata. The more deeply infiltrating lesions are the most common cause of pelvic pain.

The pathogenesis of endometriosis is still poorly understood; it is probably related to retrograde menstruation, but other factors must be involved, since retrograde menstruation is extremely common (occurring in about 90% of fertile women[3]), and endometriosis is much rarer.

Maney molecules are involved in the adhesion processes of endometrial cells. Furthermore, recent studies have pointed out the role of peritoneal response to chronic stimulation by ectopic cells. Macrophagic activation[4], autocrine and paracrine production of cytokines and growth factors[5], and finally peritoneal neovascularization[6], have all been demonstrated to be involved in implantation and maintenance of pelvic endometriosis.

Smith and co-authors in 1997[7] hypothesized a key role for angiogenesis in endometriosis progression; indeed neovascularization may produce the required blood supply to allow endometrial implantation. It is now generally accepted that the pathogenesis of peritoneal endometriosis involves the implantation of exfoliated endometrium. Essential for its survival is the generation and maintenance of an extensive blood supply both within and surrounding the ectopic tissue[8].

Angiogenesis is the process of formation of new blood vessels; in adults it occurs only in the reproductive tract of females, regulated day to day by activation and inhibition processes[9]. Specific angiogenic molecules are involved in the activation process, and other highly specific molecules are responsible for its inhibition. It is a dynamic equilibrium[9].

The most important angiogenic factor is vascular endothelial growth factor (VEGF)[9] but many cytokines are also involved in neovascularization, the most relevant being interleukin-8 (IL-8)[10]. VEGF is a 34–46 kD homodimeric glycoprotein, which is a highly specific mitogen for vascular endothelial cells. It is capable of inducing angiogenesis[11], is a potent inducer of vascular permeability[12] and is a survival factor for newly formed blood vessels[13]. Peritoneal fluid concentrations of VEGF have been demonstrated to be significantly higher in women with endometriosis than in control patients[14], and a positive correlation between the severity of endometriosis and the levels of VEGF in peritoneal fluid has been observed[6].

IL-8 is a chemoattractant for neutrophils and angiogenic agents, and is a potent angiogenic factor[15,16] produced by a wide variety of cell types including monocytes, neutrophils, endothelial cells and mesothelial cells[10]. The levels of this cytokine in peritoneal fluids of patients with endometriosis have been demonstrated to be significantly greater than in patients without the disease and a significant correlation between such levels and the extent of active endometriosis has been noted[17].

Aim of the study

We performed a study to investigate the presence of VEGF and IL-8 in ovarian endometriomata. We investigated if there were differences between the concentrations found in endometriomata and control cysts, and then we determined whether there was a correlation between the levels of VEGF and IL–8 and cyst volume.

Material and methods

Patients

We carried out a retrospective randomized study, enrolling 40 premenopausal non-pregnant women; 25 of these patients were admitted to our clinic with an ultrasonographic diagnosis of endometriosis. The remaining 15 women were admitted to our IVF unit for operative laparoscopy for the investigation of an adnexal mass.

All 40 patients were free from any kind of therapy for at least 3 months before laparoscopy and had not suffered pathologic conditions such as other ovarian tumors or pelvic inflammatory disease. There were no significant differences between the clinical characteristics of patients with and without endometriosis (Table 1).

Patients were classified as endometriotic following laparoscopic investigation and all those with endometriosis presented advanced disease according to the criteria of the revised American Fertility Society (AFS) classification[18].

Samples

The cystic fluid of ovarian endometriomata or follicular cysts of those without endometriosis was aspirated using a Verres needle immediately after enucleation and just before the removal of the cyst. After collection, each sample was immediately centrifuged at 2000g for 10 minutes at room temperature; the supernatant was separated and stored at $-20°C$ until assayed.

VEGF

VEGF levels were detected in cystic fluid samples using an enzyme immunoassay that measures its 'free' form (CYT$Elisa$™ VEGF; Peninsula Laboratories Inc., Belmont, CA, USA), having a sensitivity of 12.5 pg/ml, an intra-assay variability of ± 7.7% and an inter-assay variability of ± 10.7%[19].

IL-8

IL-8 levels were detected in cystic fluid samples using an enzyme immunoassay (PREDICTA® IL-8 Kit; Genzyme Diagnostic, Cambridge, MA, USA), having a sensitivity of 16 pg/ml, an intra-assay variability of ± 5.5% and an inter-assay variability of ± 8%.

Statistical analysis

Comparisons between the VEGF and IL-8 levels present in the cystic fluids were made using a non-parametric analysis of variance by ranks (Mann-Whitney U test). The correlations between VEGF and IL-8 cystic levels and the diameter of the adnexal mass were analyzed by linear regression analysis using the GraphPad Prism™ software package (GraphPad Software Inc., USA).

Results are expressed as the mean ± SD. A p value < 0.05 was considered to represent statistical significance.

Results

VEGF was detected in the cystic fluid of all the patients studied, with significantly higher

Table 1 Clinical characteristics and laboratory data of patients recruited to the study

Endometriosis	Patients (n)	Age (years)	Parity	Cyst diameter (mm)
No	15	33.9 ± 5.9	1.0 ± 0.2	42.0 ± 5.1
Yes	25	32.5 ± 6.5	0.2 ± 0.1*	48.7 ± 14.7

*$p < 0.001$ compared with patients without endometriosis

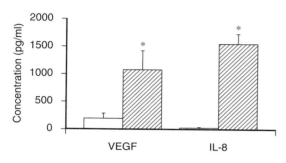

Figure 1 Concentration of vascular endothelial growth factor (VEGF) and interleukin-8 (IL-8) in follicular cysts (□) and ovarian endometriomata (▨); *$p < 0.001$, compared with follicular cysts

($p < 0.001$) concentrations seen in ovarian endometriomata (1080 ± 345 pg/ml) than in follicular cysts (195 ± 92 pg/ml) (Figure 1).

The levels of IL-8 in cystic fluid were also significantly higher ($p < 0.001$) in ovarian endometriomata (1553 ± 181 pg/ml) than in follicular cysts (28 ± 11 pg/ml) (Figure 1).

On analyzing these data, we found an inverse correlation between the VEGF levels and the diameter of the ovarian endometriomata ($p < 0.05$) and a direct correlation with the diameter of the follicular cysts ($p < 0.05$). In contrast, the correlations between IL-8 cystic fluid levels and the diameter of the adnexal masses did not reach statistical significance either for the ovarian endometriomata or for the follicular cysts.

Discussion

This is the first study to show that immunoreactive VEGF and IL-8 are present in the cystic fluids of ovarian endometriomata. It demonstrates statistically significant differences in the concentrations of these two proteins in ovarian endometriomata with respect to those detected in the adnexal masses of controls.

The hypothesis that angiogenic phenomena play an active role in the pathogenesis of the ovarian cyst formation is supported by much evidence. Guerriero et al.[20], in 1998, reported an intratumoral arterial blood flow, detected by color Doppler energy imaging, in 94% of benign ovarian tumors. Furthermore a VEGF immunostaining has been demonstrated in the epithelial lining of benign ovarian neoplasms[21].

The previous evidence that high concentrations both of VEGF[14] and IL-8[17] are present in the peritoneal fluid of women affected by endometriosis has led to the hypothesis that the peritoneum plays an important role in the maintenance of this disease by the promotion of neovascularization. Recently, Donnez et al.[22] have clearly demonstrated significantly lower VEGF levels in black lesions, compared with ectopic endometrium of women affected by endometriosis and red lesions, the values of which were similar. These data support the idea that high VEGF levels provoke an increase in the subperitoneal vascular network, facilitating implantation and viability in the earlier attachment phases of the ectopic endometrium[22].

A new model of the genesis of the ovarian endometriomata has been recently proposed based on histological data. Donnez and collaborators[23] have demonstrated that the mesothelium covering the ovary can invaginate into the ovarian cortex and that some of the invaginations are continuous with endometrial tissue; this evidence strongly suggests that metaplastic histogenesis of ovarian endometriotic lesions occurs. Once the process has become invasive, the lesion internalizes, with compression of normal ovarian stroma beneath it, and the normal tissue becomes compressed against the ovarian surface as the cyst enlarges.

The clinical trend observed in women affected by ovarian endometriotic masses seems to be biphasic: in the first active and painful phase, the cyst undergoes a rapid enlargement and increase in volume; subsequently, as the size increases, the ovarian endometriomata appear to achieve a relative 'steady state'.

To establish the importance of the angiogenic process in the development of ovarian endometriomata, we chose to investigate stage III of the disease for obtaining a model in which VEGF was likely to be produced by the cyst and not by inflammation produced by the peritoneal endometriotic lesions present in stage IV[14,18]. Our results, demonstrating that VEGF levels are inversely correlated with the diameter of the endometriotic cysts, could indicate that this growth factor is mainly important in the early phases of ovarian endometriomata progression. In contrast, although the consistently high concentrations of IL-8 detected in the chocolate cysts seem to be more involved in the non-specific pathways of inflammation, this cytokine could play an important role in supporting the vascularization of the larger and less active ovarian endometriomata.

In this later phase of the disease, in fact, all the types of cells known to produce IL-8 are present in the endometriotic cyst, i.e. monocytes, lymphocytes, neutrophils, endothelial cells, fibroblasts, macrophages, peritoneal mesothelial cells[10] and endometriotic cells[24]. This potential abundant source of IL-8 could explain the high concentrations of this cytokine in large endometriomata, whose production would be strongly stimulated by the reduced microenvironmental oxygen pressure present[16].

Conclusion

Our results, demonstrating that the levels of VEGF and IL-8 in the fluid of ovarian endometriomata are significantly higher than those detected in the adnexal masses of control subjects, would indicate that the angiogenic process may be considered a peculiarity of endometriotic cysts and not simply part of the inflammatory dynamics commonly observed in cyst formation. Furthermore, we propose different roles of these two proteins in stimulating the neovascularization of the ovarian endometriomata, with VEGF being important in the early progression and IL-8 in the maintenance of such cysts.

References

1. Strathy JH, Molgaard CA, Coulman CB. Endometriosis and infertility: a laparoscopic study of endometriosis among fertile and infertile women. *Fertil Steril* 1982;38:667–72

2. Jenkins S, Olive DL, Haney AF. Endometriosis: pathogenic implications of this anatomic distribution. *Obstet Gynecol* 1986;67:335

3. Halme J, Hammond M, Hulka J, *et al.* Retrograde menstruation in healthy women and in patients with endometriosis. *Obstet Gynecol* 1984;64:151–54

4. Halme J, Becker S, Hammond MG, *et al.* Increased activation of pelvic macrophages in infertile women with mild endometriosis. *Am J Obstet Gynecol* 1988;145:333–7

5. Tseng JF, Ryan IP, Milam TD, *et al.* Increased interleukin-6 secretion *in vitro* is up-regulated in ectopic and eutopic endometrial stromal cells from women with endometriosis. *J Clin Endocrinol Metab* 1996;81:1118–22

6. Shifren JL, Tseng JF, Zaloudek CJ, *et al.* Ovarian steroid regulation of vascular endothelial growth factor in the human endometrium: implications for angiogenesis during the menstrual cycle and in the pathogenesis of endometriosis. *J Clin Endocrinol Metab* 1996;81:3112–18

7. Smith SK. Angiogenesis. *Semin Reprod Endocrinol* 1997;15:221–7
8. McLaren J. Vascular endothelial growth factor and endometriotic angiogenesis. *Hum Reprod Update* 2000;6(1):45–55
9. Folkman J, Shing Y. Angiogenesis. *Biol Chem* 1992;267(16):10931–4
10. Arici A, Tazuke SI, Attar E, *et al.* Interleukin-8 concentration in peritoneal fluid of patients with endometriosis and modulation of inter-leukin-8 expression in human mesothelial cells. *Mol Hum Reprod* 1996;2:40–5
11. Leung DW, Cachianes G, Kuang WJ, *et al.* Vascular endothelial growth factor is a secreted angiogenic mitogen. *Science* 1989;246:1306–9
12. Keck PJ, Hauser SD, Krivi G, *et al.* Vascular per-meability factor, an endothelial cell mitogen related to PDGF. *Science* 1989;246:1309–12
13. Benjamin LE, Keshet E. Conditional switching of vascular endothelial growth factor (VEGF) expression in tumors: induction of endothelial cells shedding and regression of heman-gioblastoma-like vessels by VEGF withdrawal. *Proc Natl Acad Sci USA* 1997;94:8761–6
14. McLaren J, Prentice A, Charnock-Jones DS, *et al.* Vascular endothelial growth factor is pro-duced by peritoneal fluid macrophages in endometriosis and is regulated by ovarian steroids. *J Clin Invest* 1996;98:482–9
15. Koch AE, Polverini PJ, Kunkel SL, *et al.* Interleukin-8 is a macrophage-derived media-tor of angiogenesis. *Science* 1992;258:1798–801
16. Desbaillets I, Diserens AC, Tribolet N, *et al.* Upregulation of interleukin 8 by oxygen-deprived cells in glioblastoma suggests a role in leukocyte activation, chemotaxis, and angiogenesis. *J Exp Med* 1997;186:1201–12
17. Iwabe T, Harada T, Tsudo T, *et al.* Pathogenetic significance of increased levels of interleukin-8 in the peritoneal fluid of patients with endometriosis. *Fertil Steril* 1998;69:924–30
18. American Fertility Society. Revised American Fertility Society Classification of Endometrio-sis. *Fertil Steril* 1985;43:351–2
19. Artini PG, Fasciani A, Monti M, *et al.* Changes in vascular endothelial growth factor and the risk of ovarian hyperstimulation syndrome in women enrolled in an *in vitro* fertilization pro-gram. *Fertil Steril* 1998;70(3):560–4
20. Guerriero S, Ajossa S, Risalvato A, *et al.* Diagnosis of adnexal malignancies by using color Doppler energy imaging as a secondary test in persistent masses. *Ultrasound Obstet Gynecol* 1998;11:277–82
21. Gordon JD, Mesiano S, Zaloudek CJ, *et al.* Vascular endothelial growth factor localization in human ovary and fallopian tubes: possible role in reproductive function and ovarian cyst formation. *J Clin Endocrinol Metab* 1996; 81:353–9
22. Donnez J, Smoes P, Gillerot S, *et al.* Vascular endothelial growth factor (VEGF) in endo-metriosis. *Hum Reprod* 1998;13:1686–90
23. Donnez J, Nissole M, Gillet N, *et al.* Large ovarian endometriomas. *Hum Reprod* 1996;11: 641–6
24. Arici A, Head JR, MacDonald PC, *et al.* Regulation of interleukin-8 gene expression in human endometrial cells in culture. *Mol Cell Endocrinol* 1993;94:195–204

ART in patients with endometriosis 21

P.-N. Barri, B. Coroleu, F. Martinez, R. Tur and M. Boada

Introduction

Endometriosis is a disease with multi-factorial etiology that seriously compromises the fertility of patients who suffer from it. Many treatments have been proposed and applied to overcome the infertility usually associated with this disease. However, whatever therapeutic option is applied, more than half of patients remain infertile after treatment.

This group of infertile patients with residual endometriosis was classically considered as resorting to assisted reproductive techniques (ART) to solve their reproductive problem. From the beginning of the application of these techniques to these patients an important controversy arose over the hypothetically worse result in this group of patients in comparison with other pathologies such as tubal pathology, male factor, etc. The early works suggested that when these patients underwent *in vitro* fertilization (IVF) they had worse fertilization and implantation rates[1–3]. Recently, a meta-analysis has been published of this subject, which evaluated 660 IVF cycles and reinforced this hypothesis[4].

However, since the beginning of ART, other groups have simultaneously published studies that came to the opposite conclusion. That is to say, infertile patients with endometriosis have the same chance of becoming pregnant when they undergo IVF as do patients with other pathologies[5]. Moreover, there are ample national registers, especially in France and the UK, which confirm that infertility associated with endometriosis is a good indication for the application of ART[6,7].

There are also sufficient data in the literature to suggest that infertile patients with endometriosis have an abnormal follicular micro-environment that translates into defects of steroidogenesis on the part of the granulosa cells[8,9]. Most of the studies suggest that there is a reduced secretion of luteinizing hormone (LH), an increase in levels of interleukin (IL)-6, and a decrease in levels of vascular endothelial growth factor (VEGF)[10,11]. There is also evidence for the abnormal function of the granulosa cells from a greater presence of apoptosis phenomena and this translates into a notable reduction of blood levels of inhibin B[12,13].

Material and methods

In the Institut Universitari Dexeus, endometriosis is the fourth etiological indication (7.7% of our IVF cycles) for treating women with IVF. Other indications are more important: male factor (30.5%), tubal pathology (17.5%) and unexplained infertility (8.3%).

For this study we analyzed the results obtained in women in our IVF program who were treated in 1999 for the following infertility factors: tubal ($n = 205$ cycles), male ($n = 334$ cycles), unexplained ($n = 99$ cycles) and endometriosis ($n = 86$ cycles).

The group of infertile women with endometriosis was considered as the study group and we compared the results obtained in it with those obtained in patients who underwent IVF for other indications.

Results

As far as age is concerned, most women were in similar age groups except in the tubal factor group, whose mean age was higher. Moreover, we found that basal levels of FSH (day 3 of the cycle) were significantly higher in the group

Table 1 IVF results 1999: demographic characteristics

	Tubal	Male	Unexplained	Endometriosis
Cycles (n)	205	334	99	86
Age*	36.07 ± 5	34.3 ± 4	35.5 ± 5	34.6 ± 5
FSH (mIU/ml)**	7.9 ± 4	7.5 ± 3	8.6 ± 3	9.3 ± 6
Cancellation (%)	9.8	8.4	13.1	15.1
Oocyte pick-up (n)	185	306	86	73

$*p < 0.001$; $**p < 0.005$

Table 2 IVF results 1999: response to stimulation

	Tubal	Male	Unexplained	Endometriosis
Ampoules of gonadotropin	42.6 ± 9	43.2 ± 9	42.1 ± 9	42.6 ± 10
Follicles ≥ 15 day hCG*	9.9 ± 6.2	11 ± 5	9.5 ± 4	7.8 ± 4
Estradiol (pg/ml)**	1673 ± 986	1889 ± 981	1744 ± 920	1537 ± 1040
M-II oocytes***	9.2 ± 6	10.3 ± 6	8.9 ± 5	7.9 ± 5

$*p < 0.001$; $**p < 0.02$; $***p < 0.005$. hCG, human chorionic gonadotropin

Table 3 IVF results 1999: embryo quality

	Tubal	Male	Unexplained	Endometriosis
Fertilization (%)	68.4	68.2	71.9	71.8
Embryos	6.8 ± 1	7.2 ± 0.9	6.5 ± 0.6	6.1 ± 1.1
Embryos replaced	2.8 ± 0.8	2.8 ± 0.8	2.8 ± 0.8	2.6 ± 0.8
Embryo score	8.1 ± 1	8.4 ± 1	8.4 ± 1	8.2 ± 1
Survival after thawing (%)	71	58	68	75

of patients with endometriosis. Cancellation rates tended to be higher in the endometriosis group but without reaching a statistically significant level (Table 1).

Response to ovarian stimulation presented evidence of notable differences between the group of patients with endometriosis and the other groups. Our data confirm that with identical consumption of gonadotropins, the cycles of the endometriosis groups reached lower estradiol levels on the day of human chorionic gonadotropin (hCG) administration, fewer follicles were recruited and fewer mature oocytes were recovered (M-II) in follicular aspiration (Table 2).

With regard to fertilization and pregnancy rates, we found no difference between the groups, all of them remaining in their normal percentages within our program (Table 3). It is important to bear in mind that in order to evaluate embryo quality we included not only the usual morphological scores but also functional parameters such as implantation rate, miscarriage rate and survival of the freezing and thawing processes (Table 4).

We also wanted to analyze the results of our program of prolonged cultivation in order to evaluate whether women with endometriosis had worse blastocyst rates and lower pregnancy rates with this type of transfer. Our results in the study group were comparable with those obtained in the control groups, thus showing that embryo quality and endometrial receptivity of these women is not affected by endometriosis (Table 5).

Discussion

There is now sufficient scientific information to try to clarify ideas and concepts on the

Table 4 IVF results 1999: pregnancy

	Tubal	Male	Unexplained	Endometriosis
Oocyte pick-up (OPU) (n)	185	306	86	73
Pregnancies (n)	67	145	36	32
Pregnancy/OPU (%)	36.2	47.4	41.9	43.8
Implantation rate (%)	20	25	21	24
Multiple pregnancy (%)	46	45	30	43
Miscarriages (n)	6	19	8	3
Miscarriage rate (%)	10.5	13.8	20.8	9.4

Table 5 Results of blastocyst transfers (1995–1999) Vero cells – G1/G2 infertility factor

	Tubal	Male	Endometriosis	AID	Unexplained
Cycles (n)	156	175	58	22	67
Cultured embryos (n)	1189	1296	472	174	446
Blastocysts replaced (n)	253	255	124	24	88
Blastocysts frozen (n)	229	198	68	14	58
Blastocyst rate (%)*	40.5	35.0	40.7	21.8	32.7
Mean blastocyst/replacement	2	1.9	2.3	1.7	1.8
Pregnancies (n)	42	43	17	4	15
Pregnancy/cycle (%)	26.9	24.6	29.3	18.2	22.4
Pregnancy/replacement (%)	33.1	31.4	30.9	28.6	31.3
Gestational sacs	59	56	27	6	21
Implantation rate (%)	23.3	22.0	21.8	25	23.9
Miscarriage (%)	14.3	16.3	23.5	25.0	13.3

*$p < 0.001$

possible yield of embryos that will be presented by infertile women affected by endometriosis when they undergo IVF techniques.

It is obvious that women who have suffered frequent surgical interventions in their ovaries to extirpate endometriotic cysts have a reduced pool of ovarian follicles suitable to be recruited in an ovulation stimulation cycle[14]. As was the case in our series, there are numerous studies that indicate that these women should be treated with IVF if more than a year passes after the surgical intervention and no pregnancy has occurred[15]. It is also admitted that even if they have not undergone a surgical intervention, women with endometriosis have diminished ovarian stimulation and tend to respond less readily to normal stimulation protocols, that is to say there is a certain consensus to accept that the follicular physiology of these women is altered. It is probable that they need more stimulation and produce fewer oocytes[16]. For this reason, many of the studies that present worse results in the endometriosis group attribute the results more to the reduction in the number of available oocytes than to the reduction in fertilization rates[17] or to systemic problems such as the potential auto-immune compromise that these patients can present[18].

Nor does our study confirm the existence of lower embryo quality and worse implantation ability. Our rates of continuing clinical pregnancy, of implantation and of miscarriage are normal and totally comparable to those obtained in other indications. Another variable that is currently accepted is the absence of a relationship between the stage of the disease, the possible existence of endometriosis, and the final achieved pregnancy rate[15,19]. It is thus worth thinking that the potential of the oocytes and embryos of these women should be considered as normal. Finally, their normal implantation ability is demonstrated when these women receive donated oocytes and implant correctly, just as women affected by other pathologies do[20].

In conclusion, it is important to emphasize that infertile women who suffer from endometriosis are as good candidates to undergo IVF as women with infertility of any other origin. Moreover, even if they do have a poor prognosis in IVF, would we not accept them in IVF programs when this is unarguably their last therapeutic chance of achieving a pregnancy?

References

1. Simon C, Gutierrez A, Vidal A, *et al.* Outcome of patients with endometriosis in assisted reproduction: results from *in vitro* fertilization and oocyte donation. *Hum Reprod* 1994;9: 725–9
2. Arici A, Oral E, Bukulmez O, *et al.* The effect of endometriosis on implantation: results from the Yale University IVF-ET program. *Fertil Steril* 1996;65:603–7
3. Hull M, Williams JAC, Ray B, *et al.* The contribution of subtle oocyte or sperm dysfunction affecting fertilization in endometriosis-associated or unexplained infertility: a controlled comparison with tubal infertility and use of donor spermatozoa. *Hum Reprod* 1998; 13:1825–30
4. Barnhart KT, Dunsmoor R, Coutifaris C. The effect of endometriosis on IVF outcome. *Fertil Steril* 2000;74(Suppl. 1):Abstract O-203
5. Barri PN, Coroleu B, Martinez F, *et al.* IVF and endometriosis. *Presented at the XIV IFFS World Congress*, Proceedings of the Congress PS-2, Caracas, 1992;abstr.
6. Bachelot A, Povly JL, Devecchi A, *et al.* Bilan general FIVNAT 1997. *Contracept Fertil Sex* 1998;26:463–5
7. Templeton A, Morris JK, Parslow W. Factors that affect outcome of *in-vitro* fertilization treatment. *Lancet* 1996;348:1402–6
8. Cahill DJ, Wardle PG, Maile LA, *et al.* Pituitary-ovarian dysfunction as a cause for endometriosis-associated and unexplained infertility. *Hum Reprod* 1995;10:3142–6
9. Harlow CR, Cahill DJ, Maile LA, *et al.* Reduced preovulatory granulosa cell steroidogenesis in women with endometriosis. *J Clin Endocrinol Metab* 1996;81:426–9
10. Garrido N, Navarro J, Remohí, *et al.* Follicular hormonal environment and embryo quality in women with endometriosis. *Hum Reprod Update* 2000;6:67–74
11. Cahill DJ, Hull MGR. Pituitary-ovarian dysfunction and endometriosis. *Hum Reprod Update* 2000;6:56–66
12. Toya M, Saito H, Ohta N, *et al.* Moderate and severe endometriosis is associated with alterations in the cell cycle of granulosa cells in patients undergoing *in vitro* fertilization and embryo transfer. *Fertil Steril* 2000;73:344–50
13. Dokras A, Habana A, Giraldo J, *et al.* Secretion of inhibin B during ovarian stimulation is decreased in infertile women with endometriosis. *Fertil Steril* 2000;74:35–40
14. Nargund G, Cheng WC, Parsons J. The impact of ovarian cystectomy on ovarian response to stimulation during *in vitro* fertilization cycles. *Hum Reprod* 1995;11:81–3
15. Olivennes F, Feldberg D, Liu HC, *et al.* Endometriosis: a stage by stage analysis – the role of *in vitro* fertilization. *Fertil Steril* 1995;64:392–8
16. Al-Azemi M, Lopez Bernal A, Steele J, *et al.* Ovarian response to repeated controlled stimulation in *in vitro* fertilization cycles in patients with ovarian endometriosis. *Hum Reprod* 2000; 15:72–5
17. Azem F, Lessing JB, Geva E, *et al.* Patients with stages III and IV endometriosis have a poorer outcome of *in vitro* fertilization and embryo transfer than patients with tubal infertility. *Fertil Steril* 1999;72:1107–9
18. Domowski WP. Endometriosis and *in vitro* fertilization. *Assist Reprod Rev* 1995;5:74–81
19. Geber S, Paraschos T, Atkinsom G, *et al.* Results of IVF in patients with endometriosis: the severity of the disease does not affect the outcome, or the incidence of miscarriage. *Hum Reprod* 1995;10:1507–11
20. Díaz I, Navarro J, Blasco L, *et al.* Impact of stage III and IV endometriosis on recipients of sibling oocytes: matched case-control study. *Fertil Steril* 2000;74:31–4

Endocrine regulation of tubal function

22

M. Dayal, G. Kovalevsky and L. Mastroianni, Jr

Introduction

The fallopian tube has a critical role in reproduction, being the site of gamete transport and fertilization. A precisely timed sequence of events allows the gametes to travel in opposite directions, interact with one another, continue development, and be transported to the uterus in a controlled manner. Different portions of the fallopian tube appear to have specialized functions: the fimbrial ends are needed for ovum pick-up at the time of ovulation; the isthmus is capable of transporting spermatozoa and ova in opposite directions; and the ampulla is the principal site of fertilization.

Fallopian tube cilia and musculature are essential to these events. The fallopian tubes are lined by an epithelium that undergoes cyclic changes in response to the hormonal changes of the menstrual cycle. The epithelium is composed of ciliated and nonciliated cells. The nonciliated cells exhibit a secretory function during the follicular phase of the cycle and contribute to the intralumenal environment in which spermatozoa, ova and the zygote survive and function.

In rats and mice, the ovary and the distal portion of the fallopian tube are covered by a common fluid-filled sac that ensures direct transport of the ovulated egg into the fimbriated end of the tube. In primates, including humans, the ovulated eggs adhere to the surface of the ovary with their sticky cumulus mass. The fimbriated end of the tube sweeps over the ovulated egg, where entry into the tube is facilitated by the action of its densely ciliated fimbria. In humans and monkeys, the cilia beat synchronously in the direction of the uterus in the ampullary and isthmic portions of the tube in order to aid in egg transport[1]. This process of ovum transfer is a finely tuned event that is in part hormonally controlled. In the discussion to follow, we will focus on the endocrine regulation of tubal function during the early phases of reproduction.

Ciliary height

Egg transport is a quick and efficient process, largely secondary to ciliary action. Ciliary height undergoes cyclic changes in the setting of fluctuating hormone levels during the menstrual cycle. In 1928, Novak and Everett observed that the ciliated and secretory epithelial cells increase in height to a maximum near midcycle and then decrease in height to a minimum in the premenstrual and menstrual stages of the menstrual cycle[2].

A more recent review by Verhage et al.[3] noted inconsistent reports of the behavior of the ciliated cells in the human oviduct. Some investigators reported no change in the number of ciliated cells during the menstrual cycle while others stated that ciliogenesis could consistently be observed during the follicular phase of the cycle.

Verhage's group went on to study the ciliation–deciliation process in the human oviduct by analyzing the oviducts of 24 normally cycling women, six each during the early follicular, late follicular, early luteal and late luteal phases of the menstrual cycle[3]. Additional samples were taken from six pregnant women and six postpartum women. It was noted that hypertrophy and ciliogenesis began during the early follicular phase. The epithelial cells attained their maximum height during the late follicular stage in both the ampulla and the fimbria. By the end of the luteal phase, atrophy and deciliation took place, especially in the fimbria. Further atrophy and deciliation was noted during pregnancy and the postpartum period. Atrophy and deciliation was associated with elevated serum progesterone levels while hypertrophy and ciliation were associated with low progesterone levels and moderate estradiol levels.

The cyclic changes in ciliary height in the human were further confirmed by the observation of an increase in mitotic activity during the follicular phase and a decrease in mitotic activity as well as ciliary height coinciding with high levels of progesterone[4]. The same investigators observed estrogen-induced ciliogenesis even in postmenopausal women.

Crow et al.[5] observed that the proportion of ciliated cells varies along the length of the tube. A systematic increase in the proportion of ciliated cells was seen from the isthmus outwards, with the highest number observed in the fimbria. These same investigators compared postmenopausal sections of tube with premenopausal ones. No significant difference was found in the number of ciliated cells between the follicular and the luteal phases of the menstrual cycle but there were fewer ciliated cells in all sections of the postmenopausal tube. This effect of decreased ciliation in the postmenopausal tube was readily reversed by the administration of estrogen, suggesting tubal responsiveness to hormonal change.

Additional studies of oviductal cycles have been performed in several nonhuman primates including the rhesus and cynomolgus macaque. As in the human, estrogen is the hormone responsible for differentiation of the oviductal epithelium in the rhesus monkey. The oviducts of the adult rhesus monkey atrophy and deciliate after oophorectomy and reciliation occurs after estrogen treatment[6]. In both the cynomolgus and rhesus monkey, ciliogenesis and development of secretory activity is observed at estradiol levels of 100–200 pg/ml. Atrophy, deciliation and cessation of secretion take place when progesterone levels are above 1 ng/ml even with estradiol levels at 200 pg/ml[7]. In all these species, the hormonal regulation of ciliation and deciliation is qualitatively similar to that seen in the human.

Thus, during menstruation, when progesterone is withdrawn, the endometrium sloughs while the fimbrial epithelium begins ciliogenesis. After menses, as the endometrium proliferates due to increasing levels of estradiol, the degree of tubal ciliary proliferation increases as well. After ovulation, as the progesterone level increases, the endometrium hypertrophies while the oviductal epithelium regresses. All of these changes are most evident in the fimbria, less so in the ampulla, and least in the isthmus.

Ciliary beat frequency

Another possible factor involved in the transport function of the fallopian tube is ciliary beat frequency (CBF). CBF also changes cyclically during the menstrual cycle. Mahmood et al.[8] showed that progesterone at concentrations of 10 μg/l in vitro caused a significant reduction in CBF in the fimbrial, ampullary and isthmic portions of the human tube. Paltieli et al.[9] also investigated the effects of different levels of hormones on the ciliary activity of human oviducts. Twenty-four hours after addition of progesterone (in concentrations of 0.5 or 1 ng/ml) to fallopian tube epithelial samples, a decline of the CBF to 63% of control levels was observed; a progesterone concentration of 2 ng/ml or greater resulted in paralysis of 50–70% of cilia. These effects of progesterone were reversible with estradiol. Incubation with estradiol produced a slight, but significant increase of 4% in the mean CBF ($p = 0.002$). Incubation with Metrodin, Pergonal or luteinizing hormone (LH) did not affect ciliary motility.

The variation of CBF with respect to anatomical location in the fallopian tube has not been fully established. Westrom et al.[1] found no significant difference in CBF among regions of the fallopian tube during the menstrual cycle. Critoph and Dennis[10] found that CBF was significantly increased in the fimbria compared with the isthmus and the ampulla during the follicular phase but did not find any significant difference in CBF among anatomical sites in the luteal phase. Mahmood et al.[8] however, observed a slight, but not significant, increase in CBF in the luteal phase (5.4 Hz) as compared with the follicular phase (4.9 Hz). Given the discrepancy of these investigators' findings, further studies are necessary to establish the cyclicity of CBF.

CBF is also modulated by angiotensin II, whose receptors have been identified in the ampullary segment of the fallopian tube. Preliminary observations suggest that there is an increase in angiotensin II type I receptor binding in the proliferative phase of the cycle; binding to this receptor decreases in the secretory phase of the menstrual cycle. No statistically significant differences were observed in angiotensin II binding, receptor concentration or binding affinity in the fallopian tube on the ipsilateral or contralateral side of the corpus luteum[11]. It has been recently reported that angiotensin II has a stimulatory effect on tubal CBF in the human fallopian tube; this effect is blocked by losartan, an angiotensin II type-1 receptor antagonist[12]. In this manner, angiotensin II may act as an autocrine and/or paracrine regulator at the level of the fallopian tube. The physiological role of angiotensin II involved in human fallopian tube function is not clearly understood and needs further investigation.

Kerr et al.[13] showed a reduction in the stimulatory effect of adenosine triphosphate (ATP) (in concentrations of 100 µM) on CBF after incubation with 300 nM of progesterone for 24 hours. They also observed that progesterone increased the production of nitric oxide (NO) within the tubal lumen. Blocking NO production caused an increase in CBF that was reversed with the addition of L-arginine, an NO agonist. These findings confirm that CBF in the mammalian oviduct is in part mediated by sex hormone activation of locally produced factors.

Cyclic receptor expression

Cyclicity in ciliary height and percentage ciliation paralleled changes in estrogen receptor levels; increases in ciliary height accompanied increased levels of the estrogen receptor (ER) while decreases in height corresponded to decreased levels of ER. Progesterone was found to suppress ER during the luteal phase even though estradiol was at follicular phase levels[14,15]. The possible mechanism by which progesterone antagonizes the effect of estrogen is through suppression of ER levels below the threshold required to facilitate estradiol action.

Subtypes of the estrogen receptor as well as the androgen receptor have been localized in rat fallopian tube by Pelletier et al.[16]. ER alpha was observed in nuclei of epithelial cells as well as in stromal and muscle cells of the oviduct and the uterus. Similarly, the androgen receptor was present in the nuclei of epithelial, stromal and muscle cells of the oviduct and uterus. ER beta was not localized to the oviduct or uterus but was present in granulosa cells of developing follicles.

Shah et al.[17] investigated the cellular distribution of estrogen and progesterone receptors in the human fallopian tube by immunohistochemical localization with specific monoclonal antibodies. Intense progesterone receptor (PR) immunostaining was seen in tissues obtained at midcycle and early luteal stages of the menstrual cycle, whereas it remained undetected in menopausal tissue. ER staining was enhanced in the early follicular phase and midcycle. Menopausal tissue showed negligible staining for both PR and ER. These findings suggest that ER and PR are regulated by changes in ovarian steroid hormones.

Interestingly, Zheng et al.[18] identified follicle-stimulating hormone (FSH) receptor mRNA using *in situ* hybridization and reverse polymerase chain reaction in the tubal epithelium. Prior to this, the LH receptor with its associated ligands (human chorionic gonadotrophin (hCG), LH) was identified in the tubal epithelium as well[19]. These findings suggest the likely involvement of gonadotropins and their receptors in the physiological function of the tube.

Separate investigators reported that epidermal growth factor (EGF) is expressed in human tubal epithelium in relation to menstrual cycle stages suggesting that this growth factor is induced by estrogen[20,21]. The amount of EGF mRNA was significantly greater at the late follicular and luteal stages than at the early follicular stage. Increase in the EGF receptor protein and mRNA occurred in association with an increase in estradiol but not progesterone levels. The EGF receptor was also identified in postmenopausal tubes after estrogen replacement. Thus, EGF receptor autocrine mechanisms may play a role in mediating tubal function through the effects of estrogen.

Endocrine control of smooth muscle

It has long been speculated that the contractions of the smooth muscle of the fallopian tube play some role in transport of gametes and the pre-embryo. Their actual role in the transport of the egg remains uncertain. The precise mechanism as to how the egg is held within the ampullary segment for approximately three days and then rapidly propelled into the uterus is unresolved. It stands to reason, however, that the timing of these events is controlled, as are most other events in the menstrual cycle, by ovarian hormones. A further question is whether any effect on the muscle is direct or mediated by other factors. Some studies suggest that activity of the muscle layers of the fallopian tube does play a role in ovum transport. It appears that contractions of the ampullary segment propel the egg toward the uterus, while sphincter-like action of the isthmic segment prevents this progress.

Unopposed estrogen causes increased frequency of contractions in both layers of the musculature. This effect is prolonged and lasts beyond a decrease in estrogen level. Progesterone exposure, on the other hand, at high levels, causes inhibition of contractility, regardless of the presence of estrogen. The onset of this effect appears delayed. Thus, Lindblom et al.[22] hypothesized that estrogen stimulates tubal contractility during the follicular phase, and progesterone inhibits this activity in the luteal phase after a several-day delay.

Prostaglandins appear to influence the contractions of the tubal muscle layers[23]. Initially, a simple relationship was hypothesized with prostaglandin $F_{2\alpha}$ (PGF) having a stimulatory effect and prostaglandin E_2 (PGE) an inhibitory effect[24]. Further studies have uncovered a much more complicated relationship. When studying muscle layers individually, it was shown that PGE inhibited contractions in the circular layer, while stimulating contractions in the longitudinal layer. PGF, on the other hand, caused stimulation of contractions in both layers[25]. Thus, it is probably the relative balance of the prostaglandin levels that produces a net effect on egg transport.

Prostaglandin production in the fallopian tube has also been investigated. Some studies have shown that $PGF_{2\alpha}$ is present in the isthmic segment of the tube, while PGE_1 is rarely present. On the other hand, PGE_1 is the predominant prostaglandin in the ampullary segment[24]. Other investigators have found no difference in production of prostaglandins between regions, nor was a difference identified between follicular and luteal phases of the cycle[24].

To add to the above inconsistencies, several investigations have demonstrated that indomethacin, an inhibitor of prostaglandin synthesis, failed to significantly affect the spontaneous contractility of the fallopian tube at any time[24,26]. Several other studies have demonstrated a decrease in spontaneous motility of the tube in response to indomethacin[25].

Substantial evidence exists for the role of adrenergic mechanisms in the control of tubal contractility. Both alpha and beta receptors have been identified in the tubal muscle layers[27]. Most of the studies found an unequal distribution of the two types of receptor among the muscle layers. The alpha receptor is mostly concentrated in the longitudinal layer and mediates contractility, while the beta receptor is present mainly in the circular layer and mediates muscle relaxation. Furthermore, a higher concentration of beta receptors was identified in the ampulla.

The effects of norepinephrine and isoproterenol, a beta agonist, have been studied. Norepinephrine was shown to have an inhibitory effect on the circular layer and an excitatory effect on the longitudinal layer. Isoproterenol had an inhibitory effect on both muscle layers. From these data it would appear that beta receptors mediate relaxation of the circular muscle layer, while alpha receptors are involved in activation of contractions of the longitudinal layer. Therefore, norepinephrine may play a role in egg transport by relaxing the sphincter-like effect at the ampulla isthmic junction and increasing longitudinal contractility.

Ovarian steroids may exert their influence over muscle activity by these adrenergic mechanisms. Several studies have shown a relationship between the phase of the menstrual cycle and the type of effect norepinephrine has on the muscle[28,29]. In the proliferative phase, a high contractile response to norepinephrine administration is observed, while in the secretory phase muscle contractility is inhibited. Thus, it would appear that ovarian steroids significantly alter the response of the tubal muscle to adrenergic stimulation. The physiological relevance of this process has been challenged by data demonstrating that after destruction of adrenergic nerves or depletion of norepinephrine, pregnancy still takes place.

Most recently, nitric oxide (NO) has been implicated in regulation of smooth muscle contractility in the fallopian tube. Because of the extremely short half-life of NO, most of the investigations of this mechanism have been examined by its synthase (NOS) and NOS inhibitors. Ekerhovd et al.[30] have shown that NO induces relaxation of tubal smooth muscle, an effect which has been demonstrated in various other organs. Other investigations have concluded that certain effects of estrogen on smooth muscle are mediated by NO[31]. Estrogen-induced uterine vasodilation is antagonized by an NOS-inhibitor[32]. Therefore, it is possible that NO may be a mediator of ovarian steroid control of the tubal musculature.

The endocrine control of the fallopian tube musculature is very complicated. Investigations are challenged by differences in structure and function of the various segments of the tube. At present, even the organization and structure of the muscle layers remain uncertain. The majority of the studies have demonstrated that two major layers can be delineated: an outer longitudinal layer and an inner circular layer. An innermost longitudinal layer has also been described, but, because of its small size, this layer is thought to have a minimal effect. In the earlier studies, contractility was measured in large portions of the tube without regard to this muscle layer. Since the distinct layers have different, or even opposite, functions, this would explain the often contradictory findings of those studies. Examination of the effects of various substances on these individual layers did not resolve the controversy. Finally, more recent anatomical investigations have challenged these traditional divisions. For example, Vizza et al.[33] have shown that the myosalpinx of the human ampulla is composed of a network of multidirectional smooth muscle cell bundles, rather than distinct layers. They concluded that the musculature is designed to stir the tubal contents rather than propel them in one direction[34]. Such reports challenge many conclusions on the role of endocrine mechanisms which appear to control muscle activity.

Oviductal secretion

Once within the fallopian tube, the ovum and its cumulus are under the influence of the tubal environment. During the follicular phase, the mammalian oviduct undergoes physiological and biochemical changes which optimize the tubal environment for enhancing fertilization and early embryo development. The composition of tubal fluid, its mechanism of production and its affect on gametes and embryo survival are incompletely understood. A variety of hormones and growth factors are localized to the oviduct but their particular roles remain unclear. Different methods of identifying tubal fluid constituents have included direct sampling during surgical procedures and vascular perfusion with subsequent tubal cannulation.

The morphology and ultrastructure of the human fallopian tube epithelium at different stages of the menstrual cycle and menopause have been reassessed with reference to its secretory function[5]. In the late follicular phase, dense granules become more numerous and are adjacent to the luminal cell surface. In the luteal phase, these granules are no longer seen near the surface. The addition of estrogen to postmenopausal tubes causes changes similar to those seen in the late follicular phase where granules were located adjacent to the tubal lumen. As the appearance of these granules coincides with egg transport, their components potentially could have important effects on the oocyte and conceptus.

More than four decades ago, methods were devised for the continuous collection of oviductal fluid. Initially applied to the rabbit[35], these methods were modified for use in the rhesus monkey[36] and were later utilized for brief intervals in women undergoing tubal sterilization[37]. Systems were developed for refrigeration of the fluid collected into external chambers which facilitated analysis of its contents[38]. It was established early on that the intraluminal fluid consisted of both a transudate and an active secretion, and that the rate of fluid accumulation was under endocrine control, being modulated by both estrogen and progesterone. In the castrated rabbit, estrogen increases the rate of fluid production[39]. Levels are brought to about 50% of the estrous rate by the administration of progesterone. The rate falls to about 50% of the estrous rate during the first three days of pregnancy and is maintained at that level thereafter[40]. In an interesting 1959 experiment

evaluating the effect of the estrogen antagonist MER25, a precursor of clomiphene citrate, tubal fluid production in the estrous rabbit was suppressed by MER25[41]. However, in the castrated rabbit, MER25 exerted an estrogenic effect, pointing the way to an understanding of the impact of hormone antagonists on receptor function. The contents of tubal fluid collected under refrigeration have been assessed[38]. Lactate and pyruvate levels increased dramatically in the hours following ovulation. This is particularly pertinent in that pyruvate is a key substrate during early development in most mammalian species including the human. When this system is applied to the rhesus monkey, a dramatic increase in fluid production is associated with the estrogen surge in cycling animals[36]. This relationship was most dramatic in superovulated animals[42]. As in the rabbit, lactate and pyruvate concentrations are significantly increased following ovulation.

The appearance in tubal fluid of increased levels of lactate and pyruvate is easily explained by special metabolic characteristics of the human endosalpinx itself. In a 1958 observation on metabolic properties of the human fallopian tube, the endosalpinx was observed to produce large quantities of lactate and pyruvate, providing abundant amounts of these important substrates for early development of the fertilized egg[43].

Lippes et al.[37] have collected human tubal fluid continuously for short intervals, establishing the relationship seen in rhesus monkeys between ovulation and fluid production. There was also a dramatically increased amount of total proteins in the fluid following ovulation. The protein content of tubal fluid was also assessed in the rhesus monkey[44]. A protein which was felt to be unique to the oviduct, i.e. an oviductal specific protein, was identified in the immediate postovulatory phase of the cycle. Because of the clinical importance of understanding the tubal environment, there has been a resurgence in the interest in tubal fluid and there have been further technical advances for isolation and identification of proteins, as discussed below.

Using methods for continuous collection of secretions in the rhesus monkey, levels of free steroids were evaluated[45]. Of particular interest was that the unbound progesterone was present in greater quantities in tubal fluid than was observed in serum. In recent observations on the relationship between the tubal environment and spermatozoa, it has been established that the tubal isthmus serves as a reservoir for spermatozoa, which are attached to the epithelium[46,47]. Activation and release occurs under the influence of progesterone, providing an available pool of spermatozoa as the egg is released and picked up by the fallopian tube[48].

More recently, sophisticated *in vitro* techniques have been used to assess the secretory function of the human tube. A vascularly perfused preparation of the fallopian tube was used as a model to study the formation and composition of tubal fluid[49]. Fluid was always collected from patients in the follicular phase. The mean rate of production was 48 μl/hour. There was no correlation between metabolite concentration and length of perfusion, patient's age or patient condition. This unique technique provides a controlled method with which to examine human tubal fluid in both normal and diseased tubes.

The rate of tubal fluid production is modified by adrenergic influence. In a recent study, Tay *et al.*[50] obtained tubal samples from 38 hysterectomy patients, on which perfusion studies were performed. In ten of 17 specimens, tubal fluid spontaneously formed. The mean rate of tubal fluid production was 64.78 ml/hour. Nine of these ten patients were in the follicular phase of the cycle; the other was in the immediate postmenstrual phase of the cycle. The addition of isoproterenol (1 mM) led to further increases in tubal fluid production. Dibutyryl cyclic AMP (1 mM) reduced tubal fluid formation by 66%.

Oviductal specific glycoprotein

Ovarian steroid hormones, particularly estrogen, have been implicated in regulation of the tubal environment. An estrogen-dependent oviductal secretory glycoprotein has been shown to be unique to the fallopian tube and is conserved across several mammalian species[51]. This protein interacts with the zona pellucida, perivitelline space and vitelline or blastomere membrane of ovulated eggs and preimplantation embryos. The oviductal secretory glycoprotein enhances sperm binding and penetration of oocytes as well[50].

The human oviduct synthesizes and secretes the 110–130 kDa oviductal specific glycoprotein during the periovulatory period of the menstrual cycle[52]. Immunocytochemical studies have localized these glycoproteins to secretory granules within the secretory cells of the hamster and primate oviduct[53]. The appearance of these proteins is associated with ovulation[54–60]. In rabbits[61], baboons[52], pigs[62], rodents[63–65], and sheep[62], synthesis and secretion of these glycoproteins is regulated by estrogen.

In primates, this 110–130 kDa protein is formed by two acidic (100–120 and 110 kDa respectively) proteins and one basic (120–130 kDa) protein. The fimbria contains the two acidic proteins, the isthmic portion contains mostly the basic molecule, and all three proteins are found in the ampulla where fertilization and early embryo cleavage occur[58]. Under the influence of estrogen, the oviduct secretes these oviductal-specific proteins into the lumen as the gametes travel through the tube and interact with one another.

O'Day-Bowman *et al.*[66] further characterized the hormonal regulation of the oviductal-specific glycoprotein synthesis and secretion throughout the menstrual cycle and in all regions of the tube. They observed that the glycoprotein was found primarily in oviductal fluid during the follicular phase of the cycle, but not in serum, follicular fluid or endometrium. During the late follicular phase, mRNA expression for the human oviductal-specific glycoprotein is elevated in all regions of the tube. Although the function of this oviductal-specific protein is unknown, its appearance at the time of ovulation has led to the hypothesis that it may play a role in fertilization or preimplantation embryo development.

Similarities are apparent between species, especially in the cow, sheep and pig, where estrogen-associated oviductal proteins are of similar molecular weight. Gandolfi et al.[67] observed that these common proteins share immunocytochemical localization and glycosylation in cows, sheep and goats. This suggests a good degree of phylogenetic conservation and a significant functional role.

Murray et al.[68] have shown that the oviductal-specific protein in the mouse is synthesized and released by the oviduct in a temporal- and regional-specific manner while the fertilized egg is traveling through the fallopian tube and before a rise in progesterone levels. The 90–92 kDa protein in the mouse is intensely synthesized and released at the time of estrus until the fourth day of pregnancy in the ampulla and isthmus of the tube. This suggests differential roles of segments of tube in reproduction and a unique role for the oviductal-specific protein.

In all examined species, except mice, these oviductal-specific proteins are associated with the zona pellucida. In addition, these molecules are found in the perivitelline space in sheep[69], baboons[55], hamsters[65], mice[69–71], cows[72] and pigs[62]; and in the vitelline membrane and, in some cases, the embryonic cytoplasm, in several species. No data, however, are available on the precise function of these molecules during early development. Suggested hypotheses of the role of oviductal-specific proteins include immunological protection to the zygote[60,61], gamete recognition[73] or activation of the embryonic genome[74].

References

1. Westrom L, Mardh P, Mecklenberg C, et al. Studies on epithelia of the human genital tract. II. The mucociliary wave pattern of the fallopian tube epithelium. Fertil Steril 1977;28:955–61
2. Novak E, Everett HS. Cyclical and other variations in the tubal epithelium. Am J Obstet Gynecol 1928;516:499–530
3. Verhage HG, Bareither ML, Jaffe RC, et al. Cyclic changes in ciliation, secretion, and cell height of the oviductal epithelium in women. Am J Anat 1979;156:505–21
4. Donnez J, Casanas-Roux F, Caprasse J, et al. Cyclic changes in ciliation, cell height, and mitotic activity in human tubal epithelium during reproductive life. Fertil Steril 1985;43:554–59
5. Crow J, Amso NN, Lewin J, et al. Morphology and ultrastructure of Fallopian tube epithelium at different stages of the menstrual cycle and menopause. Hum Reprod 1994;9:2224–33
6. Allen E. Reactions of immature monkey (Macaca rhesus) to injections of ovarian hormone. J Morphol 1928;46:479–520
7. Brenner RM, Resko JA, West NB. Cyclic changes in oviductal morphology and residual cytoplasmic estradiol binding capacity induced by sequential estradiol–progesterone treatment of spayed rhesus monkeys. Endocrinology 1974; 95:1094–104
8. Mahmood T, Saridogan E, Smutna S, et al. The effect of ovarian steroids on epithelial beat frequency in the human Fallopian tube. Hum Reprod 1998;13:2991–4
9. Paltieli Y, Eibschitz I, Ziskind G, et al. High progesterone levels and ciliary dysfunction – a possible cause of ectopic pregnancy. J Assist Reprod Genetics 2000;17:103–6
10. Critoph FN, Dennis KJ. Ciliary activity in the human oviduct. Br J Obstet Gynaecol 1977;84: 216–18
11. Johnson MC, Castro A, Troncoso JL, et al. Presence of angiotensin II and expression of angiotensin II type-2 receptor in human fallopian tube. Fertil Steril 1998;70:740–6
12. Saridogan E, Djahanbakhch O, Puddefoot JR, et al. Angiotensin II receptors and angiotensin II stimulation of ciliary activity in human fallopian tube. J Clin Endocrinol Metab 1996; 81:2719–25
13. Kerr B, Martinez SP, Villalon M. Progesterone modulates the stimulatory effect on ciliary activity produced by ATP through nitric oxide pathway. Presented at the 33rd Annual Meeting of the Society for the Study of Reproduction, 2000; abstr.601
14. Press MF, Xu S, Wang J, et al. Subcellular distribution of estrogen receptor and progesterone

receptor with and without specific ligand. *Am J Pathol* 1989;135:857–64

15. Amso NN, Crow J, Shaw R. Comparative immunohistochemical study of oestrogen and progesterone receptors in the Fallopian tube and uterus at different stages of the menstrual cycle and the menopause. *Hum Reprod* 1994; 9:1027–37

16. Pelletier G, Labrie C, Labrie F. Localization of oestrogen receptor alpha, oestrogen receptor beta and androgen receptors in rat reproductive organs. *J Endocrinol* 2000;165:359–70

17. Shah A, Nandedkar TD, Raghavan VP, *et al*. Characterization and localization of estrogen and progesterone receptors of the human fallopian tube. *Ind J Exp Biol* 1999;37:893–9

18. Zheng W, Magid MS, Kramer EE, *et al*. Follicle-stimulating hormone receptor is expressed in human ovarian surface epithelium and fallopian tube. *Am J Pathol* 1996;148:47–52

19. Lei ZM, Toth P, Rao CV, *et al*. Novel expression of human chorionic gonadotropin/human luteinizing hormone receptors and ligand hCG in human fallopian tubes. *J Clin Endocrinol Metab* 1993;77:863–72

20. Adachi K, Kurachi H, Adachi H, *et al*. Menstrual cycle specific expression of epidermal growth factor receptors in human fallopian tube epithelium. *J Endocrinol* 1995;147: 553–63

21. Lei ZM, Rao CV. Expression of epidermal growth factor (EGF) receptor and its ligands, EGF and transforming growth factor-alpha, in human fallopian tubes. *Endocrinology* 1992; 131:947–57

22. Lindblom B, Hamberger L, Ljung B. Contractile patterns of isolated oviductal smooth muscle under different hormonal conditions. *Fertil Steril* 1980;33:283–7

23. Lindblom B, Wilhelmsson L, Wikland M, *et al*. Prostaglandins and oviductal function. *Acta Obstet Gynecol Scand* 1983;113(Suppl.):43–6

24. Elder MG, Myatt L, Chaudhuri G. The role of prostaglandins in the spontaneous motility of the fallopian tube. *Fertil Steril* 1977;28:86–90

25. Lindblom B, Hamberger L, Wiquist N. Differentiated contractile effects of prostaglandins E and F on the isolated circular and longitudinal smooth muscle of the human oviduct. *Fertil Steril* 1978;30:553–9

26. Laszlo A, Nadasy GL, Manos E, *et al*. Effect of pharmacological agents on the activity of the circular and longitudinal smooth muscle layers

of human fallopian tube ampullar segments. *Acta Physiologica Hungarica* 1988;72:123–33

27. Paton DM, Widdicombe JH, Rheaume DE, *et al*. The role of the adrenergic innervation of the oviduct in the regulation of mammalian ovum transport. *Pharmacologic Reviews* 1978; 29:67–102

28. Korenaga M, Kadota T. Changes in mechanical properties of the circular muscle of the isthmus of the human fallopian tube in relation to hormonal domination and postovulatory time. *Fertil Steril* 1981;36:343–50

29. Coutinho EM, Maia H, Filho JA. Response of the human fallopian tube to adrenergic stimulation. *Fertil Steril* 1970;21:590–4

30. Ekerhovd E, Brannstrom M, Alexandersson M, *et al*. Evidence for nitric oxide mediation of contractile activity in isolated strips of the human fallopian tube. *Hum Reprod* 1997;12:301–5

31. Martinez SP, Viggiano M, Franchi AM, *et al*. Effect of nitiric oxide synthase inhibitors on ovum transport and oviductal smooth muscle activity in the rat oviduct. *J Reprod Fertil* 2000; 118:111–17

32. Van Buren GA, Yang D, Clark EC. Estrogen-induced uterine vasodilatation is antagonized by L-nitroarginine methyl ester, an inhibitor of nitric oxide synthesis. *Am J Obstet Gynecol* 1992; 167:828–33

33. Vizza E, Correr S, Muglia U, *et al*. The three-dimensional organization of the smooth musculature in the ampulla of the human fallopian tube: a new morpho-functional model. *Hum Reprod* 1995;10:2400–5

34. Pulkkinen MO, Talo A. Tubal physiologic consideration in ectopic pregnancy. *Clin Obstet Gynecol* 1987;30:164–72

35. Clewe TH, Mastroianni L Jr. A method for continuous volumetric collection of oviduct secretions. *J Reprod Fertil* 1960;l:146–52

36. Mastroianni L Jr, Shah U, Abdul-Karim R. Prolonged volumetric collection of oviduct fluid in the rhesus monkey. *Fertil Steril* 1961; 12:417–21

37. Lippes J, Krasner J, Alfonso LA, *et al*. Human oviductal fluid proteins. *Fertil Steril* 1981;36: 623–9

38. Holmdahl T, Mastroianni L Jr. Continuous collection of rabbit oviduct secretions at low temperature. *Fertil Steril* 1965;16:587

39. Mastroianni L Jr, Beer F, Shah U, *et al*. Endocrine regulation of oviduct secretions in the rabbit. *Endocrinology* 1961;68:92–7

40. Mastroianni L Jr, Wallach RC. Effect of ovulation and early gestation on oviduct secretions in the rabbit. *Am J Physiol* 1961; 200:815–21

41. Mastroianni L Jr, Abdul-Karim R, Shah U, *et al*. Changes in the secretion rate of the rabbit oviduct following oral administration of 1-(p-2-diethylaminoethoxphenyl)-1-phenyl-2-anisylethanol. *Endocrinology* 1961;69: 396–401

42. Mastroianni L Jr, Urzua M, Avalos M, *et al*. Some observations on Fallopian tube fluid in the monkey. *Am J Obstet Gynecol* 1969;103:703–9

43. Mastroianni L Jr, Winternitz WW, Lowi NP. The *in vitro* metabolism of the human endosalpinx. *Fertil Steril* 1958;9:500–5

44. Mastroianni L Jr, Urzua M, Stambuagh R. Protein patterns in monkey oviductal fluid before and after ovulation. *Fertil Steril* 1970;21: 817–20

45. Wu CH, Mastroianni L Jr, Mikhail G. Steroid hormones in monkey oviductal fluid. *Fertil Steril* 1977;28:1251–6

46. DeMott RP, Lefebvre R, Suarez SS. Carbohydrates mediate the adherence of hamster sperm to oviductal epithelium. *Biol Reprod* 1995;52:1395–403

47. Lefebvre R, Suarez SS. Effect of capacitation on bull sperm binding to homologous oviductal epithelium. *Biol Reprod* 1996;54:575–82

48. Aitken RJ, Harkiss D, Knox W, *et al*. On the cellular mechanisms by which the bicarbonate ion mediates the extragenomic action of progesterone on human spermatozoa. *Biol Reprod* 1998;58:186–96

49. Dickens CJ, Maguiness SD, Comer MT, *et al*. Human tubal fluid: formation and composition during vascular perfusion of the fallopian tube. *Hum Reprod* 1995;10:505–8

50. Tay JI, Rutherford AJ, Killick S, *et al*. Human tubal fluid: production, nutrient composition and response to adrenergic agents. *Hum Reprod* 1997;12:2451–6

51. Buhi WC, Alvarez IM, Kouba AJ. Secreted proteins of the oviduct. *Cells Tissues Organs* 2000; 166:165–79

52. Verhage HG, Fazleabas AT. The *in vitro* synthesis of estrogen-dependent proteins in the baboon (*Papio anubis*) oviduct. *Endocrinology* 1988;123:552–8

53. Verhage HG, Mavrogianis P, Boice ML, *et al*. Oviductal epithelium of the baboon: hormonal control and the immuno-gold localization of oviduct-specific glycoprotein. *Am J Anat* 1990; 187:81–90

54. Boice ML, McCarthy TJ, Mavrogianis PA, *et al*. Localization of oviductal glycoproteins within the zona pellucida and perivitelline space of ovulated ova and early embryos in baboons (*Papio anubis*). *Biol Reprod* 1990;43:340–6

55. Buhi WC, Vallet JL, Bazer FW. De novo synthesis and release of polypeptides from cyclic and early pregnant porcine oviductal tissue in explant culture. *J Exp Zool* 1989;252:79–88

56. Buhi WC, Alvarez IM, Sudhipong V, *et al*. Identification and characterization of *de novo*-synthesized porcine oviductal secretory proteins. *Biol Reprod* 1990;43:929–38

57. Buhi WC, Bazer FW, Alvarez IM, *et al*. In vitro synthesis of oviductal proteins associated with estrus and 17-estradiol-treated ovariectomized ewes. *Endocrinology* 1991;128:3086–95

58. Fazleabas AT, Verhage HG. The detection of oviduct specific proteins in the baboon (*Papio anubis*). *Biol Reprod* 1986;35:455–62

59. Oliphant G, Ross PR. Demonstration of production and isolation of three sulfated glycoproteins from the rabbit oviduct. *Biol Reprod* 1982;26:537–44

60. Gandolfi F, Brevini TAL, Richardson L, *et al*. Characterization of proteins secreted by sheep oviduct epithelial cells and their function in embryonic development. *Development* 1989; 106:303–12

61. Oliphant G, Cabot C, Ross P, *et al*. Control of the humoral immune system within the rabbit oviduct. *Biol Reprod* 1984;31:205–12

62. Buhi WC, Ashworth CJ, Bazer FW, *et al*. In vitro synthesis of oviductal secretory proteins by estrogen-treated ovariectomized gilts. *J Exp Zool* 1992;262:426–35

63. Abe H, Oikawa T. Ultrastructural evidence for an association between an oviductal glycoprotein and the zona pellucida of the golden hamster egg. *J Exp Zool* 1990;256:210–21

64. Kan FWK, St-Jacques S, Bleau G. Immuno-electron microscopic localization of an oviductal antigen in hamster zona pellucida by use of a monoclonal antibody. *J Histochem Cytochem* 1988;36:1441–7

65. Kan FWK, Roux E, Bleau G. Immunolocalization of oviductin in endocytic compartments in blastomeres of developing embryos in the golden hamster. *Biol Reprod* 1993;48:77–88

66. O'Day-Bowman MB, Mavrogianis PA, Fazleabas AT, et al. A human oviduct-specific glycoprotein: synthesis, secretion, and localization during the menstrual cycle. *Micro Res Tech* 1995;32:57–69

67. Gandolfi F, Passoni L, Modina S, et al. Interspecific similarities between proteins secreted by the oviduct epithelium. *Reprod Fertil Dev* 1993;5:433–43

68. Murray MK, DeSouza MM, Messinger SM. Oviduct during early pregnancy: hormonal regulation and interactions with the fertilized ovum. *Micro Res Tech* 1995;31:497–506

69. Gandolfi F, Modina S, Brevini TAL, et al. Oviduct ampullary epithelium contributes a glycoprotein to the zona pellucida, perivitelline space and blastomere membrane of sheep embryos. *Eur J Basic Appl Histochem* 1991;35:383–92

70. Kapur RP, Johnson LV. Selective sequestration of an oviductal fluid glycoprotein in the perivitelline space of moose oocytes and embryos. *J Exp Zool* 1986;238:249–60

71. Kapur RP, Johnson LV. Ultrastructural evidence that specialized regions of the murine oviduct contribute a glycoprotein to the extracellular matrix of mouse oocytes. *Anat Rec* 1988;221:720–9

72. Wegner CC, Killian GJ. *In vitro* and *in vivo* association of an oviduct estrus-associated protein with bovine zone pellucida. *Mol Reprod Dev* 1991;29:77–84

73. Brown CR, Jones R. Binding of the zona pellucida proteins to a boar sperm polypeptide of Mr. 53 000 and identification of zona moieties involved. *Development* 1987;99:183–91

74. Crosby IM, Gandolfi F, Moor RM. Control of protein synthesis during early cleavage of sheep embryos. *J Reprod Fertil* 1988;82:769–75

Premature ovarian failure: an autoimmune disease?

23

P. Fénichel

Introduction

Premature ovarian failure (POF), a secondary amenorrhea occuring in women under the age of 40, characterized by elevated gonadotropins, sex steroid deficiency and infertility, is present in 2% of women[1]. Incipient ovarian failure with normal spontaneous cycles, infertility, high levels of follicle-stimulating hormone (FSH) and poor responses to menotropins, as described by Cameron *et al.*[2], represents one particular aspect of this syndrome. Physiological menopause is the result of a progressive reduction of the ovarian follicular pool. It occurs subsequent to a continuous atretic/apoptotic process which begins as early as fetal life and leads around the age of 50 years to a complete depletion. POF does not exactly represent a premature menopause since half the women with POF still present follicles on their ovaries, may ovulate or may become spontaneously pregnant more than 6 years after occurrence of the hypergonadotropic amenorrhea[3]. In fact, premature ovarian failure can occur as a result of three different factors: (1) a primitive reduced pool of oocytes; (2) an accelerated follicular atresia; or (3) an impaired folliculogenesis. Abnormalities of X chromosome and iatrogenic factors such as surgery, chemo- and radiotherapy are the most frequent causes of POF. However, more than half of the karyotypically normal, spontaneous POF cases remain unexplained. In these 'idiopathic' cases, a genetic or an autoimmune origin has been suggested.

Recent studies have indeed implicated genetic factors in the pathogenesis of idiopathic POF. Different genes involved in migration and proliferation of ovogonia have been characterized in mice, and could be appropriate candidates for investigation of human POF with a reduced initial follicular pool as in ataxia telegiectasia[4]. Several as yet unidentified genes residing on the long arm of the X chromosome control the ovarian preservation against accelarated atresia, which for example, is observed in Turner's syndrome.

Some autosomal genes seem also to be important for this preservation, as illustrated by the blepharophimosis syndrome with POF, associated with mutation of a chromosome 3-located gene[5]. Mutations of the FSH receptor gene have been recently described[6], allowing for the first time an explanation for resistant ovarian syndrome (ROS), which is characterized by multiple primordial follicles present on ovarian biopsy and a disturbed folliculogenesis[7]. It is likely that dissection of POF heterogeneity will lead to the discovery of new genes regulating germ cell migration or proliferation, meiosis, oocyte maturation and survival, and follicular atresia.

Autoimmune involvement in POF

An exaggerated autoimmune reaction involved in atretic accalaration, oocyte wastage or impaired folliculogenesis is one hypothesis that has been formulated since Irvine *et al.*[8] first described an association between an autoimmune adrenal deficiency and POF. Several pieces of evidence, including association with multiple autoimmune endocrine disorders, clinical reversibility, histological and immunogenetic features, experimental studies and the demonstration of circulating ovarian antibodies in serum samples from women with POF, have suggested such an origin, leading to proposals of immunosuppressive treatment[9–11]. However, the reality of such an autoimmune process, its exact role in ovarian failure, the antigenic determinant(s) of ovarian antibodies and cellular immunity, and the efficiency of corticosteroid treatment, are still far from clarified. Here, we discuss the possible role of such an autoimmune process as a cause or consequence of POF.

Physiological role of the immune system in ovarian function

Unlike the testis, the ovary is not an immunologically privileged site. Several immune cells are recruited by the ovaries during the menstrual cycle such as macrophages, lymphocytes and polymorphonuclear granulocytes[12]. These cells are able to secrete cytokines, which participate in the paracrine regulation of follicle development, ovulation and luteal function. Cytokines modulate gonadotropin-mediated control of ovarian function[13]. During the follicular phase, cytokines generally act in an inhibitory fashion, controlling the stimulatory action of FSH on the thecal and granulosa cells of the developing follicle[13]. For example tumor necrosis factor-α (TNFα) secreted by resident ovarian macrophages is an inhibitor of steroidogenesis in thecal and granulosa cells from immature follicles[13,14]. Ovulation has been considered an inflammatory process including both leukocytes and cytokines. Neutrophilic granulocytes and macrophages are particularly abundant during formation of the corpus luteum. Neutrophil phagocytosis and secreted proteases seem to be essential to the evolution of the corpus luteum; TNFα, interleukin-2 (IL-2) and interferon-γ (IFNγ) decrease progesterone secretion and act in a cytotoxic manner[13]. Therefore, it is logical to consider that abnormalities of this process could perturb ovarian function and be involved in POF by accelerating follicular atresia or by disturbing folliculogenesis.

Experimental studies

The tight relationship between the immune system and ovarian function is supported by the neonatal thymectomy model, which in the mouse leads to sterility with an autoimmune oophoritis, including a T cell infiltration and production of ovarian autoantibodies[15,16]. This oophoritis can be induced by transfering normal T cells to athymic nude mice[17]. In humans, athymic girls present dysgenetic atrophic ovaries devoid of follicles[18], which illustrates the relationship between the immune system and ovarian function.

Clinical aspects of POF

As for other autoimmune disease, psychological stress has been reported frequently at the beginning of POF[19]. Spontaneous recovery of ovarian cycles and/or spontaneous pregnancies, under hormonal replacement therapy or without any treatment, suggest indeed a partial, reversible autoimmune attack[20], as observed during the 'honeymoon period' of patients with type I insulin-dependent diabetes[21]. Association with another autoimmune disease, especially adrenal deficiency, represents the strongest evidence for an immunologic origin of POF. Autoimmune adrenal deficiency seldom occurs in isolation, and is part of the type I autoimmune polyendocrinopathy (APE-I) when associated with hypoparathyroidism and mucocutaneous candidiasis. In this autosomal recessive syndrome linked to chromosome 21 and without any association with a specific HLA (human leukocyte antigen) haplotype, POF is present in 60% of cases[22]. In APE-II, an autosomic dominant disease linked to chromosome 6 and associated to HLA B8DR3, with adrenal deficiency and hypothyroidism POF is present in 25%[23]. In all cases of idiopathic POF, combined adrenal deficiency is found in 2 to 10%[24]. Several other associations with autoimmune diseases (insulin-dependent diabetes, myasthenia, systemic lupus erythematosus) have been reported[25].

Histological findings of POF

Multiple observations[25] have been made of oophoritis occurring with T lymphocyte infiltration of the mature follicles, the steroid-producing cells being the main target of the immune attack. Most of these reported cases, however, included an autoimmune adrenal disease (clinical signs and/or autoantibodies). In the absence of adrenal autoimmunity/adrenal deficiency, lymphocytic oophoritis was only found in six of 215 cases[26]. However, immunoglobulins were frequently detected (30 to 50%) in the vascular wall staining or in the stroma and follicular cells[26]. Another interesting finding in the systematic histological screening of POF is the presence in 40% of cases of detectable ovarian follicles varying from few to numerous[25].

Immunogenetic aspects of POF

Organ-specific autoimmune diseases have been associated with specific haplotypes of HLA class II. Serological determinations of HLA class II in POF have been studied by several teams, whether adrenal deficiency was present or not. An association with HLA-DR3 was found by Walfish et al.[27] and a weak association with HLA-DR4 was reported by Jaroudi et al.[28]; however Anasti et al.[29] did not find any association. In our own cohort of 42 POF cases we confirmed a significant relationship with HLA-DR3 and a weak relationship with HLA-DR4[30]. HLA class II genes include those encoding for HLA-DR, DQ, and DP molecules, which are expressed on the cell surface participating in the presentation of the antigenic peptide to T lymphocytes. Exhibiting a high degree of polymorphism, it has been suggested that they could determine the ability to bind peptides and therefore influence specific autoimmune diseases. Recently, an association with HLA-DQ B1-0301 and -0603 has been reported[31] in POF, with autoantibodies raised against 3β-hydroxysteroid dehydrogenase (a steroid cell enzyme).

Antiovarian antibodies in POF

The presence of circulating antiovarian antibodies (AOA) is usually considered to be a suitable marker in the identification of immunological involvement. In POF, they were characterized long ago using immuno-fluorescence in animal ovaries. More recently, human ovary extracts were used in an enzyme-linked immunosorbent assay (ELISA). Circulating AOA were found in 30 to 60% of cases of karyotypically normal spontaneous POF[30,32–34]. An ELISA against whole-tissue homogenate from human ovaries at different ages was performed at the Immunology Laboratory of University of Nancy[35]. We were able to detect at least one of the three subclasses of immunoglobulins (IgG, IgM, IgA) in 59% (27 out of 46) of patients with idiopathic POF[30].

Specificity of these AOA was attested by the mean values of the three subclasses of immunoglobulins, which were significantly higher in POF patients than in all control groups tested[30] including a group of young fertile women, a group of women with Grave's disease and a group with positive antinuclear antibodies. In our POF group, sera positive for AOA were tested against other tissues, and only six out of 27 showed positive cross-reactivity corresponding to an autoimmune polyendocrinopathic state, including two cases of Addison's disease[30]. It has recently been clearly established that in the case of association with adrenal disease and/or an autoimmune polyendocrinopathy, the antigenic determinants involved in ovarian autoimmunity are represented by the steroidogenic enzymes cytochrome p450c21-hydroxylase[36], p450c17α-hydroxylase[36], p450scc cholesterol side-chain cleavage steroid enzyme[36] and 3β-hydroxysteroid dehydrogenase[37]. These antibodies are able to cross-react with all the endocrine targets that possess steroidogenic enzymes such as the adrenal gland, testis, ovary (stromal, thecal or granulosa cells) and placenta, and correspond to the steroid-producing cell antibodies earlier reported[25]. Such antibodies were differently distributed in APE-I and APE-II with or without adrenal deficiency, and were only seldom found in the absence of adrenal deficiency or in association with an other autoimmune disease[38]. In such a situation, which is generally the most frequent in AOA-positive idiopathic POF, the specific antigens have not yet been identified even using SDS-PAGE and Western blotting[34]. Several candidates have been proposed. It was first suggested that FSH or luteinizing hormone (LH) receptors could be targets for antibodies involved in POF[39,40]. Systematic screening of such antibodies using recombinant antigens has been disappointing[41]. Determination of these antigens would be useful for understanding POF cases associated with AOA.

The significance of circulating AOA remains an essential question. Do they represent a marker of a primary or secondary immune dysfunction process against the ovaries? Elevated FSH has been considered to be a potential factor able to stimulate ovarian autoimmunity through overexpression of HLA-DR antigen on granulosa cells, allowing the presentation of specific antigens to the T lymphocytes[42]. However, in our studies we did not find high AOA levels in aging women or in postmenopausal women with elevated FSH as in POF patients[30]. Mechanical aggression such as *in vitro* fertilization repetitive punctures[35] or post-traumatic castration (surgery, chemo- or radiotherapy) may also result in the production of differentiation antigens and stimulate an autoimmune reaction. We did not find such an influence of ovarian biopsy on AOA levels in our studies of idiopathic POF[30]. Several reports have also suggested that an autoimmune reaction could be associated with polycystic ovarian syndrome (PCOS) following inappropriate secretion of cytokines[43], or with Turner syndrome secondary to accelerated atresia[33]. In our studies, we were surprised to discover particularly high levels of AOA in pure PCOS women[44] and positive AOA in 50% of our Turner group[45]. These results highlight the possibility of a secondary autoimmune reaction in several ovarian diseases.

Therapeutic aspects of POF

Up to now, no specific treatment has been demonstrated to be efficient in POF except hormone replacement therapy and oocyte donation. However, histological screening has revealed that 40% of POF ovaries still contain a substantial pool of follicles[25]. This result was corroborated by ultrasonography[46,47]. Conway *et al.*[47] were able to identify follicles by endovaginal ultrasonography in 60% of cases of idiopathic POF, whether or not there were other autoimmune signs. Spontaneous cycles and/or pregnancies have frequently been reported in POF especially in patients taking hormone replacement therapy, which is likely to help this form of remission. In our own study, five pregnancies occurred under estrogen therapy among 26 POF patients who wished to conceive, including four AOA-positive women[30]. Luborsky *et al.*[32] reported a decrease in AOA after steroid treatment in two cases of POF. Several studies have examined the possible benefit of corticosteroids in POF patients[9,10,48,49]; however, they can have serious secondary effects as reported by Kalantaridou *et al.*[50]. Recently, Van Kasteren *et al.*[11] reported the results of a randomized, placebo-controlled trial using corticosteroids in premature ovarian failure. They were unable to identify any influence of corticosteroids on ovarian response to gonadotropins in their patients. However, a 15-day low-dose (9 mg daily) treatment regimen in an unselected population of POF patients may not be the best way to evaluate this immunosuppressive treatment in autoimmune POF.

Conclusion

Many clinical (psychological stress at onset, spontaneous remissions, association with autoimmune endocrinopathies), histological (oophoritis), biological (circulating antiovarian antibodies and association with HLA-DR haplotypes) and experimental (induced oophoritis) observations support the theory of participation of an autoimmune reaction raised against the ovaries in the pathogenesis of idiopathic POF. The main problems are to identify the mechanisms involved, to consider it a primary or a secondary immune reaction, and to determine its involvement in ovarian destruction. Antigenic targets of circulating AOA in the absence of autoimmune poly-endocrinopathy need to be determined. These AOA may be simple markers or may participate in functional impairment, for example AOA raised against steroidogenic enzymes. In this case, there could be cross-reaction involvement in the initiation of the process. More likely, they appear after cellular immune responses, mediated by cytotoxic T lymphocytes, leading to the destruction of the cells expressing these cytoplasmic enzymes[36]. Overexpression of HLA class II on the surface of these cells facilitates the immune process by presenting specific antigens. Abnormal ovarian production of cytokines during accelerated atresia[51], for example, contributes to this overexpression.

One should consider three different situations. In the first situation, POF is associated with an autoimmune polyendocrinopathy including adrenal deficiency; circulating AOA raised against steroidogenic enzymes are present; association with specific HLA type II is possible; lymphocytic oophoritis can be found on the ovarian biopsy. In this case, the autoimmune origin of POF is clear. In the second situation, there is no adrenal disease, nor any antiadrenal antibodies or association with clinical autoimmune disease; however, circulating antiovarian antibodies are present. These AOA may produce an immune reaction against the ovaries, but the real significance remains unknown. In the third situation, when there are none of these autoimmune signs, such a reaction is unlikely.

In idiopathic POF much attention must be given to the investigation of indirect autoimmune signs, such as association with autoimmune diseases (clinical aspects, hormone levels, antibodies). Evaluation of the ovarian follicular pool can be performed by ultrasonography rather than by ovarian biopsy. Currently, hormone replacement therapy and oocyte donation are the only effective treatments. However, corticosteroid trials should be considered in selected patients with autoimmune characteristics and a partially preserved follicular pool, in a randomized, placebo-controlled trial, to determine efficacy and optimal dosage regimen of this treatment in POF.

References

1. Coulam CB, Adamson SC, Annegera JF. Incidence of premature ovarian failure. *Obstet Gynecol* 1986;67:604–6

2. Cameron IT, O'Shea FC, Roilan JM, *et al.* Occult ovarian failure: a syndrome of infertility, regular menses, and elevated follicle-stimulating hormone concentrations. *J Clin Endocrinol Metab* 1988;67:1190–4S

3. Kalantaridou SN, Nelson LM. Premature ovarian failure is not premature menopause. *Ann N Y Acad Sci* 2000;900:393–402

4. Barlow C, Hirotsune S, Taylor R, *et al. Atm*-deficient mice: a paradigm of ataxia telegiectasia. *Cell* 1996;86:159–171

5. Nicolino M, Bost M, David M, *et al.* Familial blepharophimosis: an uncommon marker of ovarian dysgenesis. *J Pediatr Endocrinol Metab* 1995;8:127–33

6. Aittomäki K, Dieguez Lucena JL, Pakarinen P, *et al.* Mutation in the follicle-stimulating hormone receptor gene causes hereditary hypergonadotropic ovarian failure. *Cell* 1995;82:959–67

7. Jones GS, Moraes-Ruehsen M. A new syndrome of amenorrhea in association with hypergonadotropism and apparently normal ovarian follicular apparatus. *Am J Obstet Gynecol* 1969;104:597–600S

8. Irvine WJ, Cahn MMW, Scarth L, *et al.* Immunological aspects of premature ovarian failure associated with Addison's disease. *Lancet* 1968;2:883

9. Barbarino-Monnier P, Gobert B, Guillet-May F, *et al.* Ovarian autoimmunity and corticotherapy in an *in-vitro* fertilization attempt. *Hum Reprod* 1995;10:2006–7

10. Corenblum B, Rowe T, Taylor PJ. High doses, short term glucocorticoids for the treatment of infertility resulting from premature ovarian failure. *Fertil Steril* 1993;59:988–91

11. Van Kasteren YM, Braat DDM, Hemrika DJ, *et al.* Corticosteroids do not influence ovarian responsiveness to gonadotropins in patients with premature ovarian failure: a randomized, placebo-controlled trial. *Fertil Steril* 1999;71: 90–5

12. Norman RJ, Brannstrom M. White cells and the ovary-incidental invaders or essential effectors? *J Endocrinol* 1994;140:333–6

13. Brannstrom M, Norman RJ. Involvement of leucocytes and cytokines in the ovulatory process and corpus luteum function. *Hum Reprod* 1993;8:1762–75

14. Andreani CL, Payne DW, Packman JN, *et al.* Cytokine-mediated regulation of ovarian function. Tumor necrosis factor α inhibits gondotropin-supported ovarian function. *J Biol Chem* 1991;266:6761–6

15. Smith H, Sakamoto Y, Kasai K, *et al.* Effector and regulatory cells in autoimmune oophoritis elicited by neonatal thymectomy. *J Immunol* 1991;147:2928–33

16. Tong ZB, Nelson LM. A mouse gene encoding an oocyte antigen associated with autoimmune premature ovarian failure. *Endocrinology* 1999; 140:3720–6

17. Taguchi O, Takahashi T, Masao S. Development of multiple organ-localized autoimmune diseases in nude mice after reconstitution of cell function by rat fetal thymus graft. *J Exp Med* 1986;164:60–71

18. Miller ME, Chatten J. Ovarian changes in ataxia telangiectasia. *Paediatr Scand* 1967;56: 559–61

19. Letur-Körnisch H, Raoul-Duval A, Cabau A, *et al.* Stress et ménopause précoce. *CR Acad Sci Paris* 1995;318:691–8

20. Sheu BC, Ho HN, Yang YS. Spontaneous pregnancy after previous pregnancy by oocyte donation due to premature ovarian failure *Hum Reprod* 1996;11:1359–60

21. Brucker F, Harter M, Boda M, *et al.* Exploration immunitaire des diabètes de type I inauguraux. Relation avec l'insulinothérapie intensive et la survenue d'une rémission. *Rev Franc Endocrinol Clin* 1985;26:4–5

22. The Finnish-German APECED Consortium. An autoimmune disease. APECED, caused by mutations in a novel gene featuring two PHD-type zinc-finger domains. *Nat Genet* 1997;17: 399–403

23. Betterle C, Rossi A, Daélla Peria S, *et al.* Premature ovarian failure and natural history. *Clin Endocrinol* 1993;39:35–43

24. Labarbera AR, Miller MM, Ober C, *et al.* Autoimmune etiology in premature ovarian failure. *Am J Reprod Immunol* 1988;16:115–22

25. Hoeck A, Schoemaker J, Drexhage HA. Premature ovarian failure and ovarian auto-immunity. *Endocr Rev* 1997;18:107–34

26. Muechler EK, Huang KE, Schenk E. Auto-immunity in premature ovarian failure. *Int J Fertil* 1991;36:99–103

27. Walfish PG, Gottesman IS, Shewchuk AB, *et al.* Association of premature ovarian failure with HLA antigens. *Tissue Antigens* 1983;21:168–9

28. Jaroudi KA, Arora M, Sheth KV, *et al.* Human leucocyte antigen typing and associated abnormalities in premature ovarian failure. *Hum Reprod* 1994;9:2006–9

29. Anasti JN, Adams S, Kimzey LM, *et al.* Karyotypically normal spontaneous premature ovarian failure: evaluation of association with the class II major histocompatibility complex. *J Clin Endocrinol Metab* 1994;78:722–3

30. Fénichel P, Sosset C, Barbarino-Monnier P, *et al.* Prevalence, specificity and significance of antiovarian antibodies during spontaneous premature ovarian failure. *Hum Reprod* 1997;12:2623–8

31. Arif S, Underhill JA, Donaldson P, *et al.* Human leucocyte antigen - DQB1* genotypes encoding aspartate at position 57 are associated with 3β-hydroxysteroid deshydrogenase autoimmunity in premature ovarian failure. *J Clin Endocrinol Metab* 1999;84:1056–60

32. Luborsky JL, Visintin I, Boyers S, *et al.* Ovarian antibodies detected by immobilized antigen immunoassay in patients with premature ovarian failure. *J Clin Endocrinol Metab* 1990;70:69–75

33. Wheatcroft NJ, Toogood AA, Li TC, *et al.* Detection of antibodies to ovarian antigens in women with premature failure. *Clin Exp Immunol* 1994;96:122–8

34. Wheatcroft NJ, Salt C, Milford-Ward A, *et al.* Identification of ovarian antibodies by immunofluorescence, enzyme-linked immunosorbent assay or immunoblotting in premature ovarian failure. *Human Reprod* 1997;12:2617–22

35. Gobert B, Barbarino-Monnier P, Guillet-Rosso F, *et al.* Antiovary antibodies after attempts at human *in vitro* fertilization induced by follicular puncture rather than hormonal stimulation. *J Reprod Fertil* 1992;96:213–18

36. Uibo R, Aavik E, Peterson P, *et al.* Autoantibodies to cytochrome P450 enzymes p450scc, P450c17, P450c21 in autoimmune polyglandular disease type I and II and in isolated Addison's disease. *J Clin Endocrinol Metab* 1994;78:323–8

37. Arif S, Vallian S, Farzaneh F, *et al.* Identification of 3β-hydroxysteroid deshydrogenase as a novel target of steroid cell antibodies with endocrine autoimmune disease. *J Clin Endocrinol Metab* 1996;81:4439–45

38. Betterle C, Volpato M. Adrenal and ovarian autoimmunity. *Eur J Endocrinol* 1998;138:16–25

39. Chiauzzi V, Cigorrarga S, Escobar ME, *et al.* Inhibition of follicle-stimulating hormone receptor binding circulating immunoglobulins. *J Clin Endocrinol Metab* 1982;54:1221–8

40. Van Weissenbruch MM, Hoeck A, Van Vliet-Bleeker I, *et al.* Evidence for existence of immunoglobulins that block ovarian granulosa cell growth *in vitro*. A putative role in resistant ovary syndrome? *J Clin Endocrinol Metab* 1991; 73:360–7

41. Anasti JN, Flack MR, Froelich J, *et al.* The use of recombinant human gonadotropin receptors to search for immunoglobulin G-mediated premature ovarian failure. *J Clin Endocrinol Metab* 1995;80:824–8

42. Tidey GF, Nelson LM, Phillips TM, *et al.* Gonadotropins enhance HLA DR antigen expression in human granulosa cells. *Am J Obstet Gynecol* 1992;167:1768–73

43. Zolti M, Bider D, Seidman DS, *et al.* Cytokine levels in follicular fluid of polycystic ovaries in patients treated with dexamethasone. *Fertil Steril* 1992;57:501–4

44. Fénichel P, Gobert B, Carré Y, *et al.* Polycystic ovary syndrome: an autoimmune disease. *Lancet* 1999;353:2210–1

45. Fénichel P, Sosset C. Insuffisance ovarienne primitivae; apport de l'immunologie. *Ann Pediatr* (Paris) 1999;46:537–43

46. Mehta A, Matwijiw I, Lyons EA, *et al.* Non invasive diagnosis of resistant ovary syndrome by ultrasonography, *Fertil Steril* 1992;57:56–61

47. Conway GS, Kaltsas G, Patel A, *et al.* Characterization of idiopathic premature ovarian failure. *Fertil Steril* 1996;65:337–41

48. Cowchock FS, McCabe JL, Montgomery BB. Pregnancy after corticosteroid administration in premature ovarian failure (polyglandular endocrinopathy syndrome). *Am J Obstet Gynecol* 1988;58:118–9

49. Blumenfeld Z, Halachni S, Peretz BA, *et al.* Premature ovarian failure: the prognostic application of autoimmunity on conception after ovulation induction. *Fertil Steril* 1993;59:750–5

50. Kalantaridou SN, Braddock DT, Patronas NJ, *et al.* Treatment of autoimmune premature ovarian failure. *Hum Reprod* 1999;14:1777–82

51. Coulam CB, Stern JJ. Immunology of ovarian failure. *Am J Reprod Immunol* 1991;25:169–74

Preservation of fertility and ovarian function and minimalization of chemotherapy-associated gonadotoxicity and premature ovarian failure: the role of inhibin-A and -B as markers

24

Z. Blumenfeld

Introduction

As survival rates for young cancer patients continue to improve, protection against iatrogenic infertility caused by chemotherapy with or without radiotherapy assumes higher priority[1–4].

Hodgkin disease is the most common malignancy in the population aged 15–24 years[5]. Prolonged survival of almost 90% is now expected for young patients treated with cytotoxic chemotherapy for Hodgkin disease[1,5–7]. This is due to the introduction of effective chemotherapy such as mechlorethamine, vincristine, prednisone and procarbazine (MOPP) and/or adriamycin, bleomycin, vinblastine and decarbazine (ABVD) and its variants[1,5,8–10]. Similar rates of long-term survival have been reported for patients with non-Hodgkin lymphoma, as well as for patients with other types of tumor receiving chemotherapy[1,2,5–8]. Moreover, cytotoxic agents have also been used as chemotherapy for various autoimmune diseases such as systemic lupus erythematosus (SLE) and rheumatoid arthritis, and for the prevention of organ transplant rejection[1,6]. Recent advances in the understanding of the molecular biology of lymphomas permit an additional dimension – the identification of molecular characteristics associated with a poor prognosis, such as patterns of gene expression that are associated with protection against apoptosis, chemotherapy resistance, or the stimulation of angiogenesis. If such attempts prove successful, the goal of 100% cure without serious late secondary effects, despite its apparent elusiveness a few decades ago, will have been positioned clearly on the horizon[7].

Premature ovarian failure (POF) is a common long-term consequence of chemotherapy[1,6,8–12] and radiotherapy[6,13]. Whereas the cytotoxic damage is reversible in other tissues of rapidly dividing cells such as bone marrow, gastrointestinal tract and thymus[6,14], it appears to be progressive and irreversible in the ovary, where the germ cells have a limited number, fixed since fetal life, and cannot be regenerated[1,6].

Chemotherapy-associated gonadotoxicity

Breast cancer, the most common malignancy in women, affects approximately 185 000 women/year in the USA[15,16]. Almost 25% of cases occur premenopausally[15–19]. Adjuvant chemotherapy prolongs survival, but it has been shown to cause POF[15,20–25]. Premature menopause associated with vasomotor, psychosocial, genitourinary, skeletal (osteoporosis) and cardiovascular problems is usually treated effectively with hormone replacement[15,26]. However, hormone replacement therapy is contraindicated by most in breast cancer survivors[15,27]; therefore, it is of utmost clinical importance to minimize chemotherapy-associated POF in these women.

The first study of systemic adjuvant chemotherapy for breast cancer showed cessation of menses in 40% of the patients treated with thiotepa as opposed to 3% of the control group[28]. Various chemotherapeutic regimens have been in use since the late 1960s, but reports on the incidence of chemotherapy-associated amenorrhea have been erratic. Recent reviews on 15–40 studies with information on the effects of adjuvant chemotherapy on ovarian function in premenopausal women have been reported[15,29].

The reported incidence of POF ranges from 0 to 100% among different chemotherapy regimens. Most data were collected at 12 months after the beginning of treatment[15]. The average percentage of chemotherapy-associated amenorrhea in regimens based on cyclophosphamide, methotrexate and fluorouracil (CMF) given for at least 3 months was 68% (95% CI 66–70%), with a range of 20–100%[15]. This wide range can be attributed to the following variations in experimental design:

(1) Definition of amenorrhea;

(2) Definition of menopausal status;

(3) Age distribution;

(4) Therapeutic regimen (drug, dose, duration and route of administration);

(5) Population characteristics.

The risk of gonadal damage is usually directly related to the age of the patient. Patients older than 40 years experience a consistently higher rate of amenorrhea when compared with those of ≤ 40 years[15]. Rates varied from 21 to 71% in the younger age group and from 49 to 100% in the older group. The average percentage of POF for CMF-based treatments (for at least 3 months) was 40% (95% CI 36–44%) and 76% (95% CI 74–78%) for younger and older

groups, respectively. About two-thirds of premenopausal women experience POF after the CMF chemotherapy combination for breast carcinoma (95% CI 66–70%)[15].

The action of a given chemotherapeutic agent on the ovaries can occur through impairment of follicular maturation and/or depletion of primordial follicles[15,30–34]. Combination chemotherapy is used more often than single agents and it is difficult to evaluate the contribution of each individual drug. Most available information concerning the effects of chemotherapy on ovarian function has come from studies of women who received MOPP for Hodgkin disease[35].

Since the first description of drug-induced amenorrhea, many other drugs have also been implicated[34,36,37]. Alkylating agents are the most common chemotherapeutic agents associated with gonadal damage[31–35,38]. These agents are not cell-cycle specific and thus do not require cell proliferation for their cytotoxic action. It is believed that they act on undeveloped oocytes and possibly on the pregranulosa cells of primordial follicles[15,30]. Most information is available on the effects of cyclophosphamide[30,35,38]. Recent animal studies suggest that phosphoramide mustard is the main metabolite responsible for the ovarian toxicity of cyclophosphamide[15,39].

The association of doxorubicin with infertility is debatable. In a study that compared MOPP with ABVD for the treatment of Hodgkin disease, Santoro and colleagues[40] reported less ovarian toxicity in the ABVD group. However, in animal studies, doxorubicin has been shown to cause testicular damage[41]. Mitoxantrone is likely to produce amenorrhea[42].

The antimetabolites cause little ovarian toxicity when used as adjuvant treatment for breast cancer. This could be explained by their cytotoxic action on dividing cells[15]. Data available from the treatment of women with choriocarcinoma have demonstrated no adverse effects on the ovary. Schamberger and associates[43] treated seven women (aged 13–31 years) with high-dose methotrexate for osteosarcoma and found no gonadal dysfunction. Koyama and co-workers[44] observed no ovarian toxicity among nine breast cancer patients treated with adjuvant fluorouracil. Comparing melphalan (L-PAM) and fluorouracil plus L-PAM, Fisher and colleagues[45] found no difference in severity of ovarian dysfunction, which suggests that L-PAM alone was the toxic agent. Cobleigh and associates[46] confirmed these findings and presented markedly lower rates of POF in patients treated with methotrexate than in those treated with 5-fluorouracil compared with CMF.

There is not enough information available regarding which chemotherapy regimen causes the highest rate of ovarian failure. Few reports analyzed POF rates among patients who underwent different combination treatments. Cobleigh and colleagues[41] compared adriamycin and cyclophosphamide with CMF and reported a significantly lower rate of amenorrhea among those treated with the former (34% vs. 69%, respectively).

Effect of dose intensity, cumulative dose and route of administration on incidence of premature ovarian failure

It is difficult to analyze the impact of different treatment practices on the incidence of amenorrhea, in view of the multitude of confounding factors. Cyclophosphamide is the agent most commonly implicated in POF[15,30–35,38,47,48] and therefore most of the discussion will concentrate on this drug. The variables analyzed were cumulative dose, dose intensity, duration and route of administration.

Kay and Mattison[37] showed that increasing doses of cyclophosphamide caused progressive destruction of oocytes and follicles in mice. Human studies confirmed these results[1,2,15].

Padmanabhan and co-workers[49] compared the percentage of cumulative dose received by patients who developed POF with those who continued to have regular periods. Although the percentage of the cumulative dose of cyclophosphamide (at 80 mg/m^2 by mouth on days 1–14 for 12 months) received by those

who developed POF was higher (60% vs. 54%), the difference was not statistically significant.

Higher cumulative doses of cyclophosphamide cause higher POF rates[15]. Goldhirsch and colleagues[50] reported that patients treated with one preoperative cycle of CMF experienced POF rates of 10% and 33% in the younger and older age groups, respectively. The rates increased to 33% and 81% with six cycles (cumulative dose of cyclophosphamide 8400 mg/m^2) and to 61% and 95% with 12 cycles of CMF (cumulative dose of cyclophosphamide 16 800 mg/m^2). Bines and colleagues reported similar results[15]. The only discordant observation came from Moliterni and co-workers[51], who found similar POF rates regardless of cumulative dose.

Other investigators[50–55] showed different POF rates while keeping dose intensity constant. It is of note that treatment duration also varied, compromising the analysis of dose intensity as an independent variable. Wood and associates[56] analyzed variation in dose intensity while keeping cumulative dose constant, but they did not report POF rates. Brincker and colleagues[57] held duration of treatment constant and varied the cumulative dose and dose intensity. They showed that these variables were directly related to POF rates, but could not tell whether they were independent.

Thus, the preponderance of the data, with one exception[51], supports the concept of a direct correlation between dose intensity and POF. Duration of treatment and route of administration of cyclophosphamide as independent variables on POF rate remain to be determined[15].

Infertility represents one of the main long-term consequences of combination chemotherapy given for Hodgkin lymphoma, leukemia and other malignancies in young women[1,2,5,15,58]. The impairment of gonadal function after chemotherapy is much more frequent in men than in women, occurring in up to 90% of post-pubertal males[1,2,59]. Because dividing cells are known to be more sensitive to the cytotoxic effects of alkylating agents than are cells at rest, it has been suggested that inhibition of the pituitary–gonadal axis would reduce the rate of spermatogenesis and oogenesis and thereby render the germinal epithelium less susceptible to the effects of chemotherapy[1,2,6,59,60]. However, several alternatives have been attempted for preservation of fertility in young women undergoing chemotherapy treatment.

Other alternatives for fertility preservation

Although gonadotropin releasing hormone agonist (GnRH-a) treatment in parallel with chemotherapy[1] is a promising adjuvant therapy for young women, it is by no means the only option for fertility preservation. Moreover, this adjuvant treatment is not applicable to those young women undergoing very aggressive chemo- and radiotherapy for bone marrow transplantation (BMT), since POF is associated with 90% or more of those women undergoing BMT[61–66]. For these patients additional options may be available.

Cryopreservation of 'mature' metaphase II oocytes, usually after human menopausal gonadotropin (hMG)/human chorionic gonadotropin (hCG) ovarian stimulation, is an option. Although successful in rodents[65,67,68], it is still far from being a clinical alternative in humans[69,70]. Moreover, a concern of possible chromosomal aberration associated with the freezing of metaphase II oocytes has been raised[65,71]. A future possible alternative may be the retrieval of human immature oocytes for cryopreservation and in vitro maturation after thawing[65,72].

A much more clinically available option is the cryopreservation of fertilized ova, after in vitro fertilization (IVF) and before chemotherapy[73]. However, this alternative is relevant to married women or those who have a partner, and almost inapplicable to very young, single women. Moreover, the ovarian stimulation with hMG/hCG before IVF egg retrieval needs to postpone the initiation of chemotherapy, often contraindicated by hematologists and oncologists[1,65]. Furthermore, the increase in estradiol concentrations caused by hMG/hCG ovarian stimulation may possibly aggravate the clinical situation of patients with breast carcinoma or other estrogen-sensitive tumors, or that of SLE patients by inducing a flare-up of the autoimmune disease[1].

An old suggestion[74] that has recently been the focus of intense investigation is the transplantation of ovarian tissue[1–3,65,75–79]. However, a concern of possible associated malignancy in the transplanted ovary has been raised[1,3,65,79]. Therefore, future endeavors may concentrate on cryopreservation of ovarian fragments before chemotherapy, followed by thawing of these fragments, dispersion of the primordial/primary follicles, in vitro maturation and fertilization. Although this is not yet clinically available, the enormous progress of assisted reproductive technology (ART) in the past two decades lends hope that in the next few years this may indeed turn into a practical option. Until then, every effort should be made to offer all the possible options available for minimizing the gonadotoxic effect of chemotherapy.

A recent editorial in Fertility and Sterility by Oehninger[80] has discussed the pertinent question: 'Will ovarian autotransplantation have a role in reproductive and gynecological medicine?' This has successfully preserved ovarian function in rats, sheep and other animals[74–79,81,82].

Such therapy could provide a source of ovarian tissue that, when autotransplanted, would maintain an adequate estrogenic milieu that protects against heart disease and osteoporosis. It has been suggested that it may be best to restrict ovarian transplantation to women whose ovaries are disease free, because cancer can be transmitted with ovarian tissue grafts in animals[79].

A second role for this therapy could be in the form of 'oocyte banking' as a strategy to preserve the reproductive potential of younger women or girls before cancer therapy[65,76,79,81–84]. Cryopreservation of ovarian tissue before initiation of oncological treatment, followed by autologous transplantation after remission, could provide a means of protecting fertility[80,85]. Obviously, an option for these cases involves oocyte retrieval (today probably better accomplished with gonadotropin stimulation, although the natural cycle will be preferable when improved oocyte *in vitro* maturation protocols become available), followed by IVF and embryo cryopreservation[80].

Oocyte banking could have a role also in women of advancing age who elect to delay conception into the years of diminished ovarian reserve[80,82]. The feasibility of this approach has been reported in the rat[86].

The potential therapeutic use of ovarian autotransplantation mandates continued efforts to achieve better results with ovarian tissue cryopreservation (i.e. freezing of the isolated germ cell at different stages of maturity, cumulus-encased oocytes, follicles and sliced tissue) and with *in vitro* oocyte maturation procedures. Ovarian tissue can be recovered at the time of laparotomy, or ovarian biopsy specimens can be taken by laparoscopy. When autografting to an orthotopic site succeeds in restoring ovulatory menstrual cycles, hormonal replacement therapy and medical intervention in the process of conception may not be needed[76,80]. Restoration of fertility to oophorectomized sheep by ovarian autografts stored at −196°C has been reported[75]. Alternatively, oocytes could be recovered from an ectopically located graft and matured *in vitro* or, after gonadotropin stimulation, mature oocytes could be retrieved and used in ART[80].

The study of von Eye Corleta and associates[82] confirmed that ovarian grafts with sliced tissue resulted in a lower degree of ischemic or degenerative changes than intact, transplanted ovaries. In different animal models (rat, rabbit, monkey) it has been demonstrated that autotransplantation of ovaries can result in a prompt revascularization of the gland. The transplanted ovary is (or becomes after grafting) able to produce substances that promote and direct angiogenesis[86]. Recent studies have shown that the increase in gonadotropin secretion after ovarian transplantation in the rat contributes to revascularization of the graft by up-regulating the gene expression of two major angiogenic factors: vascular endothelial growth factor (VEGF) and transforming growth factor β_1

(TGF-β_1)[86]. More information is needed to determine whether the oocytes from autotransplanted ovarian tissue are competent to achieve full maturation, fertilization and embryo development.

Interesting, perplexing and challenging questions arise:

(1) Could the addition of angiogenic and other growth factors (such as VEGF, TGF-β, or others) to the transplanted ovary enhance the anchorage and number of functionally competent cells?

(2) What is the survival rate of the grafts?

(3) Could the functional longevity be prolonged by the addition of survival factors?

(4) Is the developmental potential of the female gamete preserved after transplantation (with or without an intermediate cryopreservation step)?

(5) Could gene expression (regulatory genes of growth, steroidogenesis, oocyte maturation) be manipulated before transplantation (or after) to achieve better results or to treat specific abnormalities of the germ cell line[80]?

All these questions and concerns about ovarian autotransplantation in the human need to be addressed in preclinical animal studies. Better cryopreservation methods of human ovarian tissue and oocytes must be sought. Only then should clinical studies be considered. Appropriate discussions not only at the scientific but also at the ethical level are mandatory to establish whether these techniques will benefit patients treated by reproductive and gynecological medicine[80].

Chemotherapy and co-treatment with gonadotropin releasing hormone agonists (GnRH-a)

The possibility of administering an adjuvant treatment that might limit the gonadal damage caused by an otherwise successful treatment program is attractive[4,5,87]. Glode and co-workers[88] tested this hypothesis using a murine model and concluded that an agonistic analog of GnRH appeared to protect male mice from the gonadal damage normally produced by cyclophosphamide. It may be that decreased secretion of the pituitary gonadotropin, by decreasing gonadal function, could protect against the sterilizing effects of chemotherapy. Although previous suggestions have been made[89,90], claiming that primordial germ cells fare better than germ cells that are part of an active cell cycle, this hypothesis has not been seriously tested clinically, until recently[1,91,92]. Whereas several investigators have demonstrated that GnRH-a inhibit chemotherapy-induced ovarian follicular depletion in the rat[88,91], uncertainty remains about the human application[1,91,92]. The human ovary has lower concentrations of ovarian GnRH receptors and may not necessarily exhibit the same response as rats[1,91]. Ataya and colleagues[91] found that GnRH-a protected the ovary against cyclophosphamide-induced damage in rhesus monkeys by significantly decreasing the total amount of follicle loss during the chemotherapeutic insult, and by decreasing the daily rate of follicular decline. Chapman and associates[10] found that, of their female patients treated for Hodgkin disease, 69% developed POF if they were younger than 29, while 96% developed POF if their age was more than 30 years.

Advances in the treatment of all stages of Hodgkin and non-Hodgkin lymphoma with chemotherapy and irradiation have led to long-term survival of 90% or even more in several groups of patients[1,15,16,93–95]. The improved long-term survival of relatively young patients treated for lymphoma focused attention on the gonadal toxicity of combined chemo- and radiotherapy. Whereas 86% of men had azoospermia after the COPP/ABVD regimen[94], only 48–77% of women receiving chemotherapy for lymphoma exhibited hypergonadotropic amenorrhea and ovarian failure[94–96]. Moreover, a long-term follow-up of 240 children, 15 years of age or younger, treated by MOPP for Hodgkin disease showed azoospermia in 83% of the boys, although only 13% of the girls suffered ovarian failure[92,97]. The chances of maintaining gonadal function following combined modality treatment are significantly greater among girls than boys[97]. At variance with the results reported in adults, the MOPP chemotherapy in girls with Hodgkin disease did not induce ovarian failure[98]. Since ovarian function was preserved in most long-term survivors who were treated prepubertally for lymphoma[97–99], but only in a minority of similarly treated adult patients[94], it is clinically logical and therefore tempting temporarily to create a prepubertal milieu in women of reproductive age before and during the chemotherapeutic insult[1,92].

It has been reported that 64% of adult female patients undergoing cancer therapy experienced one or more of the symptoms of ovarian failure[15,100]. Previous studies[15,59,101] suggested profound gonadal toxicity in men after adjuvant chemotherapy in patients with and without GnRH-a protection, treated for either malignant lymphoma[59] or germ-cell tumors[101], but the situation in females may be completely different. Ataya and colleagues[91] have shown, in female rhesus monkeys, that GnRH-a may protect the ovary from cyclophosphamide-induced gonadal damage. Administration of GnRH-a in parallel with cyclophosphamide has significantly decreased the daily rate of follicular decline and the total number of follicles lost during the chemotherapeutic insult, as compared to cyclophosphamide alone (without GnRH-a)[91]. This preliminary experience in rhesus monkeys is in keeping with the clinical results whereby only two of the 46 evaluable surviving women in our study group became menopausal after the GnRH-a/chemotherapy co-treatment (4.3%) as compared to a 56.5% (26/46) rate of POF in the chemotherapy alone (control) group[1,92] (Table 1).

This preliminary experience is encouraging. Although most of the survivors of the chemotherapy (with or without radiotherapy) who received the GnRH-a co-treatment resumed ovulatory menses (> 95%, 44/46),

Table 1 Comparison of clinical data and the rate of premature ovarian failure (POF) in two groups of young women undergoing chemotherapy with or without gonadotropin releasing hormone agonist (GnRH-a) co-treatment

	GnRH-a/chemotherapy	Chemotherapy	p Value
Patients (n)	51	48	NS
Evaluable patients	46	46	NS
Hodgkin disease	31/51 (61%)	29/48 (60.5%)	NS
Non-Hodgkin lymphoma	20/51 (39%)	19/48 (39.5%)	NS
Age (years)	15–40	14–40	NS
Radiotherapy	30/46 (65%)	29/46 (63%)	NS
Radiation dose (cGy)	2320 ± 1521	1882 ± 1993	NS
Pregnancies	15 in 9 women	12 in 7 women	NS
Age of pregnant women at chemotherapy (years)	18–30	16–21	NS
Cyclic ovarian function	44/46 (95.5%)	20/46 (43.5%)	< 0.01
POF	2/46 (4.3%)	26/46 (56.5%)	< 0.01

NS, not significant

only 20 of the 46 women (43.5%) who were treated with chemotherapy with or without mantle irradiation (control group) had normal ovarian function and more than half of these women (26/46) had POF and hypergonadotropic amenorrhea[1,92]. Buserelin, another GnRH-agonistic analog, administered by others[101] in a small group of young male patients in parallel with chemotherapy with or without irradiation, failed to protect from azoospermia associated with chemotherapy. As opposed to young girls, most prepubertal boys receiving chemo- and radiotherapy suffered gonadal failure (azoospermia in the boys), therefore there is little rationale to expect a significant benefit from the GnRH-a co-treatment in men[92,97–99,102]. In keeping with this hypothesis, Johnson and colleagues[59] found that no improvement in post-treatment fertility could be demonstrated by GnRH-a co-treatment in six men receiving chemotherapy for advanced lymphomas. Contrary to the apparent protective effect of GnRH-a co-treatment with chemotherapy, no protection from ovarian damage caused by irradiation in rats was provided by a GnRH-a[103].

Neither the age of the patients nor the dosages of the various cytotoxic drugs were significantly different between the study and control groups[92]. The only significant difference between the two groups was the incidence of POF and hypergonadotropic amenorrhea (56.5% vs. 4.3%; $p < 0.01$, Table 1)[1,2,92]. However, one should be very cautious about drawing long-term conclusions from these promising but still preliminary data, since our study was neither randomized nor double blind, and the follow-up in the study group was only 8 years as compared to up to 11 years in some of the patients in the control group[1,92]. This difference is attributed to the nature of the control group (retrospective historical control), whereas the study protocol was prospective[92]. Although the follow-up in the control group is longer than in the study group, the observations within the first 3 years in both groups suggest that longer follow-up will not significantly affect these results[92]. Future prospective, double-blind, randomized studies will be needed to resolve this problem, although some ethical questions may be raised upon initiation of such studies. Notwithstanding all the above, two recent studies in the *New England Journal of Medicine*[104,105] report that observational studies have given results similar to those of randomized controlled trials. They 'found little evidence that estimates of treatment effects in observational studies reported after 1984 are either consistently larger than or quantitatively different from those obtained in randomized, controlled trials'[104]. Moreover, 'the results of well-designed observational studies do not systematically overestimate the magnitude of the effects of treatment as compared with those in random-ized, controlled trials on the same topics'[105].

Two of our young patients, one in the study group, and one in the control group, who later underwent high-dose chemotherapy and autologous BMT owing to recurrence of the disease, have become prematurely meno-pausal. This is in keeping with recent experi-ence that such intensification regimens carry a high risk of permanent infertility and POF[58,61–66,92,106]. It has been well established that chemotherapy with total body irradiation followed by allogeneic or autologous BMT causes permanent elevation of gonadotropin levels, hypoestrogenism and amenorrhea in 92–100% of female patients[1,58,61,63,92]. Future endeavors are needed to challenge the long-term infertility problem of young women treated with chemotherapy.

Future studies may also use GnRH anta-gonists instead of, or in combination with, agonists for achievement of faster pituitary–ovarian desensitization, eliminating the waiting period of 7–14 days needed by the GnRH-a to achieve down-regulation[1,92,107].

What are the reasons for discrepancy between various studies?

While it is convenient to perform prelimi-nary and mating studies in rodents, owing to their availability and low cost, rat oocytes may respond to the GnRH-a/chemotherapy co-treatment protocol differently from those in humans or non-human primates[1,6]. An estrous cycle duration is 4 days in rats vs. a 28-day menstrual cycle in women or rhesus monkeys. Moreover, rats have estrous cycles without endometrial shedding, whereas women and monkeys menstruate by shed-ding the endometrial lining[1,6]. Lastly, rat ovaries have been shown to contain GnRH receptors whereas the existence and pres-ence of these receptors in human ovaries is equivocal[1,6]. Except for one report[108], most investigators conclude that GnRH receptors are not present in the human ovary[6,109,110].

Similar to the human, but different from rodents, the rhesus monkey has ovaries that also lack GnRH receptors[6].

Another point of possible concern is the dif-ferent length of waiting period between start-ing the GnRH-a and the administration of the gonadotoxic chemotherapy. In the clinical perspective, the issue of the waiting period required to establish the pituitary–gonadal suppression becomes critical in light of the obvious pressure to start chemotherapy as soon as possible after the diagnosis has been made. Indeed, before pituitary–ovarian desensitiza-tion, a 'flare-up' period of 1–2 weeks occurs during which the stimulated ovaries may be more vulnerable to the gonadotoxic effect of chemotherapy, possibly owing to increased gonadotropic and follicular stimulation[6]. In order to minimize this possible shortcoming of a GnRH-a 'flare-up', future efforts should prefer the use of GnRH antagonists rather than agonists (or their combination) for similar purposes, at least for the starting period. The discrepancy between the results of different clinical studies appears to be influenced by the inadequate time interval between the GnRH-a administration and the intiation of chemother-apy, since a short interval may possibly render the gonad hypersensitive to the cytotoxic effect of chemotherapy[6]. Another problem account-ing for the divergence among the results of dif-ferent studies may be the inadequacy of the used agonist dosage, and possibly also inter-species differences[1,6].

Inhibin measurements

We have reported[1,92] that temporary increased follicle stimulating hormone (FSH) concen-trations were experienced in about a quarter of the young women who ultimately resumed ovarian cyclic function, suggesting reversible ovarian damage in a proportion of women in addition to those experiencing POF.

Inhibin is a dimer of two subunits desig-nated α and β, of which the latter appears in several forms: βA and βB (and most recently also βC, βD and βE in non-human

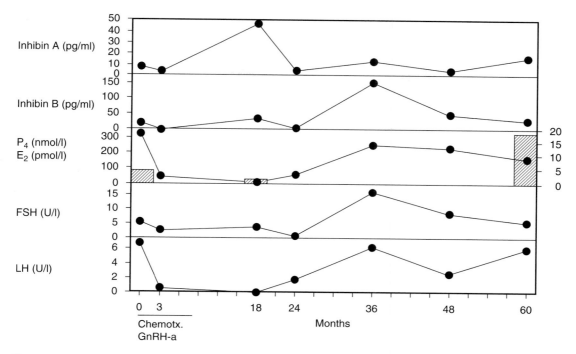

Figure 1 Longitudinal profile of inhibin A, inhibin B, progesterone (P_4) (bars), 17β-estradiol (E_2), follicle stimulating hormone (FSH) and luteinizing hormone (LH) in a young woman undergoing co-treatment with chemotherapy and a gonadotropin releasing hormone agonist (GnRH-a; Chemotx) for non-Hodgkin lymphoma. After a decrease in all hormones during chemotherapy/GnRH-a co-treatment, an increase in inhibin A and B in parallel with the return of sex hormones to normal ovulatory levels is detected

species)[92,111–113]. The dimers are thus termed inhibin A and B, respectively[111,112]. The α-β dimers, in contrast to the free α subunit or β-β subunits, are biologically active in suppressing FSH secretion[111].

Intensive research has been undertaken to characterize the biological activities of the 30–32 kDa inhibin A. In addition, a number of immunoassays have been developed, including two site methods for specific measurement of the 30–32 kDa inhibin A dimer in biological fluids[111–113]. Dimeric inhibin A-specific assays were found to detect bioactive inhibin forms in human follicular fluid and in serum[111].

Inhibin-A concentrations in the sera of the patients in the present study were, therefore, measured before, during, and following the gonadotoxic chemotherapy[93]. Inhibin-A immunoactivity was measured by commercial enzyme-linked immunosorbent assay (ELISA)

kits (Serotec) employing the method of Groome and O'Brien[114].

Longitudinal individual follow-up measurements of inhibin-A concentrations in the study group patients have shown a decrease during chemotherapy and GnRH-a treatment with a subsequent increase to normal levels within 1–2 months after the completion of the chemotherapy/GnRH-a protocol in all the treated patients, except in the older patient who developed POF (Figure 1). The mean ± SE inhibin-A concentration was 40.73 ± 10 pg/ml before starting the GnRH-a/chemotherapy treatment, decreasing to 4.77 ± 1.4 and 1.83 ± 0.5 pg/ml at 1–3 and 4–6 months of the treatment protocol, respectively[93]. The mean inhibin-A concentration increased to 26.5 ± 20 pg/ml at 2 months after the protocol, 96.4 ± 47.6 at 6 months, 69.4 ± 17 at 1 year and 177 ± 134.7 pg/ml at 2 years after treatment[93].

The high variation at 2 years was generated by two pregnant women in the study group[93]. The mean inhibin-A concentrations in the patients who developed POF after chemotherapy was below 4 pg/ml, compared to 300 ± 200 pg/ml in women undergoing hMG/hCG superovulation, and 170 ± 05 pg/ml in those patients who spontaneously conceived after the GnRH-a/ chemotherapy co-treatment protocol[93].

Inhibin is secreted by the ovarian granulosa cells in the female and by testicular Sertoli cells in the male. The fully processed form of inhibin has a molecular weight of approximately 32 kDa. Higher molecular weight forms, with precursor forms of the α subunit, also occur in follicular fluid and serum[114–120]. In addition, free α subunit forms, not associated with a β subunit, and lacking inhibin bioactivity, are also present[118]. Until the recent development of Serotec's inhibin-A assay by Nigel Groome[117,118], it was not possible accurately to distinguish between circulating functional dimeric inhibin and the free α subunit in the normal human menstrual cycle, as the previously widely used Monash radioimmunoassay[121–124] was unable to make this distinction[111–121].

Immunoreactive inhibin was undetected during perimenopausal cycles in which FSH concentrations were elevated, yet it was within the normal range during cycles with normal FSH levels[125]. Moreover, in cross-sectional studies of women approaching menopause, immunoreactive (ir)-inhibin decreased progressively in both serum and follicular fluid[124,126]. We thought, therefore, that measuring the concentrations of ir-inhibin A and B, reflecting the function and reserve of ovarian granulosa cells, may possibly aid our attempts at predicting the probability of the return of cyclic ovarian function in young women after the chemotherapeutic gonadotoxic insult. Not unexpectedly, the levels of ir-inhibin A and B were low, compatible with menopausal levels in those women who experienced hypergonadotropic amenorrhea, whereas those who resumed cyclic ovarian function had ir-inhibin A and B concentrations within normal levels[1,93].

Immunoreactive inhibin A and B concentrations decreased to menopausal levels during the chemotherapy/GnRH-a co-treatment, increasing thereafter in parallel with returning ovarian cyclic activity. In those who spontaneously conceived, the ir-inhibin A and B levels were higher than in those who did not. However, owing to the small number of the pregnancies (15) and since most of those who did not conceive were young unmarried women who were not yet interested having children, it is premature to draw any conclusion, at this time, whether the level of ir-inhibin A and B after chemotherapy is predictive of future fertility. Further experience is needed to resolve this clinically practical question.

Whereas 15 pregnancies spontaneously occurred in nine patients in the treatment group (receiving GnRH-a in parallel with chemotherapy), 12 pregnancies also spontaneously occurred in seven women in the control group (treated by chemotherapy without GnRH-a). However, all the patients who conceived in the control group were younger than 21 (16–21 years at chemotherapy), and those who spontaneously conceived in the treatment group were between 18 and 30 years old at the GnRH-a/chemotherapy co-treatment. Therefore, we believe the GnRH-a adjuvant treatment may possibly extend the 'ovarian rescue' and fertile period by almost 10 years, or possibly even more.

Inhibin-A, and possibly also -B, immunoactivity as measured by the recently developed ELISA may serve as an additional means for the evaluation of ovarian activity, besides estrogen, progesterone and gonadotropins. It is premature to conclude whether the role of inhibin A and B as markers is unequivocally superior to that of the traditional markers of ovarian function (FSH, luteinizing hormone and sex steroids). Moreover, the decrease of inhibin concentration during treatment may be attributed to either the GnRH-a treatment, or the gonadotoxicity of chemotherapy, or possibly to both. The exact mechanism for the GnRH-a/chemotherapy-associated inhibin decrease needs further investigation[1,122–126].

Future study is needed for long-term assessment of the positive and negative predictive value of these gonadal peptides (inhibins and activins) in young women undergoing gonadotoxic chemotherapy for various indications (e.g. lymphoma, leukemia, breast cancer, SLE, organ transplantation).

Future endeavors

If the protective effect observed in our preliminary study of GnRH-a and chemotherapy on future ovarian function is confirmed in larger and prospective randomized studies, it may become mandatory to use this co-treatment protocol in every woman undergoing chemotherapy. Thus, ovarian protection may enable the preservation of future fertility in survivors and prevent the bone demineralization and osteoporosis associated with hypoestrogenism and ovarian failure[1,2,6,92,94,96,107,109].

This GnRH-a co-treatment may also be applied to young women receiving cytotoxic chemotherapy for non-cancerous, benign diseases. Since almost one-quarter of young women with SLE of reproductive age may develop premature ovarian failure after cyclophosphamide pulse therapy[6,127,128], the GnRH-a co-treatment may possibly be offered to these young women in parallel with the cytotoxic treatment, as well as to any woman with an autoimmune disorder treated by gonadotoxic chemotherapy, mainly alkylating agents[1,2,128].

Until now, women undergoing aggressive cytotoxic therapy, such as that experienced in BMT, could preserve their future fertility potential only by undergoing egg retrieval and IVF with embryo cryopreservation for future thawing and embryo transfer after several years of no evidence of the malignant disease[1,81,83]. However, this ART is pertinent to female patients who have a partner. Owing to the high prevalence of lymphoma and leukemia at young ages, many of these young women may be single. Unfortunately, although the technology of sperm cryopreservation is widely utilized and successful, the technology for cryopreservation of unfertilized ova is not yet successful. It may be possible to freeze unfertilized eggs, but upon thawing the fertilizability is very low, and therefore unpractical for clinical use at present. Although intense investigational efforts are being conducted in several medical centers[1,77,78,81,83], it may take at least a few years before such technology is clinically available. Furthermore, retrieving an egg in a natural, unstimulated cycle may generate only one or two metaphase II oocytes. To increase the yield of egg retrieval by follicular aspiration, controlled ovarian hyperstimulation by hMG/hCG with or without GnRH-a co-treatment needs to be in experienced hands, and is usually practiced in IVF programs[129]. This may further postpone the initiation of cytotoxic chemotherapy for another 2 weeks or more and may be relatively contraindicated in breast cancer or other sex hormone-sensitive tumors. Owing to these shortcomings, the possibility of ART by IVF combined with embryo cryopreservation for future embryo transfer may not be applicable to all the young women with malignant diseases who have not fulfilled their fertility potential. Therefore, for all these young patients, the GnRH-a co-treatment, and possibly in the future antagonists as well, in parallel with the gonadotoxic chemotherapy, may offer an increased chance of preserving their fertility potential. This practical option may be widely experienced clinically, until the technology of cryopreservation of immature prophase I or unfertilized, metaphase II oocytes is available for young women undergoing gonadotoxic chemotherapy for various clinical indications[77,78,81,83]. The use of GnRH antagonists instead of or in combination with GnRH agonists awaits future clinical testing.

Recently, Morita and co-workers[130] have identified several molecules that are required for chemotherapy-induced oocyte apoptosis. While much of their work has relied on gene knockout mice, they have identified a small lipid antagonist of the pro-apoptotic second messenger ceramide, termed sphingosine-1-phosphate (S-1-P), as a potent protective molecule *in vitro*. They have also found that *in vivo* S-1-P pre-treatment, in mice, resulted in a dramatic dose-dependent protection of oocytes following radiotherapy[131]. Whether the positive GnRH-a adjuvant co-treatment effect is direct or possibly associated with an intraovarian increase in S-1-P is a question of tremendous scientific interest and clinical impact. It awaits further investigation.

Since most of the methods involving ovarian or egg cryopreservation are not yet clinically established and successful, one should be careful to provide these young patients with all the information concerning the various modalities to minimize gonadal damage and preserve ovarian activity and future fertility. Furthermore, combining the various modalities for a specific patient may increase the odds of preservation of future fertility. There is no contraindication to ovarian biopsy for cryopreservation combined with GnRH-a administration and follicular aspiration for IVF and embryo freezing where the patient has a spouse/partner. In cases where the chemotherapy has caused POF, as is frequently the case in BMT, the patient has cryopreserved primordial follicles and/or frozen embryos to fall back upon. However, in cases where conventional chemotherapy regimens such as are commonly used for young lymphoma patients are applied, the GnRH-a co-treatment may preserve ovarian function without necessitating the use of cryopreserved ova or embryos.

We hope that in the future many of the unanswered questions may receive appropriate scientific answers. Until then, let us be very conscientious in supplying our patients with all the possibly relevant information. Holding back on all the available information may violate the ancient dictum *primum non nocere*.

Acknowledgements

The help of Professor J. M. Rowe, Dr I. Avivi and the staff of the Hematology Institute and that of Mrs Ruth Blumenfeld, Batia Navar, Ruth Tal and Dr M. Ritter is thankfully acknowledged. This research was supported by grants from the Technion-Israel Institute of Technology, Ministry of Health and the A. Tufeld Cancer Research Fund. Presented in part at the *46th Annual Meeting of the Society for Gynecologic Investigation*, Atlanta, GA, 10–13 March 1999.

References

1. Blumenfeld Z, Avivi I, Ritter M, *et al*. Preservation of fertility and ovarian function and minimizing chemotherapy-induced gonadotoxicity in young women. *J Soc Gynecol Invest* 1999;6:229–39

2. Blumenfeld Z, Haim N. Prevention of gonadal damage during cytotoxic therapy. *Ann Med* 1997;29:199–206

3. Gosden RG, Rutherford AJ, Norfolk DR. Debate: ovarian banking for cancer patients – transmission of malignant cells in ovarian grafts. *Hum Reprod* 1997;12:403

4. Shaw J, Trounson A. Oncological implications in the replacement of ovarian tissue. *Hum Reprod* 1997;12:403–5

5. Glaser SL. Reproductive factors in Hodgkin disease in women: a review. *Am J Epidemiol* 1994; 139:237–46

6. Ataya K, Moghissi K. Chemotherapy induced premature ovarian failure: medications and prevention. *Steroids* 1989;54:607–26

7. Magrath I. Limiting therapy for limited childhood non-Hodgkin's lymphoma. *N Engl J Med* 1997;337:1304–6

8. DeVita VT Jr, Simon RM, Hubbard SM, *et al*. Curability of advanced Hodgkin's disease with chemotherapy. *Ann Intern Med* 1998;92:587–95

9. Chapman RM. Effect of cytotoxic therapy on sexuality and gonadal function. *Semin Oncol* 1982; 9:84–93

10. Chapman RM, Sutcliffe SB, Malpas JS. Cytotoxic induced ovarian failure in women with Hodgkin's disease. I. Hormonal function. *J Am Med Assoc* 1979;242:1877–81

11. Kreuser ED, Xirus N, Hetzel WD, Himpel A. Reproductive and endocrine gonadal capacity

in patients treated with COPP chemotherapy of Hodgkin's disease. *J Cancer Res Clin Oncol* 1987;113:260–6

12. Rivkees SA, Crawford JD. The relationship of gonadal damage. *J Am Med Assoc* 1988;259:2123–5

13. Shafet SM, Beardwell CG, Morris PH, *et al.* Ovarian failure following abdominal irradiation in childhood. *Br J Cancer* 1976;33:655–8

14. Ataya KM, McKanna JA, Weintraub AM, *et al.* Prevention of chemotherapy-induced ovarian follicular loss in rats. *Cancer Res* 1985;45:3651–6

15. Bines J, Oleske DM, Cobleigh MA. Ovarian function in premenopausal women treated with adjuvant chemotherapy for breast cancer. *J Clin Oncol* 1996;14:1718–29

16. Parker SL, Tong T, Bolden S. Cancer statistics, 1995. *Cancer J Clin* 1996;46:5–27

17. Hankey BF, Miller B, Curtis R, *et al.* Trends in breast cancer in younger women in contrast to older women. *Monogr Natl Cancer Inst* 1994;16:7–14

18. Higgins S, Haffty BG. Pregnancy and lactation after breast-conserving therapy for early stage breast cancer. *Cancer* 1994;73:2175–80

19. Theriault RL, Sellin RV. Estrogen-replacement therapy in younger women with breast cancer. *Monogr Natl Cancer Inst* 1994;16:149–52

20. Early Breast Cancer Trialists' Collaborative Group. Systemic treatment of early breast cancer by hormonal, cytotoxic, or immune therapy: 133 randomized trials involving 31 000 occurrences and 24 000 deaths among 75 000 women. *Lancet* 1992;339:1–15, 71–85

21. Rose DP, Davis TE. Ovarian function in patients receiving adjuvant chemotherapy for breast cancer. *Lancet* 1977;1:1174–6

22. Rose DP, Davis TE. Effects of adjuvant chemo-hormonal therapy on the ovarian and adrenal function of breast cancer patients. *Cancer Res* 1980;40:4043–7

23. Samaan NA, deAsis DN Jr, Buzdar AU, *et al.* Pituitary–ovarian function in breast cancer patients on adjuvant chemoimmunotherapy. *Cancer* 1978;41:2048–87

24. Mehta RR, Beattie CW, Das Gupta TK. Endocrine profile in breast cancer patients receiving chemotherapy. *Breast Cancer Res Treat* 1991;20:125–32

25. Dnistrian AM, Schwartz MK, Fracchia A, *et al.* Endocrine consequences of CMF adjuvant therapy in premenopausal and postmenopausal breast cancer patients. *Cancer* 1983;51:803–7

26. Speroff L, Glass RH, Kase NG. Menopause and postmenopausal hormone therapy. In Speroff L, Glass RH, Kase NG, eds. *Clinical Gynecologic Endocrinology and Infertility*, 5th edn. Baltimore, MD: Williams & Wilkins, 1994:583–636

27. Food and Drug Administration. *Labeling Guidance for Estrogen Drug Products*. Patient package insert. Rockville, MD: Food and Drug Administration, 1992

28. Fisher B, Ravdin RG, Ausman RK, *et al.* Surgical adjuvant chemotherapy in cancer of the breast: results of a decade of cooperative investigation. *Ann Surg* 1968;168:337–56

29. Collichio F, Pandya K. Amenorrhea following chemotherapy for breast cancer. Effect on disease-free survival. *Oncology* 1994;8:45–52

30. Sobrinho LG, Levine RA, DeConti RC. Amenorrhea in patients with Hodgkin's disease treated with antineoplastic agents. *Am J Obstet Gynecol* 1971;109:135–9

31. Warne GL, Fairley KF, Hobbs JB, *et al.* Cyclophosphamide-induced ovarian failure. *N Engl J Med* 1973;289:1159–62

32. Schilsky RL, Lewis BJ, Sherins RJ, *et al.* Gonadal dysfunction in patients receiving chemotherapy for cancer. *Ann Intern Med* 1980;93:109–14

33. Chapman RM. Effect of cytotoxic therapy on sexuality and gonadal function. *Semin Oncol* 1982;9:84–94

34. Gradishar WJ, Schilsky RL. Ovarian function following radiation and chemotherapy for cancer. *Semin Oncol* 1989;16:425–36

35. Morgenfeld MC, Goldberg V, Parisier H, *et al.* Ovarian lesions due to cytostatic agents during the treatment of Hodgkin's disease. *Surg Gynecol Obstet* 1972;134:826–8

36. Sherins RJ. Gonadal dysfunction. In De Vita VT Jr, Hellman S, Rosenberg SA, eds. *Cancer Principles and Practice of Oncology*, 4th edn. Philadelphia, PA: JB Lippincott, 1993:2295–406

37. Kay HH, Mattison DR. How radiation and chemotherapy affect gonadal function. *Contemp Obstet Gynecol* 1985;26:109–27

38. Averette HE, Boyce GM, Girl MA. Effects of cancer chemotherapy on gonadal function and reproductive capacity. *Cancer* 1990;40:199–209

39. Plowchalk DR, Mattison DR. Phosphoramide mustard is responsible for the ovarian toxicity of cyclophosphamide. *Toxicol Appl Pharmacol* 1991;107:472–81

40. Santoro A, Bonadonna G, Valagussa P, et al. Long-term results of combined chemotherapy–radiotherapy approach in Hodgkin's disease: superiority of ABVD plus radiotherapy versus MOPP plus radiotherapy. J Clin Oncol 1987; 5:27–37

41. Cobleigh MA, Bines J, Harris D, et al. Amenorrhea following adjuvant chemotherapy for breast cancer. Proc Am Soc Clin Oncol 1995;14:A158 (abstr.)

42. Shenkenberg TD, Von Hoff DD. Possible mitoxantrone-induced amenorrhea. Cancer Treat Rep 1986;70:659–61

43. Shamberger RC, Rosenberg SA, Seipp CA, et al. Effects of high-dose methotrexate and vincristine on ovarian and testicular functions in patients undergoing postoperative adjuvant treatment of osteosarcoma. Cancer Treat Rep 1981;65:739–46

44. Koyama H, Wada T, Nishizawa Y, et al. Cyclophosphamide-induced ovarian failure and its therapeutic significance in patients with breast cancer. Cancer 1977;39:1403–9

45. Fisher B, Sherman B, Rockette H, et al. L-Phenylalanine mustard (L-PAM) in the management of premenopausal patients with primary breast cancer: lack of association of disease-free survival with depression of ovarian function. Cancer 1979;44:847–57

46. Cobleigh MA, Bines J, Lincoln ST, et al. Amenorrhea following adjuvant chemotherapy for breast cancer. Proc Am Soc Clin Oncol 1994; 13:A55 (abstr.)

47. Miller JJ III, Williams GF, Leissring JC. Multiple late complications of therapy with cyclophosphamide, including ovarian destruction. Am J Med 1971;50:530–5

48. Damewood MD, Grochow LB. Prospects for fertility after chemotherapy or radiation for neoplastic disease. Fertil Steril 1986;45:443–59

49. Padmanabhan N, Wang DY, Moore JW, et al. Ovarian function and adjuvant chemotherapy for early breast cancer. Eur J Clin Oncol 1987; 23:745–8

50. Goldhirsch A, Gelber RD, Castiglione M. The magnitude of endocrine effects of adjuvant chemotherapy for premenopausal breast cancer patients. Ann Oncol 1990;1:183–8

51. Moliterni A, Bonadonna G, Valagussa P, et al. Cyclophosphamide, methotrexate and fluorouracil with and without doxorubicin in the adjuvant treatment of resectable breast cancer with one to three positive axillary nodes. J Clin Oncol 1991;9:1124–30

52. Tancini G, Valagussa P, Bajetta E, et al. Preliminary 3-year results of 12 versus 6 cycles of surgical adjuvant CMF in premenopausal breast cancer. Cancer Clin Trials 1979;2: 285–92

53. Bianco AR, Del Mastro L, Gallo C, et al. Prognostic role of amenorrhea induced by adjuvant chemotherapy in premenopausal patients with early breast cancer. Br J Cancer 1991;63:799–803

54. Reyno LM, Levine MN, Skingley P, et al. Chemotherapy induced amenorrhea in a randomized trial of adjuvant chemotherapy duration in breast cancer. Eur J Cancer 1993; 29A:21–3

55. Levine MN, Gent M, Hryniuk WM. A randomized trial comparing 12 weeks versus 36 weeks of adjuvant chemotherapy in stage II breast cancer. J Clin Oncol 1990;8:1217–25

56. Wood WC, Budman DR, Korzun AH, et al. Dose and dose intensity of adjuvant chemotherapy for stage II, node-positive breast carcinoma. N Engl J Med 1994;330:1253–9

57. Brincker H, Rose C, Rank F, et al. Evidence of castration-mediated effect of adjuvant cytotoxic chemotherapy in premenopausal breast cancer. J Clin Oncol 1987;5:1771–8

58. Muller U, Stahel RA. Gonadal function after MACOP-B or VACOP-B with or without dose intensification and ABMT in young patients with aggressive non-Hodgkin lymphoma. Ann Oncol 1993;4:399–402

59. Johnson DH, Linde R, Hainsworth JD, et al. Effect of a luteinizing hormone releasing hormone agonist given during combination chemotherapy on post-therapy fertility in male patients with lymphoma: preliminary observations. Blood 1985;65:832–6

60. Sutcliffe SB. Cytotoxic chemotherapy and gonadal function in patients with Hodgkin's disease. J Am Med Assoc 1979;242:1898–9

61. Nademanee A, Schmidt GM, O'Donnell MR, et al. High dose chemoradiotherapy followed by autologous bone marrow transplantation as a consolidation therapy during first complete remission in adult patients with poor-risk aggressive lymphoma: a pilot study. Blood 1992; 80:1130–4

62. Carey PJ, Proctor SJ, Hamilton PJ. Autologous bone marrow transplantation for high grade lymphoid malignancy using melphalan/irradiation conditioning without bone marrow purging or cryopreservation. Blood 1991;77: 1593–9

63. Sanders J, Buckner CD, Leonard JM, et al. Late effects on gonadal function of cyclophosphamide, total-body irradiation, and marrow transplantation. Transplantation 1983;36:252–5

64. Keilholtz U, Korbling M, Fehrentz D, et al. Long-term endocrine toxicity of myeloablative treatment followed by autologous bone marrow/blood derived stem cell transplantation in patients with malignant lymphohematopoietic disorders. Cancer 1989;64:641–5

65. Meirow D, Schenker JG. Cryopreservation and transplantation of ovarian tissue: a mode of preserving female fertility. Harefuah 1998;134: 461–4

66. Sanders JE, Buckner CD, Amos D, et al. Ovarian function following marrow transplantation for aplastic anaemia or leukaemia. J Clin Oncol 1988;6:813–17

67. Carroll J, Wood MJ, Whittingham DG. Normal fertilization and development of frozen thawed mouse oocytes: protective action of certain macromolecules. Biol Reprod 1993;48:606–12

68. Bos-Mikkich A, Wood MJ, Candy CJ, et al. Cytogenetic analysis and developmental potential of vitrified mouse oocytes. Biol Reprod 1995;53:780–5

69. Parks JE, Ruffing NA. Factors affecting low temperature survival of mammalian oocytes. Technology 1992;37:59–72

70. Trounson AO, Bongso A. Fertilization and development in humans. Curr Topics Dev Biol 1996;32:59–101

71. Vincent C, Johnson MH. Cooling, cryoprotectants and the cytoskeleton of the mammalian oocyte. Oxford Rev Reprod Biol 1992;14:72–100

72. Barnes FL, Kausche A, Tiglias J, et al. Production of embryos from in-vitro matured primary human oocytes. Fertil Steril 1996;65:1151–6

73. Apperly JF, Reddy N. Mechanism and management of gonadal failure in recipients of high dose chemoradiotherapy. Blood Rev 1995; 9:93–116

74. Biskind GR, Kordan B, Biskind MS. Ovary transplanted to spleen in rats: the effect of unilateral castration, pregnancy and subsequent castration. Cancer Res 1950;10:309–18

75. Gosden RG, Baird DT, Wade JC, et al. Restoration of fertility to oophorectomized sheep by ovarian autografts stored at −196°C. Hum Reprod 1994;9:597–603

76. Newton H, Aubard Y, Sharma V, et al. The low temperature storage and grafting of human ovarian tissue into SCID mice. Hum Reprod 1996;11:1487–91

77. Wade JC, Gosden RG. Assessment of oocyte survival in ovarian cortical grafts after frozen storage and xenografting. In Schats R, Schoemaker J, eds. Ovarian Endocrinopathies (The 8th Reinier de Graaf Symposium). Carnforth, UK: Parthenon Publishing, 1994:67–70

78. Gosden RG. Transplantation of ovaries and testes. In Edwards RG, ed. Fetal Tissue Transplants in Medicine. Cambridge: Cambridge University Press, 1992:253–79

79. Shaw JM, Bowels J, Koopman P. Fresh and cryopreserved ovarian tissue samples from donors with lymphoma transmit the cancer to the graft recipient. Hum Reprod 1996;11:1668–73

80. Oehninger S. Will ovarian autotransplantation have a role in reproductive and gynecological medicine? Fertil Steril 1998;70:20–1

81. Meirow D, Ben-Yehuda D, Prus D, et al. Ovarian tissue banking in patients with Hodgkin's disease: is it safe? Fertil Steril 1998;69:996–8

82. von Eye Corleta H, Corleta O, Capp E, Edelweiss MI. Subcutaneous autologous ovarian transplantation in Wistar rats maintains hormone secretion. Fertil Steril 1998;70:16–19

83. Moomjy M, Rosenwaks Z. Ovarian tissue cryopreservation: the time is now. Transplantation or in vitro maturation: the time awaits. Fertil Steril 1998;69:999–1000

84. Hovatta O, Silye R, Krausz T, et al. Cryopreservation of human ovarian tissue using dimethylsulphoxide and propanediol-sucrose as cryoprotectants. Hum Reprod 1996;11:1268–72

85. Gunasena KR, Villines PM, Critser ES, et al. Live births after autologous transplant of cryopreserved mouse ovaries. Hum Reprod 1997; 12:101–6

86. Dissen GA, Lara HE, Fahenbach WH, et al. Immature rat ovaries become revascularized rapidly after autotransplantation and show a gonadotropin-dependent increase in angiogenic factor gene expression. Endocrinology 1994;134:1146–54

87. Waxman JH, Ahmed R, Smith D, et al. Failure to preserve fertility in patients with Hodgkin disease. Cancer Chemother Pharmacol 1987;19: 159–62

88. Glode LM, Robinson J, Gould SF. Protection from cyclophosphamide induced testicular damage with an analogue of gonadotropin-releasing hormone. Lancet 1981;1:1132–4

89. Chapman RM, Sutcliffe S. The effects of chemotherapy and radiotherapy on fertility and their prevention. Recent Adv Clin Oncol 1986;2:239–51

90. Krepart GV, Lotocki RJ. Chemotherapy during pregnancy. In Allen HH, Nisker JA, eds. *Cancer in Pregnancy, Therapeutic Guidelines*. Mount Kisco, NY: Futura Publishing, 1986:69–88

91. Ataya K, Rao LV, Laurence E, *et al.* Luteinizing hormone-releasing hormone agonist inhibits cyclophosphamide induced ovarian follicular depletion in Rhesus monkeys. *Biol Reprod* 1995;52:365–72

92. Blumenfeld Z, Avivi I, Linn S, *et al.* Prevention of irreversible chemotherapy-induced ovarian damage in young women with lymphoma by a gonadotropin-releasing hormone agonist in parallel to chemotherapy. *Hum Reprod* 1996;11:1620–6

93. Blumenfeld Z, Ritter M, Shariki K, Haim N. Inhibin-A concentrations in sera of young women during and following chemotherapy for lymphoma – correlation with ovarian toxicity. Presented at the *44th Annual Meeting of the Society for Gynecologic Investigation*, San-Diego, CA, March 20–22, 1997. *J Soc Gynecol Invest* (Suppl.). *Am J Reprod Immunol* 1998;39:33–40

94. Kreuser ED, Felsenberg D, Behles C, *et al.* Long-term gonadal dysfunction and its impact on bone mineralization in patients following COPP/ABVD chemotherapy for Hodgkin's disease. *Ann Oncol* 1992;3(Suppl. 4):S105–10

95. Longo DL. The use of chemotherapy in the treatment of Hodgkin's disease. *Semin Oncol* 1990;17:716–35

96. Ratcliffe MA, Lanham SA, Reld DM, *et al.* Bone mineral density (BMD) in patients with lymphoma: the effects of chemotherapy, intermittent corticosteroids and premature menopause. *Hematol Oncol* 1992;10:181–7

97. Ortin TT, Shoshlak CA, Donaldson SS. Gonadal status and reproductive function following treatment for Hodgkin's disease in childhood: the Stanford experience. *Int J Radiol Oncol Biol Phys* 1990;19:873–80

98. Backshine H, Brauner R, Thibaud E, *et al.* Chemotherapy and ovarian function. Retrospective analysis in 17 girls treated for malignant tumor of hematologic disease. *Arch Fr Pediatr* 1986;43:611–16

99. Wallace WH, Shalet SM, Tellow LJ, *et al.* Ovarian function following the treatment of childhood acute lymphoblastic leukemia. *Med Pediatr Oncol* 1993;21:333–9

100. Kreuser ED, Hetzel WD, Billia DO, *et al.* Gonadal toxicity following cancer therapy in adults: significance, diagnosis, prevention and treatment. *Cancer Treat Rev* 1990;17:169–75

101. Krause W, Pfluger KH. Treatment with the gonadotropin-releasing hormone agonist buserelin to protect spermatogenesis against cytotoxic treatment in young men. *Andrologia* 1989;21:265–70

102. Byrne J, Mulvihill JJ, Myers MH, *et al.* Effects of treatment on fertility in long-term survivors of childhood or adolescent cancer. *N Engl J Med* 1987;317:1315–21

103. Jarrell JF, McMahon A, Barr RD, Young Lai EV. The agonist (d-leu-6, des-gly-10)-LHRH-ethylamide does not protect the fecundity of rats exposed to high dose unilateral ovarian irradiation. *Reprod Toxicol* 1991;5:385–8

104. Benson K, Hartz AJ. A comparison of observational studies and randomized, controlled trials. *N Engl J Med* 2000;342:1878–86

105. Concato J, Shah N, Horwitz RI. Randomized, controlled trials, observational studies and the hierarchy of research designs. *N Engl J Med* 2000;342:1887–92

106. Hinterberger-Fischer M, Kier P, Kalhs P, *et al.* Fertility, pregnancies and offspring complications after bone marrow transplantation. *Bone Marrow Transplantation* 1991;7:5–9

107. Linde R, Doelle GC, Alexander N, *et al.* Reversible inhibition of testicular steroidogenesis and spermatogenesis by a potent gonadotropin-releasing hormone agonist in normal men. *N Engl J Med* 1981;305:663–8

108. Bramley T, Menzies G, Baird D. Specific binding of gonadotropin-releasing hormone and an agonist to human corpus luteum homogenate: characterization properties and luteal phase levels. *J Clin Endocrinol Metab* 1985;61:834–40

109. McLachlan R, Healy D, Burger H. Clinical aspects of LHRH analogues in gynecology: a review. *Br J Obstet Gynaecol* 1986;93:431–54

110. Clayton R, Huhtaniemi I. Absence of gonadotropin releasing hormone receptors in human gonadal tissue. *Nature (London)* 1982;299:56–9

111. Robertson D, Burger HG, Sullivan J, *et al.* Biological and immunological characterisation of inhibin forms in human plasma. *J Clin Endocrinol Metab* 1996;81:601–76

112. Burger HG. Inhibin. *Reprod Med Rev* 1992;1:1–20

113. Porcelet E, Franchimont P. Two site enzymoimmunoassays of inhibin. *Ares-Serono Symposia Series – Frontiers in Endocrinology* 1994;3:45–54

114. Groome NP, O'Brien M. Two-site immunoassays for inhibin and its subunits. Further

applications of synthetic peptide approach. *J Immunol Methods* 1993;165:167–76

115. Groome NP, Illingworth PJ, O'Brien M, *et al.* Detection of dimeric inhibin throughout the human menstrual cycle by two-site enzyme immunoassys. *Clin Endocrinol* 1994;40: 717–23

116. Lambert-Messerlan GM, Hall JE, Sluss PM, *et al.* Relatively low levels of dimeric inhibin circulate in men and women with polycystic ovarian syndrome using a specific two-site enzyme-linked immunosorbent assay. *J Clin Endocrinol Metab* 1994;79:45–50

117. Muttukrishna S, Fowler PA, Groome NP, *et al.* Serum concentrations of dimeric inhibin during the spontaneous human menstrual cycle and after treatment with exogenous gonadotropin. *Hum Reprod* 1994;9:1634–42

118. Groome NP, Illingworth PJ, O'Brien M, *et al.* Quantification of inhibin pro-αC-containing forms in human serum by a new ultra sensitive two-site enzyme-linked immunosorbent assay. *J Clin Endocrinol Metab* 1995;80:2926–32

119. Groome NP, Lawrence M. Preparation of monoclonal antibodies reactive with the beta-A subunit of human ovarian inhibin. *Hybridoma* 1991;10:309–16

120. Groome NP, Hancock J, Betteridge A, *et al.* Monoclonal and polyclonal antibodies reactive with the 1-32 amino terminal peptide of 32 kD human ovarian inhibin. *Hybridoma* 1990;9:31–42

121. Knight PG, Muttukrishna S, Groome NP. Development and application of a two-site enzyme immunoassay for the determination of 'total' activin-A concentrations in serum and follicular fluid. *J Endocrinol* 1996;148: 267–79

122. McLachlan RI, Robertson DM, de Kretser DM, *et al.* Advances in the physiology of inhibin and inhibin-related peptides. *Clin Endocrinol* 1988;29:77–112

123. McLachlan RI, Robertson DM, Healy DL, *et al.* Circulating immunoreactive inhibin level during the normal menstrual cycle. *J Clin Endocrinol Metab* 1987;65:954–61

124. Woodruff TK, Krummen L, Baly D, *et al.* Inhibin and activin-a measured in human serum. In Burger HG, ed. *Inhibin and Inhibin-related Proteins – Frontiers in Endocrinology.* Rome: Ares-Serono Symposia, 1994;3:55–68

125. Hee J, McNaughton J, Bangah M, *et al.* Premenopausal pattern of gonadotropins, immunoreactive inhibin, estradiol, and progesterone. *Maturitas* 1993;18:9–20

126. Woodruff TK, Mather JP. Inhibin, activin, and the female reproductive axis. *Ann Rev Physiol* 1995;57:219–44

127. Langevitz P, Klein L, Pras M, *et al.* The effect of cyclophosphamide pulses on fertility in patients with lupus nephritis. *Am J Reprod Immunol* 1992;28:157–8

128. Blumenfeld Z, Shapiro D, Shteinberg M, *et al.* Preservation of fertility and ovarian function and minimizing gonadotoxicity in young women with systemic lupus erythematosus treated by chemotherapy. *Lupus* 2000;9:1–5

129. Blumenfeld Z, Barkey RJ, Youdim MBH, *et al.* Growth hormone-binding protein regulation by estrogen, progesterone, and gonadotropins in human: the effect of ovulation induction with menopausal gonadotropins, GH and gestation. *J Clin Endocrinol Metab* 1992;75:1242–9

130. Morita Y, Paris F, Perez GI, *et al.* Protection of the ovary from radiation-induced damage by small molecule therapy *in-vivo. J Soc Gynecol Invest* 2000; 7(Suppl.):164 A (abstr. 429)

131. Morita Y, Perez GI, Paris F, *et al.* Oocyte apoptosis is suppressed by disruption of the acid sphingomyelinase gene or by sphingosine-1-phosphate therapy. *Nature Med* 2000;6: 1109–14

Uterine fibroids and infertility: what strategy of management?

25

M. Szamatowicz and J. Szamatowicz

Introduction

Leiomyomas appear to be the most common female pelvic tumors that can be found in women of reproductive age. Usually at this stage they are asymptomatic but in some cases they are associated with such symptoms as menorrhagia, pelvic pain, urinary symptoms and particularly infertility. They are found in almost 30% of patients diagnosed with the above abnormalities.

Although it still remains unclear whether myomas may cause infertility, they do cause repeated loss of pregnancy, for example the presence of an intracavity tumor acts very much like an intrauterine device. It causes inflammatory response in the endometrial tissue opposite the myoma, and the area of decidua covering the myoma provides inadequate blood supply for the fetus. There is some evidence that leiomyomas are associated with an increased risk of spontaneous abortion which may depend on the size and position of the myoma. The fact that larger myomas have a more important impact on pregnancy loss compared with smaller ones is demonstrated[1].

Myomectomy and infertility

Myomectomy should be considered whenever preservation of the uterus is indispensable for its childbearing function. Indications for myomectomy include a tumor's interference with fertility or predisposition to repeated pregnancy loss due to location and number of myomas. The location of leiomyomas have an especial impact on the implantation and maintenance of pregnancy. Location of tumor influences mode of interference: directly under the endometrium the tumor may interfere with implantation because of influence on embryonic nutrition; a tumor near the uterotubal junction may cause intramural obstruction, and at the broad ligament site by the distortion of the anatomical relationship between the tubal ostium and the ovary; a supracervical tumor can change the position of the cervix and interfere with the penetration of ejaculate through the cervical canal[2].

Many studies have been done on the impact of leiomyomas on infertility and on the effectiveness of myomectomy. Different operation techniques have been discussed in numerous articles. The cumulative pregnancy rate after myomectomy varies between 29 and 87%. The live births percentage is about 48% but the spontaneous abortion rate is also relatively high (32%). The data on the effect of myomectomy on fecundity are collected in Table 1[3–10].

Many publications support the usefulness of myomectomy in enhancing fertility. Some authors are not so unequivocal, and recommend counseling before operation, which should consider size, total number and place of myomas. Retrospective analysis of number and size of myomas has revealed that fecundity after operation depends rather on the number than on the size and placing of myomas[11].

Mechanisms leading to infertility

The mechanisms by which leiomyomas may cause infertility remain unclear. Some hypotheses focus on the effect of leiomyomas

Table 1 Effect of myomectomy on fecundity: collected data

Author	Operation technique	Number of patients	Cumulative pregnancy rate (%)
Babaknia et al.[3] (1978)	laparotomy	46	44
Berkeley et al.[1] (1983)	laparotomy	50	50
Gehlbach et al.[4] (1993)	laparotomy	37	57
Dubuisson et al.[5] (1996)	laparoscopy	21	33
Sudik et al.[6] (1996)	laparotomy	67	58
Klonowska et al.[7] (1998)	laparotomy	104	29
Vercellini et al.[8] (1998)	laparotomy	138	87
Li et al.[9] (1999)	laparotomy	51	57
Dubuisson et al.[10] (2000)	laparoscopy	91	53
Total		605	51

on sperm transport due to changes in uterine contour or contractility; others concentrate on impaired implantation[12].

Many studies have been done on histological changes in the endometrium associated with leiomyomas. They include atrophy, vascular alterations, hyperplasia and the above mentioned inflammatory reaction. Recently published data showed two important factors associated with myomatosus uterus. One of them is heparin binding-epidermal growth factor (HE-EGF), a membrane-associated protein which plays a role in blastocyst endometrium interactions. The studies performed to date showed a statistically significant reduction in the production of HB-EGF in the luteal phase in women with myomatosus uterus when compared with a control group. This observation may be relevant to studies on implantation in humans[13].

Another paper published recently deals with spontaneous apoptosis in human myometrium[14]. The purpose of the study was to determine whether apoptosis is decreased in the endometrial tissue of myomatosus uterus or whether an unexplained mechanism underlies infertility caused by myoma and bleeding. It concluded that spontaneous apoptosis is significantly reduced in the uterine endometrium obtained from uteri with myomas and bleeding. These findings may help us understand new pathways when evaluating the pathophysiology of infertility in women with benign uterine disorders[14].

The presence of myomas influences the contractility of the myometrium. The myometrial structure is disturbed by tumors and differs from normal tissue. The removal of myomas results in scarring on the surface and inside the myometrium. Therefore uterine contractility is different before and after surgery. A comparison of digital intrauterine pressure recordings of spontaneous contractility, as well as after oxytocin and vasopressin challenge by intravenous bolus injections before and after operation, was done during corresponding days of the menstrual cycle. Digital signals gave us an opportunity to perform not only standard analysis of contractions (area under curve; AUC) but also to apply Furier's analysis of obtained signals (deformation index). Our finding was that, after the removal of myomas, there was a statistically significant increase in spontaneous activity of the uterus expressed by AUC. A comparison of the magnitude of oxytocin-induced change in contractility parameters between the records obtained before and after operation showed a significant difference in AUC and deformation index. No such effects were seen after vasopressin administration. Although these findings do not allow us to form conclusions, we propose that removal of uterine myomas normalizes the uterine contractility pattern and that such mechanisms may explain the therapeutic effect of the procedure on bleeding disorders and infertility[15].

Indications for myomectomy

There are several situations when myomectomy should be considered. These are: submucous leiomyomas, rapidly enlarging leiomyomas, infertility secondary to leiomyomas and desire to retain fecundity. It is important to identify prognostic factors for conception after myomectomy to reverse infertility. Recently published data revealed that postoperative fertility after myomectomy was decreased when tumors were located in the posterior wall or when the uterus was sutured. The latter is probably due to postoperative adhesions. In fact these surgical procedures are associated with adhesions involving adnexa[16].

The coincidence of menometrorrhagia, myoma and infertility should be considered with caution. This relationship has not been reported in most studies, though there is one study where the link between infertility and the existence of menometrorrhagia was found. If this result were confirmed by other studies it might suggest that myomas responsible for menometrorrhagia might also be responsible for infertility. The influence of submucous myomas on fecundity has been mentioned above. The suggestion that it is a result of deformation of the uterine cavity is reasonable, but in many studies it has been shown that even intramural myomas could impair implantation without there being deformation of the intrauterine cavity.

Myomas and ART

Since assisted reproduction techniques (ART) have been widely used, there has been a revival of interest in the potential effect of uterine myomas on the outcome of *in vitro* fertilization (IVF). The pivotal problem is whether all women with uterine myomas, irrespective of size and location, should undergo myomectomy before being treated with ART. Published data have shown that if the uterine cavity is not deformed and the myomas are not large (more than 7 cm in diameter), implantation and ongoing pregnancy rate after IVF – embryo transfer (ET) are comparable to the group of patients with normal uterus[17]. Nevertheless, both spontaneous abortion and preterm labor were more frequent among women with myomas. This is why patients with myoma should be counselled very carefully and all facts related to their condition should be explained fully. Myomectomy is one of many options before patients are referred for IVF-ET and caution should be exercised when making the decision to perform myomectomy before ART. It is however certain that large myomas compressing the uterine cavity (intramural and submucosal) need to be removed before scheduling for ART. To conclude, it is difficult to define to what extent myoma causes infertility in cases where another major fertility factor is present (male, tubal or ovulatory)[18,19].

GnRH analogs pretreatment

A separate problem that should be discussed in this review is how to operate on myomas and whether it is useful to administer gonadotropin-releasing hormone (GnRH) analogs before surgery. It seems now that the introduction of minimal invasive surgery (laparoscopy) for benign gynecological pathologies such as ovarian cysts, tubal pregnancies, endometriosis and myomas has resulted in remarkable benefit to the patients; the postoperative pregnancy rate for previously infertile women is similar to that following laparotomic myomectomy. However, laparoscopic myomectomy should be performed only by an experienced surgeon familiar with laparoscopic suturing[20]. The risk of uterine rupture during pregnancy and labor is equal to that after conservative operation. The usefulness of GnRH analogs before surgery is still open to debate. According to published data, preoperative GnRH analogs treatment is effective in reducing the size of myomas, but does not seem to offer significant advantages in myomectomy. It also increases the cost of the whole procedure[21].

Conclusions

In conclusion, the answer to the question whether myomas should be treated in patients with infertility should be yes. However, very precise estimation of number, size and location of leiomyomas should be performed before treatment. Myomas bigger than 7 cm, in contact with the uterine cavity or causing menometrorrhagia should be removed. Laparoscopic myomectomy is as effective as laparotomy. Pre-treatment with GnRH analogs does not provide any significant advantages in treatment of leiomyomas.

References

1. Berkeley AS, DeCherney AH, Polan ML. Abdominal myomectomy and subsequent fertility. *Surg Gynecol Obstet* 1983;156:319–22

2. Bernard G, Darai E, Poncelet C, *et al.* Fertility after hysteroscopic myomectomy: effect of intramural myomas associated. *Eur J Obstet Gynecol Reprod Biol* 2000;88:85–90

3. Babaknia A, Rock JA, Jones HW Jr. Pregnancy success following abdominal myomectomy for infertility. *Fertil Steril* 1978;30:644–7

4. Gehlbach DL, Sousa RC, Carpenter SE, *et al.* Abdominal myomectomy in the treatment of infertility. *Int J Gynaecol Obstet* 1993;40:45–50

5. Dubuisson JB, Chapron C, Chavet X, *et al.* Fertility after laparoscopic myomectomy of large intramural myomas: preliminary results. *Hum Reprod* 1996;11:518–22

6. Sudik R, Hush K, Steller J, *et al.* Fertility and pregnancy outcome after myomectomy in sterility patients. *Eur J Obstet Gynecol Reprod Biol* 1996;65:209–14

7. Klonowska-Dziatkiewicz E, Kulikowski M, Szamatowicz M. Leczenie operacyjne mięśniaków macicy u kobiet z nieplodnoscia. *Ginekol Pol* 1998;3:128–32

8. Vercellini P, Maddalena S, De Giorgi O, *et al.* Abdominal myomectomy for infertility: a comprehensive review. *Hum Reprod* 1998;13: 873–9

9. Li TC, Mortimer R, Cooke ID. Myomectomy: a retrospective study to examine reproductive performance before and after surgery. *Hum Reprod* 1999;14:1735–40

10. Dubuisson JB, Fauconnier A, Chapron C, *et al.* Reproductive outcome after laparoscopic myomectomy in infertile women. *J Reprod Med* 2000;45:23–30

11. Fauconnier A, Dubuisson JB, Ancel PY, *et al.* Prognostic factors of reproductive outcome after myomectomy in infertile patients. *Hum Reprod* 2000;15:1751–7

12. Vefkauf BS. Myomectomy for infertility enhancement and preservation. *Fertil Steril* 1992;58:1–15

13. Ali AF, Fateen B, Ezzet A, *et al.* A new mechanism of infertility associated with myoma: decreased production of heparin-binding epidermal growth factor in the endometrium. *Obstet Gynecol* 2000;95(4 Suppl. 1):49

14. Ali AF, Fateen B, Ezzet A, *et al.* Spontaneous apoptosis in the endometrium in the impaired myomatosus uterus. *Obstet Gynecol* 2000;95 (4 Suppl. 1):32

15. Szamatowicz J, Laudański T, Bulkszas B, *et al.* Fibromyomas and uterine contractions. *Acta Obstet Gynecol Scand* 1997;76:973–6

16. Vercellini P, Maddalena S, De Giorgi O, *et al.* Determinants of reproductive outcome after abdominal myomectomy for infertility. *Fertil Steril* 1999;72:109–14

17. Ramzy AM, Sattar M, Amin Y, *et al.* Uterine myomata and outcome of assisted reproduction. *Hum Reprod* 1998;13:198–202

18. Stovall DW, Parrish SB, Van Voorhis BJ, *et al.* Uterine leiomyomas reduce the efficacy of assisted reproduction cycles: results of a matched follow-up study. *Hum Reprod* 1998;13:192–7

19. Ugur M, Turan C, Mungan T, *et al.* Laparoscopy for adhesion prevention following myomectomy. *Int J Gynaecol Obstet* 1996;53:145–9

20. Dubuisson JB, Fauconnier A, Chapron C, *et al.* Second look after laparoscopic myomectomy. *Hum Reprod* 1998;13:2102–6

21. Campo S, Garcea N. Laparoscopic myomectomy in premenopausal women with and without preoperative treatment using gonadotropin-releasing hormone analogues. *Hum Reprod* 1999;14:44–8

Surgical approaches to uterine myomas

26

A. Volpe, S. Malmusi and A. Cagnacci

Introduction

Leiomyomas are benign hormone-sensitive fibromuscular tumors of the uterus that are detected in 25–40% of women in their reproductive years. Myomectomy is advisable for women who wish to preserve their childbearing potential and it is needed when myomas are either symptomatic, causing abnormal uterine bleeding and pain, or asymptomatic but growing rapidly causing infertility or recurrent abortion[1]. Apart from vaginal myomectomy and operative hysteroscopy, which represents a valid approach for submucous myomas, four different operative techniques have been described for the surgical approach to leiomyomas: laparotomy, laparoscopy, minilaparotomy and video-assisted minilaparotomy.

Laparotomy

Laparotomy is performed with a 10–12 cm suprapubic incision. The subcutaneous fat and abdominal fascia are crosswise opened, whereas the abdominal muscle is longitudinally opened on the midline. The parietal peritoneum is visualized and it is lengthwise opened to reach the pelvic cavity. Subsequently, a separator is inserted through the abdominal breach and an intestinal compress is inserted. After examination of the uterus and adnexa, myomectomy is performed. At the end, the uterine breach is usually closed in double or triple layers with interrupted suture. After the control of hemostasis and repeated washing of the pelvic cavity, the laparotomic breach is closed in separate layers.

Laparoscopy

For laparoscopy a pneumoperitoneum is obtained with carbon dioxide insufflation through a Veress needle. A 10 mm port is inserted through the umbilicus to introduce the optic that is connected to a camera for video monitoring. Two to three further 5–15 mm ports are inserted on the right, on the left or below the umbilicus for the introduction of the surgical instruments. Diluted vasopressin is injected in multiple sites between the myometrium and the fibroid capsule. The serosa and myometrium overlying the myoma are pierced by CO_2 laser or a monopolar electrode. A myoma screw is inserted into the fibroid to apply traction. Bipolar forceps are used for coagulation. After complete myoma removal, the myometrium and serosa are approximated with a one-layer suture on a straight or curved needle. Following repair, the uterine surface is irrigated with lactated Ringer and Interceed is applied over the suture line. Removal of myomas from the abdominal cavity is performed through one of the ports. Big myomas require fragmentation by a morcellator, scalpel or scissors.

Assisted- or non-assisted minilaparotomy

Minilaparotomy is usually performed with a 5 cm incision, 1–2 cm above the pubic symphisis. The abdominal fascia is crosswise or longitudinally opened. A uterine manipulator is used to elevate the uterus toward the midline suprapubic incision. A corkscrew manipulator is transperitoneally inserted; the parietal peritoneum is opened near to the myoma; the myoma is exteriorized through the peritoneum and the minilaparotomy incision. Myomectomy and uterus reconstruction is performed directly outside the peritoneum, then the uterus is replaced in the pelvic cavity. The abdominal incision is closed in multiple layers. In the video-assisted minilaparotomy, pneumoperitoneum as in the laparoscopy technique is performed. The videocamera is used to identify the myoma and, after peritoneum closure, hemostasis is further controlled under videolaparoscopy. An accurate toilette of the pelvic cavity is performed via a suction-irrigator.

Studies comparing laparoscopy with laparotomy

Laparoscopy is a technique with substantial benefits for the patient in the early outcome: reduced postoperative pain, shorter hospital stay and faster recovery[2–4]. However, the number and size of myomas represent a limitation for this technique, particularly due to the lengthening of the surgical procedure and the difficulty of performing a valid uterine reconstruction. Indeed, uterine dehiscence during pregnancy in women conceiving after laparoscopic myomectomy has already been reported[5–8], although rare cases of this late complication have also been described after abdominal surgery[9]. On the other hand, the laparotomic approach is characterized by longer hospital stay and recovery time. Only a few authors have reported their experiences with laparoscopic myomectomy[10–13]. These studies have suggested the advantages of laparoscopic surgery over laparotomy in the management of uterine myomas[10–16], but the two techniques have not been prospectively compared in randomized trials. In a recent case–control non-randomized study the authors have reported that a laparoscopic approach may be safely chosen for patients with myomas and that it offers the benefits of less postoperative intravenous narcotic use,

a shorter hospital stay and no greater intraoperative blood loss than in abdominal myomectomy[17]. In a retrospective non-randomized study on laparoscopic versus laparotomic myomectomy, blood loss among the patients undergoing the former technique was reported to be significantly lower, but also the size of the myoma was significantly smaller (58 ± 7.16 g vs 337 ± 77.4 g respectively; $p < 0.00001$). Numbers of days of hospitalization, to resumption of normal activity, and to complete recovery were greater for the patients who underwent myomectomy by laparotomy than by laparoscopy[18]. A prospective, randomized study comparing laparoscopic with laparotomic myomectomy in a sample size of 40 selected patients reported similar advantages for laparoscopic myomectomy[19]. After laparoscopic myomectomy, at least 80% of patients were analgesic free on day 2, discharged from hospital by day 3, and feeling fully recuperated on day 15, whereas this was so only in 20% after abdominal myomectomy. Also, blood loss after laparoscopy was smaller than after laparotomy (200 ± 50 ml vs 230 ± 44 ml respectively; $p < 0.05$). In this study the mean diameter of the largest myoma was 4.4 ± 0.8 cm in the laparoscopy group and 4.7 ± 1.3 cm in the laparotomy group; consequently, accurate selection of the cases was performed and the data should be applied only to these conditions.

Studies comparing laparoscopy with minilaparotomy

There is no randomized study comparing myomectomy performed by minilaparotomy with that by laparoscopy. In a prospective, non-randomized study on laparoscopic versus video-assisted minilaparotomy, blood loss in patients undergoing laparoscopy was less, but this group was also characterized by smaller myomas (58 ± 7.16 g vs 247 ± 30.1 g; $p < 0.00001$). Instead, days of hospitalization (1.06 vs 1.28), to resumption of normal activity (11.2 vs 12.2), and to complete recovery (20.9 vs 23.1) were similar in the two groups[18].

Studies comparing minilaparotomy with laparotomy

There is no randomized study comparing the early outcome of myomectomy performed by laparotomy with that by video- or non-video-assisted minilaparotomy. These latter surgical techniques could offer as satisfactory a uterine repair as laparotomy, but may have better outcome in terms of fever, blood loss, pain, canalization and dimission time. A retrospective, non-randomized study compared myomectomy performed by laparoscopically assisted minilaparotomy with that by laparotomy. Blood loss was similar between the two techniques, but days of hospitalization (1.28 vs 3.3; $p < 0.00004$), to resumption of normal activity (12.2 vs 39.2; $p < 0.0001$), and to complete recovery (23.1 vs 70.0; $p < 0.00002$) were less in the minilaparotomy than in the laparotomy group[18].

In our institute, a prospective randomized trial evaluating the early outcome of video- or non-video-assisted minilaparotomy and laparotomy is in progress. Inclusion criteria are the presence of one myoma with a diameter less than 8 cm or 2–5 myomas with total diameter less than 16 cm. So far, 38 women have been recruited of whom 14 have undergone minilaparotomy, 16 video-assisted minilaparotomy and eight laparotomy. Age and body mass index were similar in the three groups. The maximum diameter of the myomas was similar among the groups (7.0 ± 0.6 cm for video-assisted minilaparotomy; 6.5 ± 0.7 cm for minilaparotomy; 5.2 ± 0.7 cm for laparotomy; NS), but number of myomas was higher in the laparotomy group than in the video-assisted minilaparotomy or minilaparotomy (2.5 ± 0.7 vs 1.1 ± 0.09 vs 2 ± 0.3 respectively; $p < 0.02$). Postoperative pyrexia was similar among the groups (37.9 ± 0.1°C for minilaparotomy vs 37.7 ± 0.08°C for video-assisted minilaparotomy vs 38 ± 0.2°C for laparotomy; NS). Persistence of fever was longer for laparotomy than for video-assisted minilaparotomy (87.4 ± 17.1 hours vs 42.4 ± 9.7 hours respectively; $p < 0.05$). Video-assisted minilaparotomy also resulted in a time of canalization shorter than that of laparotomy (32.6 ± 3.4 hours vs 47 ± 6.1 hours respectively; $p < 0.05$) and a time of dimission shorter than both laparotomy and minilaparotomy (79.9 ± 7.7 hours vs 165.1 ± 5.9 hours vs 117.4 ± 10.8 hours respectively; $p < 0.0001$). After laparotomy, the net change of hematocrit was greater than that after assisted and non-assisted minilaparotomy, and this was statistically significant at time 24 hours ($-9.1 \pm 1.5\%$ vs $-5.3 \pm 0.5\%$ vs $-5.6 \pm 0.9\%$; $p < 0.02$) and 48 hours ($-9.8 \pm 0.9\%$ vs $-6.1 \pm 0.7\%$ vs $-7.5 \pm 1.2\%$; $p < 0.05$). These data show that in women with one myoma less than 8 cm of diameter or with 2–5 myomas with a diameter less than 16 cm, in comparison with laparotomy, myomectomy in video-assisted minilaparotomy offers several advantages. We think that these data cannot be applied to myomas of greater volume or higher number. Consequently, accurate preoperative screening to determine the number and size of myomas is important to choose on an individual basis the approach that best suits the surgeon's capacities and to guarantee a better outcome for the woman.

References

1. Friedman AJ. The role of leuprorelin in treating leiomyomas: a critical review. *Hormonal Therapy in Obstet and Gynecol* 1998;3:22–6
2. Vermesh M, Silva PD, Rosen GF, *et al.* Management of unruptured ectopic gestation by linear salpingostomy: a prospective, randomized clinical trial of laparoscopy versus laparotomy. *Obstet Gynecol* 1989;73:400–4
3. McMahon AJ, Russell IT, Baxter JN, *et al.* Laparoscopic versus minilaparotomy cholecystectomy: a randomised trial. *Lancet* 1994;343: 135–8
4. Stoker DL, Spiegelhalter DJ, Singh R, *et al.* Laparoscopic versus open inguinal hernia repair: randomised prospective trial. *Lancet* 1994;343:1243–5

5. Pelosi M, Pelosi MA. Spontaneous uterine rupture at thirty-three weeks subsequent to previous superficial laparoscopic myomectomy. *Am J Obstet Gynecol* 1997;177:1547–9

6. Friedmann W, Maier RF, Luttkus A, *et al*. Uterine rupture after laparoscopic myomectomy. *Acta Obstet Gynecol Scand* 1996;75:683–4

7. Dubuisson JB, Chavet X, Chapron C, *et al*. Uterine rupture during pregnancy after laparoscopic myomectomy. *Hum Reprod* 1995; 10:1475–7

8. Harris WJ. Uterine dehiscence following laparoscopic myomectomy. *Obstet Gynecol* 1992; 80:545–6

9. Verkauf BS. Myomectomy for fertility enhancement and preservation. *Fertil Steril* 1992;58:1–15

10. Daniell JF, Gurley LD. Laparoscopic treatment of clinically significant symptomatic uterine fibroids. *J Gynecol Surg* 1991;7:37–40

11. Dubuisson JB, Lecuru F, Foulot H, *et al*. Myomectomy by laparoscopy: a preliminary report of 43 cases. *Fertil Steril* 1991;56:827–30

12. Nezhat C, Nezhat F, Silfen SL, *et al*. Laparoscopic myomectomy. *Int J Fertil* 1991;36:275–80

13. Hasson HM, Rotman C, Rana N, *et al*. Laparoscopic myomectomy. *Obstet Gynecol* 1992;80: 884–8

14. Semm K. New methods of pelviscopy (gynecologic laparoscopy) for myomectomy, ovariectomy, tubectomy and adnectomy. *Endoscopy* 1979;11:85–93

15. Semm K, Mettler L. Technical progress in pelvic surgery via operative laparoscopy. *Am J Obstet Gynecol* 1980;138:121–7

16. Mettler L, Semm K. Pelviscopic uterine surgery. *Surg Endosc* 1992;6:23–31

17. Silva BA, Falcone T, Bradley L, *et al*. Case-control study of laparoscopic versus abdominal myomectomy. *J Laparoendosc Adv Surg Tech A* 2000;10(4):191–7

18. Nezhat CR, Nezhat F, Bess O, *et al*. Laparoscopically assisted myomectomy: a report of a new technique in 57 cases. *Int J Fertil Stud* 1994;39:39

19. Mais V, Ajossa S, Guerriero S, *et al*. Laparoscopic versus abdominal myomectomy: a prospective, randomized trial to evaluate benefits in early outcome. *Am J Obstet Gynecol* 1996;174: 654–8

Regulation of fetal allograft survival by hormone-controlled T cell cytokines

27

M.-P. Piccinni, G. Scarselli, C. Scaletti,
A. Vultaggio, E. Maggi and S. Romagnani

Introduction

Despite the fact that the embryo is considered an allograft because of paternal major histocompatibility complex (MHC) antigens, and represents a potential target for the maternal immune system, it is not rejected. This suggests that a maternal immunological tolerance of the conceptus occurs. Some recent findings support a central role for T cell derived cytokines in the regulation of both fetal allograft survival and fetal rejection.

Role of Th1 and Th2 cells in fetal allograft survival

Human activated CD4[+] T cells can be classified on the basis of their pattern of cytokine production[1,2]. Type 1 CD4[+] T cells (Th 1) produce interleukin (IL)-2, tumor necrosis factor (TNF)-β and interferon (IFN)-γ and are the main effectors of phagocyte-mediated host defense, which is highly protective against infections sustained by intracellular parasites[1,2]. On the other hand, type 2 CD4[+] T cells (Th2) produce IL-4, which stimulates Immunoglobulin E (IgE) and IgG1 antibody production, IL-5 (promoting the growth and differentiation of eosinophils), and IL-13 and IL-10 which together with IL-4 inhibit several macrophage functions. The Th2 cell is mainly responsible for phagocyte-independent host defense, e.g. against certains nematodes[1,2].

The development of Th1- and Th2-type responses depends on several factors. Some of these factors are hormones. Progesterone, which acts in the preparation of endometrium for implantation at concentrations comparable to those present at the materno-fetal interface during pregnancy, is a potent inducer of production of Th2-type cytokines (i.e. IL-4 and IL-5)[3]. Another candidate hormone involved in the modulation of T helper cell function is relaxin, a polypeptide hormone predominantly produced by the corpus luteum and decidua during pregnancy. Recently, we showed that relaxin favors the development of T cells producing IFN-γ, without exerting any effect on the production of IL-4[4]. Relaxin may counterbalance the Th2-inducing activity of progesterone.

It appears that some Th1-dependent effector mechanisms, such as delayed-type hypersensitivity and cytotoxic T lymphocyte activity, play a central role in acute allograft rejection[5,6]. Since Th1-type cytokines promote allograft rejection and therefore may compromise pregnancy, the production at the feto-maternal interface level of Th2-type cytokines, which inhibit the Th1 responses, may improve fetal survival. There is clear evidence to suggest that maternal T lymphocytes at the feto-maternal interface play an important role in fetal survival and development. In mice, it has been reported that Th2-type cytokines IL-4, IL-5 and IL-10 are detectable at the feto-maternal interface during the whole period of gestation, whereas IFN-γ is transient, being detectable only in the first period[7]. Based on these findings, the existence of a bidirectional interaction between the maternal immune system and the reproductive system during pregnancy was hypothesized[8]. In humans, we recently showed that at the feto-maternal interface, maintenance of pregnancy is associated with IL-4 and IL-10 production by decidual T cells[9,10].

Role of leukemia inhibitory factor in successful embryo implantation and embryo development

Studies in mice suggest that the production of Leukemia inhibitory factor (LIF) is an endometrial requirement for implantation and embryo development, inasmuch as female mice lacking a functional *LIF* gene are fertile but their blastocysts fail to implant and do not develop unless the blastocysts are transferred to wild-type pseudopregnant recipients or the animals are treated locally with LIF[11].

In endometrium, besides the endometrial epithelial and stromal cells that produce LIF, LIF mRNA was detected in decidual natural killer (NK) cells and T cells[12]. Recently, we found that LIF production is mainly a property of Th2-like cells[9]. We also showed that the development of LIF-producing T cells was down- regulated by Th1 inducers, IL-12, IFN-α and IFN-γ, and up-regulated by IL-4 and progesterone[9], a hormone which promotes the differentiation of T cells into Th2 effectors[3]. Blastocysts showed the presence of mRNA for LIF β receptor mRNA[13], suggesting that it may be capable of responding to LIF stimulus at the appropriate timing for implantation.

Finally and more importantly, a concomitant defect of both LIF, IL-4 and IL-10 production was observed in decidual T cells of women suffering from unexplained recurrent abortion and undergoing spontaneous abortion during the first trimester of pregnancy, in comparison with the decidual T cells of women with normal pregnancy who underwent a voluntary abortion[9,10]. Of note is that the reduced production of LIF, IL-4 and IL-10 in women suffering from unexplained recurrent abortion was not observed at the level of peripheral blood, suggesting that this is not an inherent feature of T cells, but rather a microenvironmentally generated alteration.

Conclusions

Based on all these findings, we suggest that a hormonal–cytokine network at the level of the materno-fetal interface plays an important role in both blastocyst implantation and maintenance of successful pregnancy.

Progesterone may be at least in part responsible for a Th2 switch at the feto-maternal interface. IL-4 produced by Th2 cells can in turn promote the development of T cells producing LIF, which seems to be essential for embryo implantation and development. Both IL-4 and IL-10 can inhibit the development and function of Th1 cells and macrophages, thus preventing allograft rejection. In addition, IL-10 produced by the Th2 cells, inducing histocompatibility leukocyte antigen-group G (HLA-G) expression on human trophoblast could also play a role in protecting the fetus by inhibiting its lysis by maternal NK cells[14]. A defect in the integrity of this network may result in fetal loss.

Relaxin, rather, may counterbalance the Th2-inducing activity of progesterone and promote an adequate Th1 response when the latter could be required to protect the mother against dangerous intracellular pathogens. However, IFN-γ production induced by relaxin could also enhance the expression of HLA-G by trophoblast and down-regulate maternal NK cells' cytotoxic activity against the trophoblast[15]. IFN-γ could also induce the expression of indoleamine 2,3-dioxygenase by macrophages at the feto-maternal interface; thus IFN-γ could prevent the immunological rejection of the fetal allograft by suppressing T cell activity[16].

A direct cause-and-effect relationship between a local defect of Th2-type cytokine (IL-4 and IL-10) and LIF expression by T cells and pregnancy loss has been found, and hormonal influences seem to play a critical role in determining the T cell cytokine pattern[17–19].

References

1. Mosmann TR, Coffman RL. Th1 and Th2 cells: different patterns of lymphokine secretion lead to different functional properties. *Annu Rev Immunol* 1989;7:145–73
2. Romagnani S. Human Th1 and Th2: doubt no more. *Immunol Today* 1991;12:256–7
3. Piccinni M-P, Giudizi MG, Biagiotti R, *et al*. Progesterone favors the development of human T helper cells producing Th2-type cytokines and promotes both IL-4 production and membrane CD30 expression in established Th1 cells clones. *J Immunol* 1995;155:128–33
4. Piccinni M-P, Bani D, Beloni L, *et al*. Relaxin favors the development of activated human T cells into Th1-like effectors. *Eur J Immunol* 1999;29:2241–7
5. Suthanthiran M, Strom TB. Immunobiology and immunopharmacology of organ allograft rejection. *J Clin Immunol* 1995;15:161–71
6. Nickerson P, Steurer W, Steiger J, *et al*. Cytokines and the Th1/Th2 paradigm in transplantation. *Curr Opin Immunol* 1994;6:757–64
7. Lin H, Mosmann TR, Guilbert L, *et al*. Synthesis of T helper 2-type cytokines at maternal-fetal interface. *J Immunol* 1993;151:4562–73
8. Wegmann TG, Lin H, Guilbert L, *et al*. Bidirectional cytokine interactions in the maternal-fetal relationship: is successful pregnancy a Th2 phenomenon? *Immunol Today* 1993;14:353–6
9. Piccinni M-P, Beloni L, Livi C, *et al*. Defective production of both leukemia inhibitory factor and type 2 T-helper cytokines by decidual T cells in unexplained recurrent abortions. *Nat Med* 1998;4:1020–4
10. Piccinni M-P, Beloni L, Livi C, *et al*. The maintenance of pregnancy is associated with predominance of Th2 type-cytokines. In Colarcurci N, Cardone A, eds. *The Embryo from Gametogenesis to Implantation*. Naples: Giuseppe Nicola 1998:177–180
11. Stewart CL, Kaspar P, Brunet LJ, *et al*. Blastocyst implantation depends on maternal expression of leukemia inhibitory factor. *Nature* 1992;359:76–9
12. Jokhi PP, King A, Sharkey AM, *et al*. Screening of cytokine messenger ribonucleic acids in purified human decidual lymphocyte populations by the reverse-transcriptase polymerase chain reaction. *J Immunol* 1994;153:4427–35
13. Eckert J, Niemann H. mRNA expression of leukemia inhibitory factor (LIF) and its receptor subunits glycoprotein 130 and LIF-receptor-beta in bovine embryos derived *in vitro* or *in vivo*. *Mol Hum Reprod* 1998;4:957–65
14. Moreau P, Adrian-Cabestre F, Menier C, *et al*. IL-10 selectively induces HLA-G expression in human trophoblasts and monocytes. *Int Immunol* 1999;11:803–11
15. Lefebvre S, Moreau P, Guiard V, *et al*. Molecular mechanisms controlling constitutive and IFN-gamma-inducible HLA-G expression in various cell types. *J Reprod Immunol* 1999;43:213–24
16. Munn DH, Zhou M, Attwood JT, *et al*. Prevention of allogeneic fetal rejection by tryptophan catabolism. *Science* 1998;281:1191–3
17. Piccinni M-P, Romagnani S. Regulation of fetal allograft survival by hormone-controlled Th1- and Th2-type cytokines. *Immunol Res* 1996;15:141–50
18. Piccinni M-P, Maggi E, Romagnani S. Role of hormone-controlled T-cell cytokines in the maintenance of pregnancy. *Biochem Soc Trans* 2000;28:212–15
19. Piccinni M-P, Scaletti C, Maggi E, *et al*. Role of hormone-controlled Th1- and Th2-type cytokines in successful pregnancy. *J Neuroimmunol* 2000;109:30–3

Subset distribution and proliferative response of peripheral blood T cells from patients with recurrent spontaneous abortion

28

M. Massobrio, G. Menato, P. Castagna, V. Redoglia and F. Andresini

Introduction

Recurrent spontaneous abortion (RSA) is an infertility disease defined as three or more consecutive spontaneous miscarriages occurring within 20 weeks of gestation, with the same partner; it occurs in 1% of women. It is associated with a number of conditions: parental chromosomal anomalies (2.6–4%), anatomical factors (15–28%), endocrinological diseases (20%) and autoimmune problems (20%), but 50–60% of cases of RSA are clinically unexplained[1–3].

Pregnancy seems to modify the responsiveness of the immune system, with a decrease of maternal cell-mediated responses and an increase of humoral responses. These alterations are characterized by a shift of the T helper (Th) cell response from a Th1 to a Th2 response[4]. It has been suggested that the Th2-type cytokines may have a protective effect in fetal development, whereas Th1 cytokines have a negative effect[5–7].

Materials and methods

The aim of this study was to investigate subset distribution and the proliferative response of peripheral blood T cells in a group of pregnant women who had experienced previous unexplained RSA, and compare the findings with those of a control group of normal pregnant women.

Case/control selection

In the period January 1998 to June 2000, in the RSA-Ambulatory section of the Department of Obstetrics and Gynecology of the University of Turin, Italy, we observed 68 couples who underwent complete diagnostic assesments: hematological, immunological and endocrine assessments, a search of genetic disorders, vaginal infections and anatomical defects, and an examination of spermatic fluid. A total of 37 couples (54%) were considered to be affected by unexplained RSA, being negative to all assessments. A total of 20 patients entered this study following these selection criteria:

(1) Age ≤ 35 years;

(2) Negative to all diagnostic assessments;

(3) At least two spontaneous abortions within the first trimester;

(4) Between the 5th and 10th weeks of pregnancy;

(5) Not receiving drugs before or during gestation.

The criteria for the controls (*n* = 30) were:

(1) Age ≤ 35 years;

(2) No previous autoimmune diseases or any particular pathology;

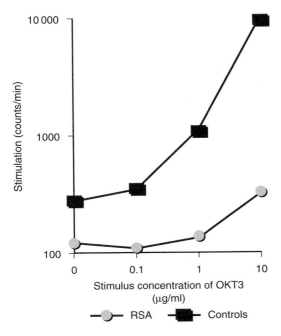

Figure 1 T-cell proliferative analysis in recurrent spontaneous abortion patients ($n = 20$) and a control group ($n = 30$). Stimulation is represented by an anti-CD3 monoclonal antibody (OKT3)

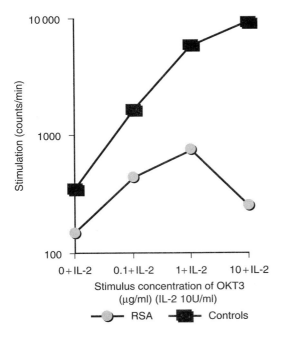

Figure 2 T-cell proliferative stimulation represented by an anti-CD3 monoclonal antibody (OKT3) + interleukin (IL)-2

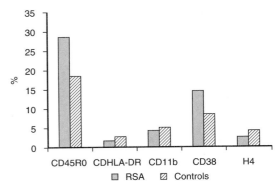

Figure 3 T-cell phenotypic analysis in recurrent spontaneous abortion patients ($n = 20$) and a control group ($n = 30$). Values are expressed as percentages of the indicated population of CD4$^+$ T cells. Differences: NS

(3) Number of successful pregnancies ≥ 1, without any previous miscarriage;

(4) Between the 5th and 10th weeks of gestation;

(5) Not receiving drugs before or during pregnancy.

Both groups were evaluated between the 7th and 10th weeks of pregnancy with a single blood sample. The clinical characteristics of RSA patients and controls were: mean age; 30.3 years (RSA) and 31.6 years (controls); abortions for RSA patients, mean 3.17 (range 2–5; pregnancies for controls, mean 1.2 (range 1–2); gestational age at evaluation, 6 weeks + 4 days (RSA) and 7 weeks + 1 day (controls).

T-cell studies

T cells from RSA patients and controls were analyzed phenotypically in both CD4$^+$ and CD8$^+$ populations by a monoclonal antibody (mAb) panel including resting/naive (CD45RA$^+$) and memory/recently activated (CD45R0$^+$) molecules and activation molecules (CD11b, CD25, CD30, CD38, CD69, HLA-DR and H4). After incubation, washing and fixation, the cells underwent cytofluorimetric analysis. The functional analyses were performed by *in vitro* stimulation with anti-CD3 antibodies, interleukin (IL)-2 and phyto-hemagglutinin (PHA) and measured by ^{3}H-Tdr incorporation.

Results and conclusions

The phenotypic analysis revealed that total leukocyte count and CD3$^+$ cell percentage were similar in the two groups. By contrast, the proportion of CD4$^+$ cells was significantly increased in RSA patients (RSA median 45.7%, range 30–55% vs. control median 24.8%, range 5.3–39%; $p < 0.0001$). Moreover, in CD4$^+$ T cells, RSA patients displayed a lower expression of HLA-DR, CD11b and H4, and a higher expression of CD45R0 and CD38 than did normal pregnant women, but the differences were only marginally significant. In CD8$^+$ T cells, both groups of women displayed a striking expression of CD11b$^+$ cells (100%), whereas the RSA women displayed a higher expression of HLA-DR and CD38 than normal pregnant women. Preliminary experiments assessing the proliferative response of peripheral blood T cells suggested that T cells from RSA patients displayed a decreased response to anti-CD3 mAb and to anti-CD3 + IL-2, but a normal response to PHA (Figures 1 and 2). These data show that RSA patients showed a T-cell pattern that was different from that displayed by normal pregnant women, which suggests that the immune system may play a role in RSA.

Considering that RSA is an uncommon pathology and that the number of cases we observed was quite limited, it is remarkable that the CD4$^+$ increase in RSA patients was so strongly statistically significant ($p < 0.0001$). The differences in other antigens can only be considered as a trend. Within the CD4$^+$ population, RSA patients showed a decrease of HLA-DR$^+$, CD11b$^+$ and H4$^+$ cells with an increase in CD45R0 and CD38 proportions, suggesting an anergic-like phenotype (Figure 3). These data are supported by functional experiments showing a decreased *in vitro* response to anti-CD3 mAb.

The evaluation of pregnancy evolution in RSA patients and controls showed a different percentage of miscarriage: 40% vs. 10% of abortions, respectively, in the new pregnancy.

Functional analysis of the T-cell subsets expanded in RSA patients may help, in the future, to elucidate the pathogenesis of RSA. The future perspectives of this study are: to assess the T-cell subset expanded; to evaluate the possible correlation between the T-cell pattern and pregnancy evolution in order to derive novel prognostic tools useful in the management of these patients; to analyze the same parameters in non-pregnant RSA patients; and to evaluate a possible immuno-regulatory role of therapy.

References

1. Plouffe L, White EW, Tho SP, *et al.* Etiologic factors of recurrent abortion and subsequent reproductive performance of couples: have we made any progress in the past 10 years? *Am J Obstet Gynecol* 1992;167:313–21
2. Clifford K, Rai R, Watson H, *et al.* An informative protocol for the investigation of recurrent miscarriage: preliminary experience of 500 consecutive cases. *Hum Reprod* 1994;9:1328–32
3. Stephenson MD. Frequency of factors associated with habitual abortion in 197 couples. *Fertil Steril* 1996;66:24–9
4. Lin H, Mosmann TR, Guilbert L, *et al.* Synthesis of T helper 2-type cytokines at the maternal–fetal interface. *J Immunol* 1993;151: 4562–73
5. Wegmann TG, Lin H, Guilbert L, *et al.* Bidirectional cytokine interactions in the maternal–fetal relationship: is successful pregnancy a Th2 phenomenon? *Immunol Today* 1993; 14:353–6
6. Hill JA, Polgar K, Anderson DJ. T helper 1-type immunity to trophoblast in women with recurrent spontaneous abortion. *J Am Med Assoc* 1995; 273:1933–6
7. Ragupathy R. Th1-type immunity is incompatible with successful pregnancy. *Immunol Today* 1997; 18:478–82

Early pregnancy-promoting actions of luteinizing hormone and human chorionic gonadotropin

29

Z. M. Lei and Ch. V. Rao

Introduction

Early pregnancy represents an extremely complex chain of events that include gamete maturation, fertilization, early embryonic growth and development, implantation, placentation and pregnancy maintenance. Coordinated actions of various hormones on the reproductive tract as well as on the pre-implantation embryo are essential. It is well known that luteinizing hormone (LH) and human chorionic gonadotropin (hCG) bind to their ovarian receptors to stimulate the synthesis of steroid hormones, which in turn play critical roles during early pregnancy. It was not clear until recently whether LH and hCG were also directly involved. Recent demonstration of LH/hCG receptors in gametes, preimplantation embryos, fallopian tubes, uterus, placenta, lymphocytes, monocytes and macrophages has raised this possibility[1-7]. There are now considerable *in vitro* and *in vivo* data which suggest that direct LH and hCG actions on non-gonadal tissues are important in early pregnancy. Elucidating these actions will have applications for improving pregnancy rates in assisted reproductive technologies, developing newer therapies against early pregnancy complications and devising new strategies for contraception. A comprehensive review on potential novel roles of LH and hCG during early pregnancy has been published[4]. Since then, substantial progress has been made and this article summarizes the progress.

LH/hCG receptors in non-gonadal tissues

A variety of studies indicate that a number of non-gonadal tissues, in addition to gonads, contain LH/hCG receptors. These include gametes, early embryo, oviduct, uterus, cervix, placenta, fetal membrane, umbilical cord, brain, spinal cord, neural retina, skin, breast, zona reticularis of adrenal cortex, urinary bladder, blood vessels in target tissues, cavernous sinus carotid rete complex, T-lymphocyte, monocyte and macrophage[1-9]. There are also many tissues that are receptor-negative: lung, liver, kidney, smooth muscle, heart and spleen. The presence of LH/hCG receptors in non-gonadal tissues was widely seen across species which include human, baboon, cattle, sheep, pig, rat, rabbit, mouse and turkey[4-10].

Receptors in non-gonadal tissues have been detected by multiple techniques such as reverse transcriptase–polymerase chain reaction, Northern blotting, Western blotting, ligand blotting, covalent receptor cross-linking, ligand binding, *in situ* hybridization, immunocytochemistry, gene transfections and laser scanning confocal microscopy[1-13]. Not all the techniques were used on all the tissues; however, more than one was used in most cases, which eliminated the possibility of a methodological artifact being responsible for the presence of receptors in non-gonadal tissues. While *cis*-acting elements are the same, *trans*-acting factors are different not only between gonadal and non-gonadal tissues, but also

185

between various non-gonadal tissues and cells[11–13]. As in gonads, non-gonadal LH/hCG receptors are subjected to both homologous and heterologous hormone regulation[14–16].

Receptor levels in non-gonadal tissues are usually much lower than in gonadal tissues. However, like gonadal tissues, all non-gonadal target tissues contain multiple receptor transcripts and usually a single receptor protein. Even though receptor processing may appear similar between gonadal and non-gonadal tissues, sequencing different LH/hCG receptor transcripts revealed that it is different between non-gonadal and gonadal tissues[10].

Non-gonadal, like gonadal LH/hCG receptors, can activate two signaling pathways[4–7,14,17]. The first is cyclic adenosine monophosphate (AMP)/protein kinase A and the second is protein kinase C. A recent study on regulation of the indoleamine 2,3-dioxygenase (IDO) gene expression in syncytiotrophoblasts by hCG revealed that hCG can also utilize the mitogen activated protein (MAP) kinase pathway, independent of protein kinase A signaling[18]. Activation of MAP kinase signaling pathway by hCG was also reported in baboon endometrial stromal cells[19].

LH/hCG effects on fertilization and early embryonic growth and development

Oviductal glycoprotein (OGP) is one of the best characterized proteins secreted by oviductal epithelium. It promotes gamete maturation, fertilization, and early embryonic growth and development[20]. Through their receptors in oviductal epithelium, LH and hCG can increase OGP synthesis by decreasing degradation of its transcripts[21]. These observations suggest that LH/hCG receptors in oviductal epithelium may be involved in promoting the early pregnancy events. These possibilities were tested in co-culture experiments with bovine oviductal epithelial cells, spermatozoa or early bovine embryos. These experiments revealed that sperm rapidly bind to oviductal epithelial cells, then are gradually released. This release is stimulated by both LH and

hCG, but not by thyroid-stimulating hormone or follicle-stimulating hormone[22]. These findings suggest that LH/hCG may act on oviductal epithelium and/or on sperm, so that they are released and available for fertilization of oocytes. In co-culture experiments with early bovine embryos, LH and hCG can stimulate their development into blastocysts in a dose- and time-dependent and hormone-specific manner[23]. This effect is mediated by OGP, as inhibition of OGP synthesis cells can prevent LH and hCG actions[23].

The presence of LH/hCG receptors in pre-implantation embryos suggests that LH and hCG can influence their growth and development[1,2]. Ji and Bavister[24] demonstrated that LH can enhance early stages of hamster embryonic growth to morulae and blastocysts.

One major oviductal function is to transport gametes to the ampullary–isthmic junction, the site of fertilization and transport of embryos to the uterus. Given the presence of LH/hCG receptors in oviductal smooth muscle[21,25] and the fact that LH/hCG can cause oviductal relaxation, especially during the periovulatory period[26], the LH/hCG effect on oviductal relaxation could be physiologically important in opening the ampullary–isthmic junction for ascent of spermatozoa, fertilization of gametes and exit of early embryo to the uterus. The LH/hCG effect could be mediated by increasing oviductal PGE_2 synthesis[27].

The pre-ovulatory LH surge could be a main source of hormone that can directly act on the oviduct by an endocrine mechanism. Another potential source is hCG made by oviductal epithelium[25]. The ectopic site of hCG synthesis in human tubal epithelium is found to be up-regulated by ovarian steroid hormones and down-regulated by LH and hCG[28]. After fertilization, embryos could become a major source as hCG can be detected as early as the 6-cell stage[2,29,30].

hCG effects on implantation and placentation

Implantation is a critical event that determines whether pregnancy succeeds. In recent years, it has become clear that cross-talk between the active blastocyst and receptive uterus is essential for implantation. hCG as an embryonic signal that promotes uterine receptivity has been described extensively[4–7]. A number of *in vitro* studies on human and animal uteri have shown that hCG can directly act on luminal and glandular epithelium and stromal cells of endometrium, and myometrial smooth muscle. Stimulation of stromal cell decidualization and proliferation of myometrial smooth muscle by hCG have been well-documented[4–7,31]. hCG can influence a broad spectrum of biochemical and molecular signals required for implantation and placentation. For instance, hCG can regulate the expression of endometrial cyclooxygenase-2[19,32,33], prolactin[34], insulin-like growth factor binding protein-1 (IGFBP-1)[35], leukemia inhibitory factor (LIF)[36], interleukin-6 (IL-6)[36,37], tumor necrosis factor-α (TNF-α)[37] and Fas ligand[38]. Many of these molecules are known to function as maternal signals to regulate implantation and placentation[39–41].

Several recent *in vivo* studies have further demonstrated the direct hCG actions on uterine receptivity. Infusion of hCG into oviducts of cycling and ovariectomized baboons in a manner that mimics blastocyst transit results in morphological and biochemical changes in all three major endometrial cell types[42]. Changes include an increase in cell proliferation, height of luminal epithelium, expression of α-smooth muscle actin, a marker of initiation of decidualization, and up-regulation of glycodelin, a secretory protein of glandular epithelial cells.

To avoid confounding indirect effects through increasing ovarian steroid hormone synthesis, hCG was administered systemically into healthy young women with inactive or absent ovaries[43]. It resulted in morphological transformation of endometrium into a decidual phenotype. Endometrial score values were consistently higher in hCG-treated cycles than in control cycles.

Direct hCG effects on biochemical changes in the uterine microenvironment were determined by an intrauterine microdialysis system to locally apply low hCG concentrations to the endometrium of women during the luteal phase of the menstrual cycle[44]. Consistent with previous observations, hCG induced pronounced changes in levels of IGFBP-1, prolactin, LIF, macrophage colony stimulating factor, vascular endothelial growth factor and matrix metalloproteinase-9[44].

hCG can influence placentation. It has been well-established that hCG can regulate its own synthesis and enhance cytotrophoblast differentiation[45]. Recent studies have demonstrated that hCG is also involved in promoting extravillous trophoblast invasion into the uterine wall, at least in part, by up-regulating trophoblast insulin-like growth factor II (IGF-II) receptors[46–48].

hCG effects on pregnancy maintenance

The ability to maintain myometrial quiescence is essential for completion of pregnancy. Previous studies have demonstrated that human myometrium contains LH/hCG receptors and hCG suppresses myometrial contractions by up-regulation of G protein subunit Gαs, down-regulation of gap junctions and decreasing intracellular Ca^{2+} levels[4–7,49]. These findings suggest that hCG could be involved in maintaining myometrial quiescence. A recent study tested whether hCG can fulfill this role *in vivo* by measuring myometrial contractions in response to intrauterine instillation of prostaglandin E_2 or $F_{2\alpha}$ and hCG in healthy non-pregnant women[50]. Results showed that prostaglandins markedly stimulated the amplitude and frequency of contractions and hCG inhibited them.

These studies suggest that hCG could be used as a tocolytic agent. In fact, this possibility was tested in a preterm labor mice model. In this model, a single intraperitoneal prostaglandin $F_{2\alpha}$ injection at day 16 of pregnancy resulted in labor and delivery in 100% of the mice within 24 hours, and it was prevented by the hCG treatment[51]. hCG appears to work by down-regulating myometrial gap junctions[52].

hCG effects on immunosuppression

The issue of maternal acceptance of the antigenically foreign embryo leading to successful pregnancy has long been a riddle. Several previous studies suggested that hCG regulates the immune system by an unknown mechanism. There were inconsistent reports on immunoregulatory roles of hCG[53,54]. The findings that lymphocytes[55], monocytes[56], macrophages[57], trophoblasts[45] and endometrium[58] contain LH/hCG receptors rekindled the interest in determining whether hCG is a fetal factor that contributes to maternal tolerance of the fetal graft.

Recent studies demonstrated that hCG suppresses IL-2 and oncostatin M secretion from phytohemagglutinin-activated peripheral blood mononuclear cells[59,60], and increases mRNA levels of monocyte chemoattractant protein-1 in the interferon-γ stimulated human monocytic cell line THP-1[57]. hCG also directly acts on endometrium to stimulate a pro-implantation cytokine, LIF, and inhibit a pro-inflammatory cytokine, IL-6[36]. These data suggest that hCG suppression of cell-mediated allogeneic reaction during early pregnancy may involve differential regulation of maternal cytokine production to favor a continuation of pregnancy. IDO is an inducible enzyme that catalyzes the rate-limiting step in tryptophan degradation. Its activity is closely related to T-lymphocyte tolerance, and is necessary to maintain effective immunological protection during gestation[61]. Syncytiotrophoblasts contain high IDO levels. Treatment of human syncytiotrophoblasts with hCG resulted in a dose- and time-dependent and hormone-specific increase in mRNA and protein levels and enzyme activity of IDO[18]. Moreover, hCG reduced a cytotoxic effect on syncytiotrophoblasts when they were co-cultured with allogenic lymphocytes, and this protective hCG effect was blocked by the specific IDO inhibitor addition[18]. These results suggest that hCG has immunoregulatory functions to prevent fetal rejection by promoting tryptophan breakdown at the fetomaternal interface.

hCG effects on blood vessels

Endothelial cells and smooth muscle of uterine, placental, umbilical and gonadal blood vessels contain LH/hCG receptors[4-7]. Regulation of uterine blood flow by hCG in laboratory animals and in women has been well demonstrated[4-7]. Recent studies indicated that the response of rat uterine vasculature to hCG depended on cycle day and pregnancy as well as the route of administration[62,63]. Vasodilation stimulated by hCG can occur in the absence of vascular endothelium, suggesting a direct action on smooth muscle[63]. Endothelial LH/hCG receptors also serve as a specific transcytotic carrier of its ligands across the endothelial barrier[64] and in vasculo- and angiogenesis through regulation of relevant cytokine synthesis[65].

The clinical importance of hCG in regulating uterine blood flow was investigated in women who showed signs of threatened abortion at six to eight weeks of gestation[66]. The abortion rate in patients given hCG and magnesium was significantly lower than in those patients treated with magnesium alone. The hCG- and magnesium-treated patients showed a decreased uterine arterial resistance index as measured by intravaginal pulsed Doppler probe. This decrease was not correlated with any changes in ovarian steroid hormone levels. Improved utero-placental perfusion could be one of the mechanisms to explain the beneficial hCG effect in the treatment of threatened and habitual abortions.

Conclusions and perspectives

LH and hCG play many critical roles during early pregnancy through both direct actions on gametes and the reproductive tract as well as indirect actions through increasing gonadal steroid synthesis. The direct actions include promoting gamete maturation, fertilization, early embryonic growth and development, implantation, placentation, protection from maternal rejection of the fetus and pregnancy maintenance. These findings suggest several potential clinical uses of hCG.

These may range from enhancement of early embryonic quality, increasing pregnancy rates, treatment of threatened and habitual abortions and the prevention of pre-term labor and delivery. Recently, targeted disruption of the LH/hCG receptor gene was accomplished[67]. Null animals are infertile with a dramatic underdevelopment of the reproductive tract organs. These animals are expected to be very useful in determining the importance of non-gonadal LH signaling in the body.

References

1. Mishra S, Lei ZM, Rao ChV. Bovine oocytes and early embryos contain luteinizing hormone/human chorionic gonadotropin receptors. Presented at the *Endocrine Society Annual Meeting*, Toronto, Canada 2000;abstr. 1335

2. Mishra S, Lin PC, Lei ZM, *et al.* Evidence for the presence of human chorionic gonadotropin/luteinizing hormone receptors in human oocytes and early embryos. *J Soc Gynecol Invest* 2000;7(Suppl.):abstr. 576

3. Eblen A, Bao S, Lei ZM, *et al.* Human sperm contains luteinizing hormone and chorionic gonadotropin receptors. *J Soc Gynecol Invest* 1998;5(Suppl.):abstr. F278

4. Rao ChV. The beginning of a new era in reproductive biology and medicine: expression of low levels of functional luteinizing hormone/human chorionic gonadotropin receptors in nongonadal tissues. *J Physiol Pharmacol* 1996;47:41–53

5. Rao ChV. Potential novel roles of luteinizing hormone and human chorionic gonadotropin during early pregnancy in women. *Early Pregnancy: Biology and Medicine* 1997;3:1–9

6. Rao ChV. Novel concepts in neuroendocrine regulation of reproductive tract functions. In Bazer FW, ed. *The Endocrinology of Pregnancy*. New Jersey: Humana Press, 1998:125–144

7. Rao ChV. A paradigm shift on the targets of luteinizing hormone/human chorionic gonadotropin actions in the body. *The Journal of the Bellevue Obstetrical & Gynecological Society* 1999; XV:26–32

8. Skipor J, Bao S, Grzegorzewski W, *et al.* The inhibitory effect of hCG on counter current transfer of GnRH and the presence of LH/hCG receptors in the perihypophyseal cavernous sinus-carotid rete vascular complex of ewes. *Theriogenology* 1999;51:899–910

9. Zheng M, Shi H, Segaloff DL, *et al.* Luteinizing hormone receptor (LHR) binding and localization in the mouse reproductive tract. *J Soc Gynecol Invest* 2000;7(Suppl. 1):abstr. 622

10. You S, Kim H, Hsu C-C, *et al.* Three different turkey luteinizing hormone receptor (tLH-R) isoforms I: characterization of alternatively spliced tLH-R isoforms and their regulated expression in diverse tissues. *Biol Reprod* 2000;62:108–16

11. Hu Y, Lei ZM, Rao ChV. *Cis*-acting elements and *trans*-acting proteins in the transcription of chorionic gonadotropin/luteinizing hormone receptor gene in choriocarcinoma cells and placenta. *Endocrinology* 1996;137:3897–905

12. Hu YL, Lei ZM, Rao ChV. Analysis of the promoter of luteinizing hormone/human chorionic gonadotropin receptor gene in neuroendocrine cells. *Life Sci* 1998;63:2157–65

13. Hu YL, Lei ZM, Huang ZH, *et al.* Determinants of transcription of the chorionic gonadotropin/luteinizing hormone receptor gene in human breast cells. *Breast J* 1999;5:186–93

14. Dufau ML. The luteinizing hormone receptor. *Annu Rev Physiol* 1998;60:461–96

15. Han SW, Lei ZM, Rao ChV. Homologous down-regulation of luteinizing hormone/chorionic gonadotropin receptors by increasing the degradation of receptor transcripts in human uterine endometrial stromal cells. *Biol Reprod* 1997;57:158–64

16. Gawronska B, Stepien A, Ziecik AJ. Effect of estradiol and progesterone on oviductal LH-receptors and LH-dependent relaxation of the porcine oviduct. *Theriogenology* 2000;53:659–72

17. Kisielewska J, Flint APF, Ziecik AJ. Phospholipase C and adenylate cyclase signaling systems in the action of hCG on porcine myometrial smooth muscle cells. *J Endocrinol* 1996;148:175–80

18. Lei ZM, Rao ChV. The immunoprotective role of human chorionic gonadotropin at fetal-maternal interface. *J Soc Gynecol Invest* 2000;7 (Suppl.):abstr. 504

19. Srisuparp S, Strakova Z, Luborsky J, *et al.* Signaling pathways activated by chorionic gonadotropin (CG) in the primate endometrium. *Biol Reprod* 2000;62(Suppl. 1):abstr. 33

20. O'Day-Bowman MB, Marvrogianis PA, Reuter LM, *et al.* Association of oviduct-specific glycoproteins with human and baboon (*papio anubis*) ovarian oocytes and enhancement of human sperm binding to human hemizonae following *in vitro* incubation. *Biol Reprod* 1996;54:60–69

21. Sun T, Lei ZM, Rao ChV. A novel regulation of the oviductal glycoprotein gene expression by luteinizing hormone in bovine tubal epithelial cells. *Mol Cell Endocrinol* 1997;131:97–108

22. Mishra S, Lei ZM, Rao ChV. Novel effect of luteinizing hormone and human chorionic gonadotropin on the release of sperm bound to oviductal epithelial cells. *J Soc Gynecol Invest* 1999;6(Suppl. 1):abstr. 45

23. Mishra S, Lei ZM, Rao ChV. A novel role for luteinizing hormone in promoting the development of early bovine embryos into blastocysts through its actions on oviductal epithelial cells. *Biol Reprod* 1999;60(Suppl. 1):abstr. 185

24. Ji WZ, Bavister BD. Direct effects of gonadotropic hormones on *in vitro* development of early cleavage stage hamster embryos. *Biol Reprod* 1998;59(Suppl. 1):abstr. 71

25. Lei ZM, Toth P, Rao ChV, *et al.* Novel co-expression of human chorionic gonadotropin (hCG)/human luteinizing hormone receptors and their ligand, hCG, in human fallopian tubes. *J Clin Endocrinol Metab* 1993;77:863–72

26. Gawronska B, Paukku T, Huhtaniemi I, *et al.* Oestrogen-dependent expression of LH/hCG receptors in pig fallopian tube and their role in relaxation of the oviduct. *J Reprod Fertil* 1999;115:293–301

27. Han SW, Lei ZM, Rao ChV. Up-regulation of cyclooxygenase-2 gene expression by chorionic gonadotropin in mucosal cells from human fallopian tubes. *Endocrinology* 1996;137:2929–37

28. Han SW, Lei ZM, Rao ChV. Hormonal regulation of ectopic human chorionic gonadotropin (hCG) synthesis by human fallopian tube epithelial cells. Presented at the *Endocrine Society Annual Meeting*, New Orleans 1998;abstr. P1-350

29. Fishel SB, Edwards RG, Evans CJ. Human chorionic gonadotropin secreted by preimplantation embryos cultured *in vitro*. *Science* 1984;223:816–18

30. Bonduelle ML, Dodd R, Liebaers I, *et al.* Chorionic gonadotropin-β mRNA, a trophoblast marker, is expressed in human 8-cell embryos derived from tripronucleate zygotes. *Hum Reprod* 1988;3:909–14

31. Horiuchi A, Nikaido T, Yoshizawa T, *et al.* hCG promotes proliferation of uterine leiomyomal cells more strongly than that of myometrial smooth muscle cells *in vitro*. *Mol Hum Reprod* 2000;6:523–8

32. Zhou XL, Lei ZM, Rao ChV. Treatment of human endometrial gland epithelial cells with chorionic gonadotropin/luteinizing hormone increases the expression of cyclooxygenase-2 gene. *J Clin Endocrinol Metab* 1999;84:3364–77

33. Munir I, Fukunaga K, Miyazaki K, *et al.* Mitogen-activated protein kinase activation and regulation of cyclooxygenase 2 expression by platelet-activating factor and hCG in human endometrial adenocarcinoma cell line HEC-1B. *J Reprod Fertility* 1999;117:49–59

34. Han SW, Lei ZM, Rao ChV. Treatment of human endometrial stromal cells with chorionic gonadotropin induces their morphological and functional differentiation into decidua. *Mol Cell Endocrinol* 1999;147:7–16

35. Peng X, Kim JJ, Fazleabas AT. Apoptosis and differentiation in baboon stromal cells. *Biol Reprod* 2000;60(Suppl. 1):abstr. 510

36. d'Hauterive SP, Hazee-Hagelstein MT, Hazout A. The materno-fetal interface: embryonic factors (hCG, IGF-2) regulate the expression of endometrial cytokines, and TGFβ-related peptides contribute to maternal tolerance of the fetal graft. Presented at the *Endocrine Society Annual Meeting*, Toronto 2000;abstr. 822

37. Uzumcu M, Coskun S, Jaroudi K, *et al.* Effect of human chorionic gonadotropin on cytokine production from human endometrial cells *in vitro*. *Am J Reprod Immunol* 1998;40:83–8

38. Selam B, Kayisli UA, Arici A. Human chorionic gonadotropin up-regulates Fas ligand expression in endometrial stromal cells: a mechanism for an immuno-privileged trophoblastic invasion. *J Soc Gynecol Invest* 2000;7(Suppl. 1):abstr. 594

39. Kim JJ, Jaffe RC, Fazleabas AT. Blastocyst invasion and the stromal response in primates. *Hum Reprod* 1999;14(Suppl.):45–55

40. Bischof P, Haenggeli L, Campana A. Effect of leukemia inhibitory factor on human cytotrophoblast differentiation along the invasive pathway. *Am J Reprod Immunol* 1995;34:225–30

41. Yang M, Lei ZM, Rao ChV. Mechanism of leukemia inhibitory factor induced differentiation of human cytotrophoblasts. Presented at the *Endocrine Society Annual Meeting*, San Diego 1999;abstr. P1–6

42. Fazleabas AT, Donnelly KM, Srinivasan S, et al. Modulation of the baboon (*Papio anubis*) uterine endometrium by chorionic gonadotropin during the period of uterine receptivity. *Proc Natl Acad Sci USA* 1999;96: 2543–8

43. Fanchin R, Peltier E, Frydman R, et al. Human chorionic gonadotropin: does it affect human endometrial morphology *in vivo*? *Sem Reprod Med* 2001;in press

44. Licht P, Russu V, Wildt L. On the role of human chorionic gonadotropin (hCG) in the embryo-endometrial microenvironment. Implications for differentiation and implantation. *Sem Reprod Med* 2001;in press

45. Lei ZM, Rao ChV. Endocrinology of trophoblast tissue. In Becker KA, ed. *Principles and Practice of Endocrinology and Metabolism*. Philadelphia: Lippincott Williams & Wilkins, 2000:180–86

46. Lei ZM, Taylor DD, Gercel-Taylor C, et al. Human chorionic gonadotropin promotes tumorigenesis of choriocarcinoma JAR cells. *Trophoblast Res* 1999;13:147–59

47. Islami D, Mock P, Bischof P. Effects of human chorionic gonadotropin on trophoblast invasion. *Sem Reprod Med* 2001;in press

48. Zygmunt M, McKinnon T, Lala P, et al. Human chorionic gonadotropin (hCG) increases externalization of IGF-II receptor (IGF-II R) in extravillous trophoblast. *J Soc Gynecol Invest* 2000; 7(Suppl. 1):abstr. 417

49. Phillips RJ, Robson SC, Europe-Finner GN. Regulation of Gαs gene expression in human myometrial cells by chorionic gonadotropin: a cAMP-mediated process. *J Soc Gynecol Invest* 2000;7(Suppl. 1):abstr. 668

50. Toppozada MK. Does hCG have a direct effect on the human myometrium? *Fertil Steril* 1998; 70(Suppl. 1):abstr. O–184

51. Kurtzman JT, Spinnato JT, Goldsmith LJ, et al. Human chorionic gonadotropin exhibits potent inhibition of preterm delivery in a small animal model. *Am J Obstet Gynecol* 1999;181: 853–7

52. Kurtzman J, Jones E, Goldsmith LJ, et al. Inhibition of preterm delivery by human chorionic gonadotropin is associated with down-regulation of myometrial gap junctions. *Am J Obstet Gynecol* 2000:182:1:Part 2; abstr. 668

53. Chaouat G, Menu E, Delage G, et al. Immuno-endocrine interactions in early pregnancy. *Hum Reprod* 1995;10(Suppl.)2:55–9

54. Chaouat G, Menu E. Maternal T cell reactivity in pregnancy. *Curr Top Microbiol Immunol* 1997; 222:103–26

55. Lin J, Lojun S, Lei ZM, et al. Lymphocytes from pregnant women express human chorionic gonadotropin/luteinizing hormone receptor gene. *Mol Cell Endocrinol* 1995;111: R13–R17

56. Zhang YM, Lei ZM, Rao ChV. Functional importance of human monocyte luteinizing hormone and chorionic gonadotropin receptors. *J Soc Gynecol Invest* 1999;6(Suppl. 1):abstr. 46

57. Zhang YM, Lei ZM, Rao ChV. Human microphages contain luteinizing hormone and chorionic gonadotropin receptors. *J Soc Gynecol Invest* 1998;5(Suppl. 1):abstr. 212

58. Reshef E, Lei ZM, Rao ChV, et al. The presence of gonadotropin receptors in nonpregnant human uterus, human placenta, fetal membranes and decidua. *J Clin Endocrinol Metab* 1990;70:421–30

59. Komorowski J, Gradowski G, Stepien H. Effects of hCG and beta-hCG on IL-2 and sIL-2R secretion from human peripheral blood mononuclear cells: a dose-response study *in vitro*. *Immunol Lett* 1997;59:29–33

60. Komorowski J, Gradowski G, Stepien H. Effects of human chorionic gonadotropin (hCG) and beta-hCG on oncostatin M release from human peripheral blood mononuclear cells *in vitro*. *Cytobios* 1997;92:159–63

61. Munn DH, Zhou M, Attwood JT, et al. Prevention of allogeneic fetal rejection by tryptophan catabolism. *Science* 1998;281: 1191–3

62. Rao ChV, Alsip NL. Use of the rat models to study hCG/LH effects on uterine blood flow. *Sem Reprod Med* 2001;in press

63. Hermsteiner M, Zoltan DR, Doetsch J, et al. Human chorionic gonadotropin dilates uterine and mesenteric resistance arteries in pregnant and nonpregnant rats. *Pflugers Arch* 1999;439:186–94

64. Ghinea N, Milgrom E. A new function for the LH/hCG receptor: transcytosis of hormone across the endothelial barrier in target organs. *Sem Reprod Med* 2001;in press

65. Zygmunt M, Herr F, Keller-Schoenwetter S, *et al.* Characterization of human chorionic gonadotropin as a novel angiogenic factor for uterine endothelial cells. 2001;in review

66. Toth P. Clinical data supporting importance of vascular LH/hCG receptors of uterine blood vessels. *Sem Reprod Med* 2001;in press

67. Lei ZM, Mishra S, Zou W, *et al.* Targeted disruption of the luteinizing hormone/human chorionic gonadotropin receptor gene. *Mol Endocrinol* 2001;15:184–200

Is there a role for aspirin in recurrent miscarriage?   30

S. Daya

Introduction

Although the prevalence of recurrent miscarriage has not been ascertained with confidence, it is generally believed that 3–5% of women of reproductive age will have had three or more miscarriages[1]. The previously used term for this condition was habitual abortion, which has been replaced by the kinder and less provocative term 'recurrent miscarriage'. In North America, the World Health Organization definition of abortion or miscarriage is used, i.e. 'the expulsion or extraction from its mother of a fetus weighing less than 500 g'. This stage in pregnancy is equivalent to a gestational age of 20 weeks. Recurrent miscarriage is further divided into a primary category, in which the woman has had three or more consecutive miscarriages with no pregnancy having gone beyond 20 weeks; a secondary category, in which the woman has had three or more consecutive miscarriages after at least one pregnancy that has progressed beyond 20 weeks and may have resulted in a live birth or stillbirth; and a tertiary category, in which a woman has had three or more miscarriages (not necessarily consecutively) interspersed with pregnancies that have progressed beyond 20 weeks[1].

It is important to use this categorization consistently so that the evidence can be more accurately evaluated to identify factors that affect outcome and to determine whether diagnostic procedures and therapeutic interventions are effective. Unfortunately, universal acceptance of this approach has not yet been reached resulting in much confusion in the literature, in which the data from women with early and late (> 20 weeks) pregnancy losses are grouped together with those from women who have recurrent early miscarriage[2]. When reviewing the evidence on recurrent miscarriage, it is important to correct for these contaminating features.

Causes of recurrent miscarriage and factors affecting outcome

Many factors (some of which are well established whereas others are supported only by anecdotal evidence) have been suggested to have a role in the etiology of recurrent miscarriage[1]. The evaluation of couples with this disorder involves extensive testing, including a search for karyotype anomalies, uterine abnormalities (including congenital uterine anomaly, fibroids, intrauterine adhesions and cervical incompetence), endocrine abnormalities (including luteal phase deficiency, diabetes mellitus and thyroid dysfunction), infections (particularly with *Ureaplasma urealyticum*), autoimmune dysfunction (particularly antiphospholipid antibody syndrome) and alloimmune dysfunction.

Female age is a well-recognized negative prognostic factor; the likelihood of miscarriage increases with female age, especially after age 35 when the risk of having a trisomic conceptus is markedly elevated. In addition to the effect of age, the number of previous miscarriages is directly correlated with the likelihood of subsequent miscarriage. Consequently, in any study evaluating the efficacy of treatment for recurrent miscarriage, it becomes necessary to stratify for female age and the number of previous miscarriages. Unfortunately, most studies to date have failed to account for these important confounding factors.

Antiphospholipid antibody syndrome

Antiphospholipid antibody syndrome (APS) involves the production of autoantibodies against protein epitopes, which form complexes with negatively charged phospholipids in cell membranes[3]. These antiphospholipid antibodies (APA), e.g. anticardiolipin and lupus anticoagulant, are associated with thrombocytopenia, thrombosis and recurrent fetal loss. The definition of APS requires the presence of any one or more of these clinical features together with lupus anticoagulant or anticardiolipin antibodies (moderately positive, at 20–80 GPL or MPL, or highly positive with greater than 80 GPL or MPL).

APA have been detected in 15% of women with recurrent miscarriage[4]. In contrast, in one study, the prevalence of APA was only 2–4% among an unselected population of pregnant women. Among women with only one miscarriage, there was no significant difference in the presence of APA compared with a control population[5]. However, in another study, the difference in prevalence of APA between controls and women with two or more consecutive miscarriages was significant[6]. It should be noted that in APA-positive women, the majority of pregnancy losses were fetal deaths that occurred after the fetus had a detectable heartbeat[7].

Although the pathogenesis of pregnancy loss is unclear, thrombosis of the utero–placental vasculature has been observed on histological examination of the placenta, suggesting a possible causal mechanism[8]. Antiphospholipid antibodies require a cofactor (β_2 glycoprotein-I) prior to binding to the platelet membrane phospholipid epitopes, activating the production and release of thromboxane A_2, or similar substances, leading to platelet aggregation, vasoconstriction

and subsequently thrombosis[3]. Alternatively, the antibodies may bind to endothelial cells and inhibit prostacyclin production, altering the thromboxane A_2 to prostacyclin ratio, resulting in platelet aggregation, vasoconstriction and intravascular thrombosis[9]. Results from murine studies have suggested that APA may directly impair trophoblast function[10]. An increase in thromboxane synthesis[11] and a decreases in the distribution of annexin V, a natural placental anticoagulant protein[12], may also play a role.

Treatment with aspirin – a critique of the evidence

In the first few weeks of pregnancy, women with recurrent miscarriage produce an excess of thromboxane A_2, whereas several weeks later, a prostacyclin deficiency is seen[13]. In contrast, non-pregnant women with recurrent miscarriage exhibit normal production of both thromboxane and prostacyclin[14]. These observations suggest that either thromboxane dominance or prostacyclin deficiency may be causally related to miscarriage. The gaining acceptance of the role of thrombosis in the pathogenesis of recurrent miscarriage has led to management of these patients with antithrombotic therapy. Aspirin inhibits platelet cyclo-oxygenase activity thereby blocking the synthesis of the vasoconstrictory and proaggregatory thromboxane A_2 without affecting the synthesis of prostacyclin, which promotes vasodilatation and antiaggregation[15]. Thus, the administration of low-dose aspirin in early pregnancy may be of benefit by suppressing thromboxane synthesis and restoring to normal the thromboxane/prostacyclin ratio.

Uncontrolled studies

In a case series of 18 women with APS and recurrent miscarriage, aspirin (100 mg daily) commenced one month before attempting conception and continued throughout the pregnancy resulted in live birth in 19 out of

21 (90%) pregnancies[16]. In six pregnancies, prednisone was also administered because of autoimmune-related thrombocytopenia.

In another case series of 28 women who were APA-positive and had a history of recurrent miscarriages, treatment with low-dose aspirin (75 mg daily) until 38 weeks gestation resulted in 20 cases (71%) with a successful outcome (although of these cases prematurity was observed in five and neonatal death in one out of 20)[17].

Controlled, non-randomized studies

Among a cohort of 22 patients with APA and two or more miscarriages, six refused treatment and served as the control group and the rest were treated with low-dose aspirin (50 mg twice daily) commenced soon after a positive pregnancy test (for all except two women who started treatment after the third month of pregnancy). In addition, in five women fluocortolone (20 mg daily) was administered. Among the 11 women receiving only low-dose aspirin, nine (89%) had a successful delivery, whereas in the untreated group only one out of six (17%) had a successful outcome[18].

Randomized controlled studies

In a small randomized study involving 19 women with APA but who were considered low risk because they had none of the associated signs or symptoms of APS (i.e. ≤ 1 prior miscarriage and no history of thrombosis or thrombocytopenia), the use of low-dose aspirin (81 mg daily) throughout the pregnancy in 11 women resulted in a similar live birth rate to that in the control group of eight women receiving usual care (89% versus 100%, respectively)[19].

In the only placebo-controlled randomized study of aspirin in women with recurrent miscarriage and detectable anticardiolipin antibodies, the use of aspirin (50 mg daily) or placebo in pregnancy was associated with an identical live birth rate of 71%[20]. Interestingly, in women with recurrent miscarriage and normal anticardiolipin antibody levels, the live birth rates in the aspirin and placebo groups were also identical at 22 out of 29 (76%). These observations indicate that the presence of anticardiolipin antibodies is a negative prognostic factor for successful pregnancy only in women with recurrent miscarriage and administration of aspirin in pregnancy is not efficacious.

Randomized controlled studies of co-administration of heparin

The use of heparin has been advocated on the basis of its anticoagulant activity, which counteracts the thrombotic events caused by the binding of APA to phospholipid or other cross-reactive substance[21,22]. Furthermore, the addition of heparin to APA-positive serum from women with recurrent pregnancy was associated with a dose-dependent decrease in IgG binding to cardiolipin and phosphatidylserine[23–25].

There are now two randomized trials in the literature evaluating the benefit of adding heparin to low-dose aspirin in the treatment of APA-associated recurrent miscarriage. In the first trial, 50 women with at least three previous consecutive spontaneous pregnancy losses and APA were assigned to continue with low-dose aspirin (81 mg daily, commenced before conception) alone or to receive, in addition, twice-daily subcutaneous injections of heparin 5000 IU at the first confirmed pregnancy test (at approximately 5 weeks' gestation). The proportion of live births in the experimental group (heparin plus aspirin) was 20 out of 25 (80%) compared with 11 out of 25 (44%) in the control (aspirin only) group, a difference that was statistically significant (odds ratio (OR) 5.09, 95% confidence interval (CI) 1.45–17.92)[26].

In the second trial, 90 women with a history of recurrent miscarriage and persistently positive APA were randomly allocated to receive either low-dose aspirin (75 mg daily) or low-dose aspirin and 5000 IU unfractionated heparin subcutaneously every 12 hours (experimental group)[27]. All women started treatment with low-dose aspirin when they

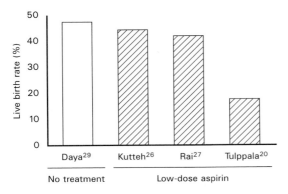

Figure 1 Miscarriage rates in women with recurrent miscarriage and antiphospholipid syndrome (APS) treated with low-dose aspirin (hatched bars) and in women with untreated, unexplained recurrent miscarriage (open bar)

had a positive urine pregnancy test. When fetal cardiac activity was confirmed by ultrasonography, the women were then randomly allocated also to receive heparin or to continue with low-dose aspirin alone. Treatment was stopped at 34 weeks' gestation. The proportion of live births in the experimental group was 32 out of 45 (71%) compared with 19 out of 45 (42%) in the group on low-dose aspirin alone, a difference that was statistically significant (OR 3.37, 95% CI 1.40–8.10).

Both studies described above confirm the superior efficacy of the combination of heparin and aspirin as treatment for women with recurrent miscarriage and persistently positive APA. In fact, in the technical bulletin on APS of the American College of Obstetricians and Gynecologists released in 1998, the recommendation for treatment of this syndrome with prior fetal death or recurrent pregnancy loss is daily administration of heparin and low-dose aspirin during pregnancy[28]. This recommendation is intriguing particularly since the efficacy of low-dose aspirin has not yet been established.

Pregnancy success with aspirin alone

When reviewing the evidence from randomized controlled trials in which aspirin alone

was administered in one arm of the trials in women with recurrent miscarriage and APS, an interesting phenomenon can be observed. These data are shown in Figure 1 and indicate that the likelihood of pregnancy success is relatively low with aspirin, ranging from 17% to 44%, a range that would be expected without treatment in women with unexplained recurrent miscarriage[29]. Furthermore, in a large cohort study of aspirin administered at a dose of 75 mg daily, the rate of success was similar to that in women not treated with aspirin[30].

In light of these low success rates and the lack of proven efficacy of low-dose aspirin alone, the recommendation that aspirin be administered to women with recurrent miscarriage and APS is questionable.

Risks of aspirin

The ability of aspirin to block the synthesis of prostaglandins also increases the risk of damage to the gastrointestinal mucosa[31]. Although the erosions are usually trivial, they may progress to ulcers, which in turn may bleed or perforate, and may even cause death. In addition, the action of aspirin to reduce thrombus formation also increases the recipient's susceptibility to bleeding. The rates of these adverse events are probably higher than many doctors like to believe[32].

In a meta-analysis of 24 randomized controlled trials (comprising almost 66 000 participants), the risk of gastrointestinal hemorrhage was significantly higher in those taking aspirin for at least one year than in placebo. The risk of hemorrhage with doses of aspirin less than 163 mg daily was 2.30% compared with 1.45% for those taking placebo (OR 1.59, 95% CI 1.40–1.81)[33]. Compared with placebo, the 'number needed to harm' for hemorrhage with aspirin was 100. Thus, for every 100 patients treated with aspirin, one more additional case of hemorrhage would be observed than with placebo.

In a large double-blind placebo-controlled trial, the likelihood of suffering bleeding disorders antenatally, intrapartum and postpartum was significantly higher in women taking low-dose aspirin (60 mg per day) during pregnancy[34]. The risk was higher among compliant aspirin takers than in the intention-to-treat analysis, suggesting that these adverse effects are real.

The consequences of exposure to aspirin for the developing fetus are not well understood. Salicylates have a common spectrum of activity in a variety of species tested, but differences in plasma protein binding affinity translate into variability in the effective dose. Thus, the results from animals cannot readily be extrapolated to human studies. Nevertheless, there is little reason to expect qualitatively different effects in different species[35].

When administered to the mother, salicylates transfer readily to the fetus[36,37], in which pharmacologic activity, such as inhibition of prostacyclin and thromboxane, is also observed[38]. Compared with the adult, the fetus and newborn have lower plasma protein binding of salicylates, reduced metabolic activity and less efficient elimination thereby leading to high plasma concentrations[35].

The epidemiologic data provide consistent evidence that the risk of bleeding in the newborn increases with maternal exposure to aspirin at analgesic doses shortly before delivery[35]. At lower doses (≤ 150 mg/day), no clinical signs of bleeding were observed. However, a smaller effect at these low doses could not be ruled out[35].

There have been case reports of preterm occlusion of the ductus arteriosus and pulmonary hypertension in the fetuses of mothers taking salicylates. None of the neonates exposed *in utero* to very low doses (< 81 mg daily) late in gestation showed evidence of these conditions[35]. However, the study groups were very small resulting in low power to detect such rare outcomes.

Aspirin consumption early in pregnancy has been extensively studied with respect to the risk of congenital malformations. The evidence for aspirin teratogenicity in animals is definitive[35]. The data for human teratogenicity are inconclusive, primarily because of inadequate information on exposure and insufficient control for potential confounders. The point estimates of risk suggest the possibility of an elevated risk of cardiac defects (including hypoplastic left ventricle, coarctation of the aorta and aortic stenosis)[35].

The central nervous system may be sensitive to exposure at dose levels too low to causes structural anomalies, yet high enough to be manifest as deficits in cognitive or behavioral development[35]. Aspirin exposure was observed in one study to be associated with a lower IQ and attention decrements[39], although these findings were not supported by another study[40]. The biological plausibility of the potential for an adverse effect can be deduced from the observation that fetal circulation to the brain is decreased by prostaglandin inhibition[41].

In a recent study of childhood cancer, prenatal use of antipyretics and analgesics were found to be associated with subsequent neoplasms in the offspring, in particular solid tumors[42]. Unfortunately, data on aspirin use could not be analyzed separately to evaluate the possibility of a causal relationship between aspirin exposure and childhood cancer.

Conclusion

Although aspirin use in women with recurrent miscarriage and APS is widely accepted as a therapeutic option, the evidence for its efficacy is lacking. What little evidence that exists from randomized trials indicates that aspirin has no value, with success rates that are not better than those one would expect without treatment. In addition, the risks of gastrointestinal and pregnancy-related hemorrhage are not insignificant. The consequences of aspirin exposure for the developing fetus are not well understood but the evidence for aspirin teratogenicity in animals is definitive. The relatively high plasma concentration that is achieved in the fetus from maternally administered salicylates is a cause for concern that adverse effects in the human fetus may occur, even though the data so far are inconclusive. The widespread use of low-dose aspirin for recurrent miscarriage should be halted until definitive evidence on its efficacy and safety has been collected from appropriately conducted randomized controlled trials involving stratification for important covariates.

References

1. Daya S. Habitual abortion. In Copeland LJ, Jarrell JF, eds. *Textbook of Gynecology.* Philadelphia: WB Saunders Company, 2000: 227–71

2. Branch DW, Silver RM. Criteria for antiphospholipid syndrome: early pregnancy loss, fetal loss, or recurrent pregnancy loss? *Lupus* 1996; 5:409–13

3. Sait KH, Van den Hof MC, Robinson KS. Antiphospholipid antibody syndrome in pregnancy. *J Soc Obstet Gynaecol Can* 1997;19:1083–92

4. Clifford K, Rai R, Watson H, *et al.* An informative protocol for the investigation of recurrent miscarriage. Preliminary experience of 500 consecutive cases. *Hum Reprod* 1994;9: 1328–32

5. Infante-Rivard C, David M, Gauthier R, *et al.* Lupus anticogulant, anticardiolipin antibodies, and fetal loss. A case control study. *N Engl J Med* 1991;325:1063–6

6. Kutteh WH, Lyde EC, Abraham SM, *et al.* Association of anticardiolipin antibodies and pregnancy loss in women with systematic lupus erythematosus. *Fertil Steril* 1993;60:449–55

7. Wechsler B, Du LTH, Piette JC. Is there a role for antithrombotic therapy in the prevention of pregnancy loss? *Haemostasis* 1999;29(Suppl 1): 112–20

8. De Wolf F, Carreras LD, Moerman P, *et al.* Decidual vasculopathy and extensive placental infarction in a patient with repeated thromboembolic accidents, recurrent fetal loss, and a lupus anticoagulant. *Am J Obstet Gynecol* 1982; 142:829–34

9. Rote NS, Walter A, Lynden TW. Antiphospholipid antibodies – lobsters or red herrings? *Am J Reprod Immunol* 1992;28:31–7

10. Shoenfeld Y, Shere Y, Blank M. Antiphospholipid syndrome in pregnancy – animal models and clinical implications. *Scand J Rheumatol* 1998;27:533–6

11. Peaceman AM, Rehnberg KA. The effect of aspirin and indomethacin on prostacyclin and thromboxane production by placental tissue incubated with immunoglublin G fractions from patients with lupus anticoagulant. *Am J Obstet Gynecol* 1995;173:1391–6

12. Rand JH, Wu XX, Anree HA, *et al.* Pregnancy loss in the antiphospholipid-antibody syndrome – a possible thrombogenic mechanism. *N Engl J Med* 1997;337:154–60

13. Tulppala M, Viinikka L, Ylikorkala O. Thromboxane dominance and prostacyclin deficiency in habitual abortion. *Lancet* 1991;337:879–81

14. Tulppala M, Viinikka L, Ylikorkala O. Non-pregnant women with a history of habitual abortion have normal and luteal function independent production of prostacyclin and thromboxane A$_2$. *Fertil Steril* 1992;57: 1216–19

15. Ylikorkala O, Viinikka L. The role of prostaglandins in obstetrical disorders. *Ballières Clin Endocrinol Metab* 1992;6:809–27

16. Balasch J, Carmona F, Lopez-Soto A, *et al.* Low-dose aspirin for prevention of pregnancy losses in women with primary antiphospholipid syndrome. *Hum Reprod* 1993;8:2234–39

17. Lima F, Khamashta MA, Buchanan NMM, *et al.* A study of sixty pregnancies in patients with the antiphospholipid syndrome. *Clin Exp Rheumatol* 1996;14:131–6

18. Passaleva A, Massai G, D'Elios MM, *et al.* Prevention of miscarriage in antiphospholipid syndrome. *Autoimmunity* 1992;14:121–5

19. Cowchock S, Reece EA. Do low risk pregnant women with antiphospholipid antibodies need to be treated? *Am J Obstet Gynecol* 1997;176: 1099–100

20. Tulppala M, Marttunen M, Soderstrom-Anttila V, *et al.* Low-dose aspirin in prevention of miscarriage in women with unexplained or autoimmune related recurrent miscarriage: effect on prostacyclin and thromboxane A$_2$ production. *Hum Reprod* 1997;12: 1567–72

21. Chamley LW, McKay EJ, Pattison NS. Inhibition of heparin/antithrombin III cofactor activity by anticardiolipin antibodies. A mechanism for thrombosis. *Thromb Res* 1993;71: 103–11

22. Shibata S, Harpel P, Bona C, *et al*. Monoclonal antibodies to heparin sulfate inhibit the formation of thrombin–antithrombin III complexes. *Clin Immunol Immunopathol* 1993;67: 264–72

23. Ermel LD, Marshburn PB, Kutteh WH. Interaction of heparin with antiphospholipid antibodies (APA) from the sera of women with recurrent pregnancy loss (PRC). *Am J Reprod Immunol* 1995;33:14–20

24. McIntyre JA, Wagenknecht DR. Interaction of heparin with α_2-glycoprotein I and antiphospholipid antibodies *in vitro*. *Thromb Res* 1992; 68:495–500

25. McIntyre JA, Taylor CG, Torry DS, *et al*. Heparin and pregnancy in women with a history of repeated miscarriages. *Haemostasis* 1993;23(Suppl 1):202–11

26. Kutteh WH. Antiphospholipid antibody-associated recurrent pregnancy loss: treatment with heparin and low-dose aspirin is superior to low dose aspirin alone. *Am J Obstet Gynecol* 1996;174:1584–9

27. Rai R, Cohen H, Dave M, *et al*. Randomized controlled trial of aspirin and aspirin plus heparin in pregnant women with recurrent miscarriage associated with phospholipid antibodies (or antiphospholipid antibodies). *BMJ* 1997;314:253–7

28. ACOG Educational Bulletin. *Antiphospholipid Syndrome*. American College of Obstetricians and Gynecologists, No. 244, February 1998

29. Daya S. Immunotherapy for unexplained recurrent spontaneous abortion. *Infertility Reprod Med Clinics of N America* 1997;8:65–77

30. Rai R, Backos M, Baxter N, *et al*. Recurrent miscarriage – an aspirin a day? *Hum Reprod* 2000;15:2220–3

31. Henry D, Lim LLY, Rodriguez LAG, *et al*. Variability in risk of gastrointestinal complications with individual non-steroidal anti-inflammatory drugs: results of a collaborative meta-analysis. *BMJ* 1996;312:1563–6

32. Tramer MR, Moor RA, Reynolds DJ, *et al*. Quantitative estimation of rare adverse events which follow a biological progression: a new model applied to chronic NSAID use. *Pain* 2000;85:169–82

33. Derry S, Loke YK. Risk of gastrointestinal hemorrhage with long term use of aspirin: meta-analysis. *BMJ* 2000;321:1183–7

34. Golding J. A randomized trial of low dose aspirin for primiparae in pregnancy. *Br J Obstet Gynaecol* 1998;105:293–9

35. Hertz-Picciotto I, Hopenhayn-Rich R, Golub M, *et al*. The risks and benefits of taking aspirin during pregnancy. *Epidemiol Rev* 1990;12: 108–48

36. Palmisano PA, Cassady G. Salicylate exposure in the perinate. *J Am Med Assoc* 1969;209: 556–8

37. Wolff, F, Berg R, Bolte A, *et al*. Perinatal pharmacokinetics of acetylsalicylic acid. *Arch Gynecol* 1982;233:15–22

38. Ylikorkala O, Makila UM, Kaapa P, *et al*. Maternal ingestion of acetylsalicylic acid inhibits fetal and neonatal prostacyclin and thromboxane in humans. *Am J Obstet Gynecol* 1986;155:345–9

39. Streissguth AP, Treder RP, Barr HM, *et al*. Aspirin and acetaminophen use by pregnant women and subsequent IQ and attention decrements. *Teratology* 1987;35:211–19

40. Klebanoff MA, Berendes HW. Aspirin exposure during the first 20 weeks of gestation and IQ at four years of age. *Teratology* 1988;37: 249–55

41. Heymann MA, Rudolph AM. Effects of acetylsalicylic acid on the ductus arteriosus and circulation in fetal lambs *in utero*. *Circ Res* 1976; 38:418–22

42. Gilman EA, Wilson LMK, Kneale GW, *et al*. Childhood cancers and their association with pregnancy drugs and illnesses. *Paediatr Perinat Epidemiol* 1989;3:66–94

Insulin-like growth factor system and fetal growth

31

E.-M. Rutanen

Introduction

The growth of the fetus is characterized by an increase in cell number and size, and elaboration of structures. This requires adequate availability of oxygen and nutrients which pass freely to the fetus from the mother's bloodstream via the placenta. From the 15th to about 30 to 34 weeks the fetus gains weight at about 5 g/day and after 34 weeks to term at 30–35 g/day. Altogether, the fetus gains two thirds of its weight during the third trimester of pregnancy. Undernutrition, placental dysfunction, hypoxia and decreased maternal blood flow may all result in restriction of fetal growth. Depending on gestational age, growth retardation is reflected as decreased number or decreased size of fetal cells.

Growth restriction due to decrease in cell size occurs in late gestation and is characterized by asymmetrical growth retardation in contrast to the condition that generally occurs in early pregnancy that produces a symmetrically small fetus (due to restriction of cellular hyperplasia).

In addition to oxygen and nutrients a great number of growth promoting or inhibiting factors on the maternal side, at the maternal–placental interface and in the fetus are involved in the regulation of fetal growth. These factors can be endocrine hormones or growth factors that act in an endocrine or auto/paracrine manner. Some of these growth factors may exert several roles during fetal development depending on their concentration and interactions with other growth factors. Others may act in a highly tissue-specific

manner. Insulin required for the metabolism of glucose is secreted by the fetal pancreas. Insulin is believed to be the major tropic hormone for fetal growth.

Fetal growth is determined partly by genetic and partly epigenetic factors. Thirty-eight per cent of variation in birth weight has been attributed to genetic factors and the remaining 62% to epigenetic factors: half of these being maternal factors and the rest unknown.

In this chapter, I focus on insulin-like growth factors (IGF) which perhaps are the most important and, at least, most studied growth factors regarding fetal growth. When addressing the role of IGFs in any biological process, the whole IGF system needs to be considered. The system includes two IGFs: IGF-I and IGF-II, their respective receptors and a family of six binding proteins (IGFBP-1–6) that have equal or greater affinity with IGFs as compared with their receptors[1]. IGFs bear structural relationship to proinsulin. They have 40% homology with insulin. In addition, there is a 60% homology between human IGF-I and IGF-II. IGFs stimulate cell proliferation and differentiation, and have insulin-like metabolic effects.

IGF-I and II both bind to type 1 IGF receptor which resembles the insulin receptor. IGF-II can bind to type 2 IGF-receptor which is identical to mannose–6-phosphate receptor. The biological action of type 2 IGF receptor remains unknown. The interaction between IGFs and their receptors is mediated either negatively or positively by IGFBPs, i.e. binding proteins can either stimulate or inhibit IGF action[2,3]. IGFs, either of them, and their receptors are present in virtually all cell types examined. The expression of individual binding proteins is more or less tissue specific and IGFBPs are of major importance in the regulation of IGF actions at the cellular level during growth and development. In the circulation IGFBP-3 is the most abundant and has a significant function as a carrier protein of IGFs with which it forms a large complex. The second most abundant IGFBP in the blood-stream is IGFBP-2, supposed to have an important role with IGF-II in early fetal growth[4]. Perhaps the most important IGFBP in placental and fetal development is IGFBP-1, which is produced in abundant amounts by maternal decidua and fetal liver, and which is present in very high concentrations in amniotic fluid[5,6].

As well as being modulators of IGF action, binding proteins may also have functions independent of IGFs. For example, IGFBP-1 binds with its RGD sequence to α5β1 integrin, a specific cellular receptor for the extracellular matrix protein, fibronectin, and also alters cellular motility[2,3]. The other IGFBPs may serve to modulate further IGF availability to IGFBP-1 and to IGF receptors. The IGFBPs themselves are modified by mechanisms such as proteolysis and phosphorylation[7,8]. Binding proteins modulate the acute metabolic effects of IGFs.

IGF system and normal fetal growth

The evidence supporting a role for the IGF system in fetal growth comes from different types of study regarding gene expression, tissue content, cellular localization and circulating levels. Finally, direct experimental evidence of the influence of the IGF system on fetal growth comes from gene manipulation studies.

In the mother, circulating levels of IGF-I and IGFBP-1 increase during pregnancy[9]. IGF-II concentrations are higher in the fetus than in the adult. Also IGF-I concentrations in the fetus rise with gestation but are low compared with the levels in the mother[10].

Concentrations of both IGFs in the fetal circulation are related to birth weight at term. The major IGFBPs in the human fetus are IGFBP-1 and IGFBP-2. At 9–12 weeks there is a striking increase in IGFBP-1 and IGFBP-2 levels in amniotic fluid[11]. Messenger RNA (mRNA) for IGFs, IGFBPs and IGF-receptors are all expressed in the developing human at very early embryonic stage and are detectable throughout gestation. Several studies have shown that changes in tissue mRNA levels may not necessarily be accompanied by corresponding changes in serum or plasma concentrations of these peptides and, therefore, the concept of the role of IGFs in fetal growth must extend into paracrinology with measurements of tissue mRNA or peptide levels.

The distribution of IGF-I, IGF-II, IGF-receptor and IGFBP gene expression and tissue content of these peptides at the feto-maternal interface, i.e. in the decidua and placenta, shows how even great changes at tissue level are not necessarily detected in circulating levels[12,13]. Even though IGF-II mRNA expression is more abundant in fetal tissues and in the placenta than in adult tissues throughout gestation as compared with IGF-I, the recent evidence supports a more important role for IGF-II only in early pregnancy[14].

IGF-I has the ability to regulate partitioning of nutrients between the placenta and the fetus. IGFs stimulate the growth of human fetal fibroblasts, myoblasts, chondrocytes, osteoblasts, hepatocytes, glial cells and adrenal cells. IGFs also affect the differentiation of fetal cells, including muscle, cartilage and the nervous system. The major regulator of IGF-I production in the fetus is insulin[4]. Fetal insulin mediates IGF-I secretion. The expression of IGFBPs varies in different fetal and maternal cell types. The trophoblast contains IGF-II mRNA but not IGF-I, suggesting a role for IGF-II and IGFBPs in cell-to-cell communication at the feto-maternal surface.

The anchoring villus of the invading fetal placenta expresses primarily α5β1 integrin[2,3]. It is speculated that this invading cytotrophoblast phenotype invading into maternal decidua is confronted by high concentrations of IGFBP-1 which interacts via its RGD sequence with α5β1 integrin on the invading intermediate trophoblast cell membrane. In this way the interactions between IGFBP-1 and the intermediate trophoblast serve to alter invasiveness of this highly invasive trophoblast phenotype. It is also of interest that during intermediate trophoblast invasion into the maternal decidua, proteolysis of extracellular matrix components occurs and that IGFBP-1 is the only IGFBP for which no binding protein-protease has yet been described. Thus, the presence of abundant IGFBP-1 in maternal decidua suggests that it may have a dual role: as a modulator of IGF action and as a modulator of decidua/trophoblast interactions. IGFBP-1 has been suggested to modulate acute metabolic effects of IGFs because it is acutely regulated by glucoregulatory hormones; insulin inhibits, and cortisol and glucagon stimulate, IGFBP-1 production.

Not only the amount but also the isoforms of IGFBP-1 in tissues and body fluids change during pregnancy. In non-pregnant serum there is a single highly phosphorylated isoform, whereas in pregnant serum, amniotic fluid and decidual tissue, IGFBP-1 is present in non-phosphorylated plus several phosphorylated forms[15]. Fetal serum also exhibits the same forms of IGFBP-1. The rise of IGFBP-1 in maternal circulation is explained by the appearance of the new phosphoisoforms.

IGF system and fetal growth disorders

IGFs and IGFBPs are not only involved in the regulation of normal growth and differentiation of the fetus, but are also involved in the pathophysiology of intrauterine growth retardation and perhaps also of macrosomia. The IGF-1 concentrations in fetal serum are low and IGFBP-1 concentrations high in growth retarded fetuses, and IGFBP-3 and IGFBP-2 are also low[10,16,17]. The alterations in blood levels seem to reflect changes in mRNA levels in fetal tissues. The reason for alterations in the IGF system during pregnancy can be maternal of fetal. Several studies have shown

that IGFBP-1 concentration in both maternal serum and fetal serum is negatively correlated with birth weight. Giudice et al.[18] compared serum IGF-I, IGF-II, and IGFBP-1 concentrations in women with normal pregnancy to those in women with severe pre-eclampsia and growth retardation. No clear difference was found in IGF-I and IGF-II levels between the study groups, whereas IGFBP-1 levels were significantly higher in women with severe pre-eclampsia. Similar data were earlier found by Iino et al.[19]. One explanation could be hypoxia at the feto-maternal interface, since hypoxia was shown to stimulate IGFBP-1 gene expression. However, opposite results have been obtained in early pregnancy. Hietala et al.[20] measured maternal serum IGFBP-1 concentrations in 1000 women at the time of second trimester Down's screening. All data were collected after delivery. Surprisingly, the women who developed pre-eclampsia in late pregnancy had significantly lower levels of IGFBP-1 than the control women in mid-trimester. The levels were lowest in women who developed both gestational diabetes plus pre-eclampsia. Hyperinsulinemia, which has been shown to be a risk factor for pre-eclampsia, may be an explanation for the decrease in maternal serum IGFBP-1 in early pregnancy in women who developed pre-eclampsia in late pregnancy. The data are in agreement with those by DeGroot et al.[21], who found that the increase in maternal serum IGFBP-1 concentrations seen in healthy women in early mid-trimester was lacking in women who developed pre-eclampsia in late pregnancy.

Gene manipulation studies

The strongest evidence for the role of IGFs and IGFBPs in fetal growth comes from gene manipulation studies. Knockout of the gene encoding IGF-I results in reduced fetal growth, organ hypoplasia, delayed ossification of cartilage and finally death[22]. Knockout of IGF-II causes growth deficit in early pregnancy, but not in late pregnancy[23]. Knockout of type 1 IGF receptor, which signals the anabolic effects of both IGF-I and IGF-II, results in even more severe growth retardation than IGF-I or IGF-II knockout, suggesting that factors other than IGFs exert effects on fetal growth through the type 1 IGF receptor. Overexpression of IGF-I enhances body growth and overexpression of IGFBP-1 gene results in low birth weight. Overexpression of IGFBP-3 is followed by organomegaly[24]. Although the gene manipulation studies are done in mice, the effects of modifying IGF action should be relevant to human physiology as well.

In summary, a great body of evidence supports a role for IGFs and their binding proteins in fetal growth, although the molecular mechanisms of their action still remains to be clarified.

References

1. Rajaram S, Baylink DJ, Mohan S. Insulin-like growth factor-binding proteins in serum and other biological fluids: regulation and function. *Endocr Rev* 1997;18:801–31
2. Hamilton GS, Lysiak JJ, Han VKM, *et al.* Autocrine-paracrine regulation of human trophoblast invasiveness by insulin-like growth factor (IGF)-II and IGF-binding protein (IGFBP)-1. *Exp Cell Res* 1998;244:147–56
3. Giudice LC, Irwin JC. Roles of the insulinlike growth factor family in nonpregnant human endometrium and at the decidual : trophoblast interface. *Semin Reprod Endocrinol* 1999;17: 13–21
4. Hill DJ, Petrik J, Arany E. Growth factors and regulation of fetal growth. *Diabetes Care* 1998; 21:(Suppl. 2):B60–B9
5. Koistinen R, Kalkkinen N, Huhtala ML, *et al.* Placental protein 12 is a decidual protein that binds somatomedin and has an identical N-terminal amino acid sequence with somatomedin binding protein from human amniotic fluid. *Endocrinology* 1986;118:1375–8
6. Rutanen E-M, Bohn H, Seppälä M. Radioimmunoassay of placental protein 12: levels in amniotic fluid, cord blood and sera of healthy adults, pregnant women and patients with trophoblastic disease. *Am J Obstet Gynecol* 1982; 144:460–3
7. Kubler B, Cowell S, Zapf J, *et al.* Proteolysis of insulin-like growth factor binding proteins by a novel 50-kilodalton metalloproteinase in human pregnancy serum. *Endocrinology* 1998; 139:1556–63
8. Jones JI, D'Ercole AJ, Camacho-Hubner C, *et al.* Phosphorylation of insulin-like growth factor (IGF)-binding protein in cell culture and *in vivo*: effects on affinity for IGF-I. *Proc Natl Acad Sci USA* 1991;88:7481–5
9. Hall K, Hansson U, Lundin G, *et al.* Serum levels of somatomedins and somatomedin binding protein in pregnant women with type 1 or gestational diabetes and their infants. *J Clin Endocrinol Metab* 1986;63:1300–5
10. Fant M, Salafia C, Baxter R, *et al.* Circulating levels of IGFs, IGF binding proteins in human cord serum: relationship to intrauterine growth. *Regulatory peptides* 1993;48:29–39
11. Verhaeghe J, Coopmans W, van Herck E, *et al.* IGF-I, IGF-II, IGF binding protein 1, and C-peptide in second trimester amniotic fluid are dependent on gestational age but do not predict weight at birth. *Pediatr Res* 1999;46:101–8
12. Giudice LC, Milkowski DA, Lamson G, *et al.* Insulin-like growth factor-binding proteins in human endometrium: steroid-dependent message ribonucleic acid expression and protein synthesis. *J Clin Endocrinol Metab* 1991;72: 779–87
13. Giudice LC, Mark SP, Irwin JC. Paracrine actions of insulin-like growth factors and IGF-binding protein-1 in non-pregnant human endometrium and at the decidual-trophoblast interface. *J Reprod Immun* 1998;39:133–48
14. Badinga L, Song S, Simmen RCM, *et al.* Complex mediation of uterine endometrial epithelial cell growth by insulin-like growth factor-II (IGF-II) and IGF-binding protein-2. *J Mol Endocrinol* 1999;23:277–85
15. Martina NA, Kim E, Chitkara U, *et al.* Gestational age-dependent expression of insulin-like growth factor-binding protein-1 (IGFBP-1) phosphoisoforms in human extra-embryonic cavities, maternal serum, and decidua suggests decidua as the primary source of IGFBP-1 in these fluids during early pregnancy. *J Clin Endocrinol Metab* 1997;82: 1894–8

16. Wiznitzer A, Reece EA, Homko C, *et al*. Insulin-like growth factors, their binding proteins, and fetal macrosomia in offspring of nondiabetic pregnant women. *Am J Perinatol* 1998; 15:23–8

17. Cianfarani S, Germani D, Rossi P, *et al*. Intrauterine growth retardation: evidence for the activation of the insulin-like growth factor (IGF)-related growth-promoting machinery and the presence of a cation-independent IGF binding protein-3 proteolytic activity by two months of life. *Pediatr Res* 1998;44:374–80

18. Giudice LC, Martina NA, De Las Fuentes L, *et al*. Insulin-like growth factor binding protein-1 (IGFBP-1) in the circulation of women with severe preeclampsia. *Am J Obstet Gynecol* 1997;176:751–7

19. Iino K, Sjöberg J, Seppälä M. Elevated circulating levels of decidual protein, placental protein 12, in preeclampsia. *Obstet Gynecol* 1986;68: 58–60

20. Hietala R, Pohja-Nylander P, Rutanen E-M, *et al*. Serum insulin-like growth factor binding protein-1 at 16 weeks gestation and subsequent preeclampsia. *Obstet Gynecol* 2000;95:185–9

21. DeGroot CJM, O'Brien TJ, Taylor RN. Biochemical evidence of impaired trophoblastic invasion of decidual stroma in women destined to have preeclampsia. *Am J Obstet Gynecol* 1996;175:24–9

22. Liu J-P, Baker J, Perkins AS, *et al*. Mice carrying null mutations of the genes encoding insulin-like growth factor-I (Igf-1) and type-1 IGF receptor (Igf1r). *Cell* 1993;75:59–72

23. Baker J, Liu J-P, Robertson EJ, *et al*. Role of insulin-like growth factors in embryonic and postnatal growth. *Cell* 1993;75:73–82

24. Murphy LJ, Rajkumar K, Molnar P. Phenotypic manifestations of insulin-like growth factor binding protein-1 IGFBP-1 and IGFBP-3 over-expression in transgenic mice. *Prog Growth Factor Res* 1995;6:425–32

Metabolic and epidemiological evidence of the association between insulin resistance and pre-eclampsia

32

O. Ylikorkala, H. Laivuori and R. Kaaja

Introduction

Pre-eclampsia is still the most common pregnancy complication and occurs in approximately 5% of nulliparous women. Its etiology has remained open, but several pathognomonic signs and changes, such as vasoconstriction, increased platelet aggregation and reduced placental perfusion imply that the basic disturbance in pre-eclampsia may primarily concern the regulation of the function of blood vessels. Pre-eclampsia can be called a pregnancy-specific occlusive vascular disorder. On the other hand, insulin resistance in men and non-pregnant women is a well-established risk factor for hypertension and ischemic heart disease[1]. This syndrome involves hypertension and several lipid abnormalities, and hyperhomocysteinemia and hyperleptinemia may be parts of insulin resistance in non-pregnant subjects[2,3]. We have studied the presence of features of insulin resistance during and after pre-eclamptic pregnancy.

Materials and methods

We studied 22 nulliparous pre-eclamptic and 16 nulliparous normotensive pregnant women, at an average of 35–36 weeks of gestation[4]. None of these subjects had gestational diabetes, as confirmed by normal findings during a 2-h oral glucose tolerance test. Insulin sensitivity was assessed by using the Bergman's minimal model. This test consists of intravenous injection of glucose (0.3 g/kg), followed by intravenous injection of insulin (0.03 IU/kg) 20 min later; frequent blood samples collected before and after glucose injection (up to 180 min) are assessed for glucose and insulin, and from their concomitant changes, insulin sensitivity can be calculated.

In another study we performed a 3-h oral glucose tolerance test (OGTT) in 44 women, at an average of 17 years after their first pregnancy; 22 women had had a pre-eclamptic and 22 a normotensive first pregnancy[5]. We also measured a number of steroid hormones and vasoactive compounds in these women[6].

Results

Insulin sensitivity was on average 37% less ($p < 0.009$) in pre-eclamptic women than in control women (Figure 1). Insulin sensitivity correlated negatively with the gestational age in pre-eclamptic women ($r = -0.53$; $p < 0.01$) but not in control women. When the same women were tested 3 months after delivery, insulin sensitivity had increased to 4–5 times the level seen during pregnancy. However, the women who had pre-eclamptic pregnancies still had reduced ($p < 0.04$) insulin sensitivity (Figure 2).

Pre-eclamptic women had higher plasma homocysteine concentrations than the controls (6.7 ± 0.4 vs. 3.8 ± 0.2 µmol/l, mean ± SD; $p < 0.001$) (Figure 3)[7]. Homocysteine showed a significant negative correlation with insulin sensitivity ($r = -0.51$; $p = 0.02$). Three months after delivery, plasma homocysteine had increased in the women with prior

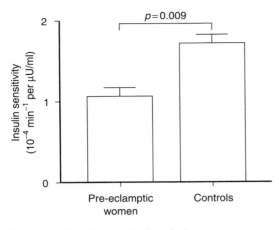

Figure 1 Insulin sensitivity during pregnancy, as assessed by the minimal model, in women with pre-eclampsia and in normotensive controls

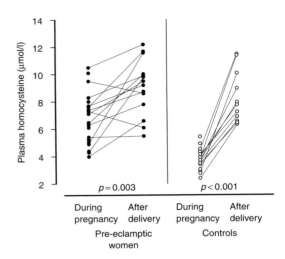

Figure 3 Homocysteine levels in pre-eclamptic and normotensive women, during pregnancy and at 3 months after delivery

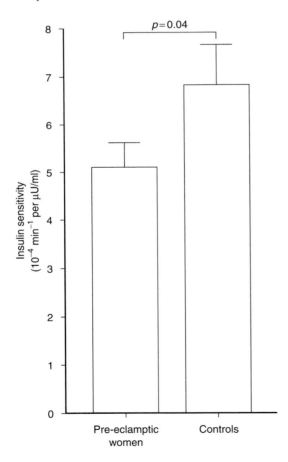

Figure 2 Insulin sensitivity at 3 months after delivery, as assessed by the minimal model, in women with pre-eclampsia and in normotensive controls

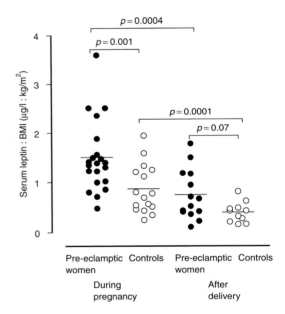

Figure 4 Leptin levels (related to body mass index, BMI) in pre-eclamptic and normotensive women, during pregnancy and at 3 months after delivery

pre-eclampsia and showed no difference between the groups.

Serum leptin, as related to body mass index, was elevated in pre-eclampsia (Figure 4)[8]. Leptin correlated with serum insulin ($r = 0.47$;

$p = 0.03$) and insulin sensitivity ($r = 0.36$; $p = 0.10$), but only in pre-eclamptic women.

In the second study of women at 17 years after their first pregnancy, blood glucose levels before and during the OGTT showed no difference between the study groups. However, to keep prior pre-eclamptic women normoglycemic, more insulin was needed both before and during the OGGT. Thus prior pre-eclamptic women showed a significant insulin resistance.

In these same women, serum free testosterone was elevated (20.6 ± 2.2 vs 15.0 ± 0.3 pmol/l, $p < 0.03$), as also were the free androgen index and the free testosterone/estradiol ratio, in the women with a history of pre-eclampsia. Endothelin-1, prostacyclin and thromboxane showed no differences between the study groups.

Discussion

We have provided evidence that acute pre-eclampsia is associated with actual insulin resistance and also with hyperhomocysteinemia and hyperleptinemia, which are themselves indicative of insulin resistance. Some of these signs persist to the late puerperium and even up to 17 years after pregnancy.

Our data do not allow us to deduce whether these changes are primary ones, and therefore possible etiologic factors in pre-eclampsia, or whether they are solely secondary reactions to the vasoconstriction, decreased plasma volume and increased sympathetic activity which characterize pre-eclamptic women and which may lead to similar metabolic changes. However, there is extensive epidemiological evidence that conditions such as obesity, polycystic ovarian disease and gestational diabetes, which manifest with insulin resistance, do predispose women to an increased risk of pre-eclampsia. These data may allow us to speculate that insulin resistance is not only a secondary change in pre-eclampsia, but may precede its onset and thus be of pathognomonic significance in pre-eclampsia.

Women with a history of pre-eclampsia showed insulin resistance 17 years after delivery. This finding may explain the epidemiological evidence that women with prior pre-eclamptic pregnancy have 1.7–2.4-fold lifetime risks of hypertension, ischemic heart disease and diabetes[9-12]. Thus pre-eclampsia may not be a pregnancy-specific phenomenon, but may be expressed many decades after the acute phase of the disease. Taking into account a vast body of evidence that estrogen replacement therapy is effective in primary prevention of cardiovascular disease, we may perhaps suggest that women with a history of pre-eclampsia may be advised to start the use of estrogen replacement when they become menopausal.

References

1. Reaven G. Role of insulin resistance in human disease. *Diabetes* 1988;37:1595–1607
2. Welsch G, Loscalzo J. Homocysteine and athero-thrombosis. *N Engl J Med* 1998;338:1042–50
3. de Courten M, Zimmet P, Hodge A, *et al.* Hyper-leptinemia: the missing link in the metabolic syndrome? *Diabetic Med* 1997;14:200–8
4. Kaaja R, Laivuori H, Laakso M, *et al.* Evidence of a state of increased insulin resistance in pre-eclampsia. *Metabolism* 1998;48:892–6
5. Laivuori H, Tikkanen MJ, Ylikorkala O. Hyperinsulinemia 17 years after pre-eclamptic pregnancy. *J Clin Endocrinol Metab* 1996;81:2908–11
6. Laivuori H, Kaaja R, Rutanen E-M, *et al.* Evidence of high circulating testosterone in women with prior pre-eclampsia. *J Clin Endocrinol Metab* 1998;83:344–7
7. Laivuori H, Kaaja R, Turpeinen U, *et al.* Plasma homocysteine levels elevated and inversely related to insulin sensitivity in pre-eclampsia. *Obstet Gynecol* 1999;93:489–93
8. Laivuori H, Kaaja R, Koistinen H, *et al.* Leptin during and after pre-eclamptic or normal

pregnancy: its relation to insulin sensitivity. *Metabolism* 2000;49:259–63

9. Hannaford P, Ferry S, Hirsch S. Cardiovascular sequelae of toxemia of pregnancy. *Heart* 1997; 77:154–8

10. Jonsdottir L, Arngrimsson R, Geirsson R, *et al.* Death rates from ischemic heart disease in women with a history of hypertension in pregnancy. *Acta Obstet Gynecol Scand* 1995;74:772–6

11. Sibai B, El-Nazer A, Gonzales-Ruis A. Severe pre-eclampsia–eclampsia in young primigravid women: subsequent pregnancy outcome and remote prognosis. *Am J Obstet Gynecol* 1986;155:1011–16

12. Chesley L, Annitto J, Csogroev R. The remote prognosis of eclamptic women; sixth periodic report. *Am J Obstet Gynecol* 1976;124:446–59

Genetics of postmenopausal complications

33

F. Massart and M. L. Brandi

Background

The menopause is the permanent cessation of menstruation resulting from the loss of ovarian follicular activity[1]. It is recognized as having occurred after 12 consecutive months of amenorrhea, for which there is no other obvious pathological or physiological cause. The menopause is of global significance to health authorities as well as being of great significance for individual women. It is estimated that in 1990 there were approximately 467 million women in the world aged 50 years and over, a number expected to increase to 1.2 billion by the year 2030[1]. It is estimated that by then perhaps 50 million women worldwide will reach the menopause annually. Atherosclerotic cardiovascular disease, osteoporotic fracture and perhaps Alzheimer's dementia are major health problems which have been linked to the occurrence of menopause. In addition, breast, colon, ovary and uterine cancer incidence increase significantly after menopause. These health consequences of the postmenopause are believed to be related to low sex steroid hormone levels, in particular estrogens and progestins, that characterize the hormonal milieu for menopausal women[2,3]. However, not only the concentrations of sex steroids but also the differential responses to these molecules represent important modulators of sex steroid bioeffects in humans. Indeed, the 'steroid response' comprises hormonal synthesis, receptors and transcriptional activities of the ligand/receptor complex (Figure 1).

In the following sections, we will review data from our own laboratory, as well as the literature suggesting that genetic variation may contribute to higher postmenopause complication risk and/or influence the outcome of disease.

Enzymes involved in progestin and estrogen metabolism

Estrogens and progestins are synthesized and metabolized from cholesterol in several steps by a number of different enzymes. Genes encoding for these enzymes have been sequenced and genetic variations in many of them have been identified.

3β-Hydroxysteroid dehydrogenase/ ketosteroid isomerase (3β-HSD/KSI)

The dual functional 3β-HSD/KSI catalyzes the formation of Δ^4-3-ketosteroids. The enzyme catalyzes two reactions, the dehydrogenation of 3β-equatorial hydroxysteroids and the subsequent isomerization of Δ^5-3-ketosteroid products to yield the α,β-unsaturated ketones. To date, two forms of the enzyme (types I and II) have been described in human encoded genes on chromosome 1p13 that are closely linked[4–7]. Type I enzyme is expressed principally in the placenta and skin, and possibly also in the breast. It is about five times more active but has very similar substrate specificity to the type II enzyme, the principal enzyme in adrenals and gonads[8]. The types I and II *3β-HSD/KSI* genes are highly homologous in structure, consisting of a 5′ untranslated exon and three coding exons for 7.8 kb length[9]. They diverge in the 5′ sequences responsible for the tissue specificity of their expression[10].

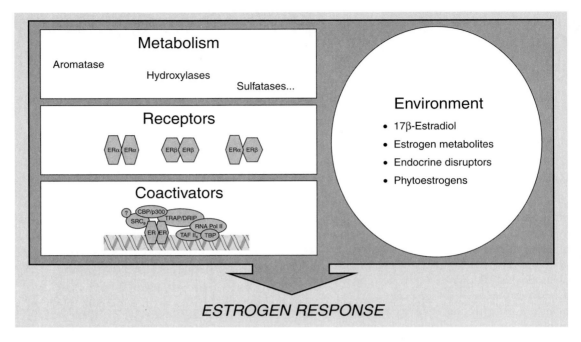

Figure 1 Polymorphisms of the estrogen response

Interest in the type II 3β-HSD/KSI exists because it catalyzes the final steps in progestin biosynthesis (i.e. the conversion of pregnenolone to progesterone)[5,11]. Therefore, a stimulating (or inhibitory) effect on 3β-HSD expression and activity is correlated with a consequent change in serum progesterone concentration. In type II *3β-HSD*, a polymorphic simple sequence microsatellite repeat is located in the third intron[9,12] approximately 250 bp from the 5′ end of exon 4[6], whose alleles present different distributions between races[13]. However, no case–control studies used *3β-HSD* polymorphisms.

17α-Hydroxylase/17,20-lyase (CYP17)

Cytochrome P450c17 is the key enzyme in the estrogen synthesis[14], and encoded by a single gene in mammals[15]. The enzyme catalyses the 17α-hydroxylation of pregnenolone and progesterone and has, in addition, a 17,20-lyase activity. Both activities are required for androgen and estrogen synthesis[15,16], but the 17,20-lyase activity (the C–C cleavage

reaction) determines what fraction of the pregnenolone and progesterone will be used in the estrogen and androgen synthesis, the remaining undergoing the cortisol synthesis pathway. It has been hypothesized that high 17α-hydroxylase/17,20-lyase activity may be at least one of the biochemical determinants of increased breast cancer risk.

CYP17, the gene coding for this enzyme, maps to chromosome 10 and contains 8 exons and 7 introns[15]. A polymorphism (a T–C substitution) in the 5′ untranslated region, at 27-bp upstream of the start of transcription, has been described[16,17]. Feigelson *et al.*[17] demonstrated that the C allele was more frequent in postmenopausal patients with advanced breast cancer than in controls and suggested this variant to be associated with an increased risk of the disease. The variant C allele was found to be associated with higher serum estradiol and progesterone levels in young healthy individuals[18]. In addition, women with homozygote C/C genotype had elevated levels of estrogens and androgens in postmenopause[19] and were about half as likely as women with the opposite genotype to be current hormone replacement therapy (HRT) users[20]. The T–C substitution has several times been suggested to create a putative Sp-1 binding site (CCAC<u>T</u>-CCACC)[17]. This would provide a mechanism for the up-regulation of transcriptional activation of the variant CCAC<u>C</u> (C) allele and higher activity of the enzyme[21]. The ability of motifs of *CYP17* 5′ untranslated region (UTR) containing the T–C polymorphic site to bind to the human transcription factor Sp-1 *in vitro* has been investigated[22]. No binding of any of the *CYP17* alleles was observed under the given experimental conditions. No other sequence within 100 bp of each of the *CYP17* alleles formed complexes with the transcription factor Sp-1 or enhanced binding to the polymorphic CACC box. Further, by genotyping 510 breast cancer patients and 201 control individuals, there was found no difference in the genotype frequencies[22]. However, a non-significant trend was observed for a higher frequency of the C/C genotype in older patients (age at diagnosis above 55 years) (15.2%) versus younger patients (age at diagnosis below 45 years) (8%). The same non-significant trend was observed for postmenopausal patients with an advanced stage of the disease (stage III and IV) (18.3%) versus premenopausal patients with stages I and II disease (9.2%)[22]. Although these above trends were in the same direction as the initial studies of Feigelson *et al.*[17], the association between the C allele and breast cancer risk has not been confirmed by others[19,23–25]. Similarly, Spurdle *et al.*[26] provided no evidence for an association between ovarian cancer risk and the genotype defined by T–C polymorphism of the *CYP17* gene.

17β Hydroxysteroid dehydrogenase (17β-HSD)

17β-hydroxysteroid dehydrogenases play essential roles in steroidogenesis. The 17β-HSD isoforms (types I–IV) catalyze the final steps in androgen and estrogen biosynthesis. Type I converts estrone to 17β-estradiol using NADPH as a cofactor and is also known to be estrogenic 17β-HSD[27–29]. Type II is a microsomal form and uses NAD^+ as cofactor. It catalyzes the oxidation of testosterone and 17β-estradiol to form androstenedione and estrone, respectively[10,30]. Its principal function is to inactivate circulating androgens and estrogens. Type III, also known as androgenic 17β-HSD, is found in the microsomes of the testis where it reduces androstenedione to testosterone[30,31]. Recently, a NAD^+ dependent type IV, similar to type II, has been cloned and shown to be principally involved in the inactivation of estrogen and androgen[32]. To date, only polymorphisms of *17β-HSD* type I gene, which is closely linked to the susceptibility gene for hereditary breast and ovarian cancer (*BRCA1* gene) on chromosome 17q21, have been studied[33,34]. There are several known polymorphisms in this gene[35]. An A–G transition at exon 6, leading to an amino acid substitution in codon 312 (Ser[312]-Gly), as well as a C–T substitution creating a *Bbv*I site in intron 5, was studied in Finnish familial and sporadic breast cancer patients, but no difference in allele distribution was observed[36]. In addition, codon 312 polymorphim, as well as codon 237 variants (Ala[237]-Val) do not affect either the catalytic or the immunological properties of the type I enzyme[37]. A polymorphic $(AAAT)_n$ repeat and a deletion of 12 bp in the 5′ flanking area of the *17β-HSD* gene have been reported[38]. The 5′ flanking regions contained consensus sequences for *cis*-acting elements that may function as regulators of *17β-HSD* gene expression. These sequences included estrogen, progesterone, and glucocorticoid response elements and a cAMP response element[39]. Responsive sequences of transcription factor GATA-3 have been identified in the 5′ flanking regulatory area of *17β-HSD* and it will, therefore, be of great interest to follow the influence of the polymorphisms in the 5′ flanking area of *17β-HSD* on GATA-3 binding and transcriptional activation of the gene.

Aromatase (CYP19)

In postmenopausal women, local aromatization of androgens to estrogens is the main source of estradiol. These local conversions of estrogens, as well as the conversion of androstenedione to estrone, are catalyzed by the aromatase cytochrome P450 complex (CYP19)[40]. This may be very important in mammary tissue, where the tumor and the surrounding tissue are the main sites of synthesis in breast cancer patients[41,42]. Moreover clinical findings in patients with aromatase deficiency, as well as in a knockout mouse (ArKO) lacking functional aromatase, illustrate the role of this enzyme for the development of the reproductive organs and mammary glands in the female and for the regulation of gonadotropins in both male and female[43,44]. The *CYP19* gene polymorphisms sites in introns 4, 5, 6, 7, the 5' regulatory area and 3' UTR have been described[45] and used in breast cancer studies: a tetranucleotide repeat polymorphism, $(TTTA)_n$, located in intron 4 of the *CYP19* gene[46]; and a $C^{826}T$ variation in exon 7 which gives rise to the amino acid substitution $Arg^{264}Cys$ and is observed by sequencing and SSCP analysis[47–49]. Sourdaine et al.[48] found one $Arg^{264}Cys$ heterozygote in five breast tumors, but no polymorphism was seen in an equal number of controls, suggesting a low Cys^{264} allele frequency in the British population. In contrast, Watanabe et al.[49] found the Cys^{264} allele frequency to be 30% in a Japanese population sample. Siegelmann-Danieli and Buetow[45] also reported the variant in US breast cancer cases. Although creating a non-conservative amino acid substitution, this polymorphism has no apparent effect on aromatase activity or response to aromatase inhibitors[48,49], nor is it associated with breast cancer risk in Japanese women[49]. There have been numerous reports of different $(TTTA)_n$ repeat alleles being associated with variation in breast cancer risk. Kristensen et al.[50] found that carrying the $(TTTA)_{12}$ allele was associated with an increased risk of breast cancer in their Scandinavian population (odds ratio (OR) 2.42, 95% confidence interval (95% CI) 1.03–5.80). This was confirmed in a study by Haiman and co-workers[51] where the $(TTTA)_{12}$

allele was over-represented in breast cancer cases (OR 1.84, 95% CI 1.02–3.32), but refuted by Siegelmann-Danieli and Buetow[45], who found that $(TTTA)_{12}$ occurred at a greater frequency in their control population. Haiman et al.[51] also found an increase in breast cancer risk associated with the $(TTTA)_{10}$ allele (OR 4.03, 95% CI 1.52–10.67) and Siegelmann-Danieli and Buetow[45] reported a greater frequency of the $(TTTA)_7$ allele measuring 171 bp in cases compared with controls (18.5 vs 13.38%, OR 1.47, 95% CI 0.99–2.17). In addition, Healey et al.[52], have identified two new polymorphisms in the *CYP19* gene: a TCT insertion/deletion in intron 4 and a G–T substitution in intron 6, which have rare allele frequencies of 0.35 and 0.45, respectively, in the British population. They found strong linkage disequilibrium between the alleles of these two loci with $(TTTA)_n$ repeats, but no significant association of any alleles with breast cancer risk. Recently, we observed that $(TTTA)_{12}$ homozygote genotype was significantly more frequent in non-osteoporotic women in comparison with osteoporotic women (72.7% vs 27.2%), while $(TTTA)_8/(TTTA)_{12}$ genotype was significantly more represented in osteoporotic women (90.48% vs 9.5%) ($p < 0.01$). In addition, women with a high number of $(TTTA)_n$ repeats had a significantly higher lumbar bone mineral density (BMD) value and lower spine fracture incidence in comparison with women with shorter $(TTTA)_n$ repeats ($p \leq 0.03$)[53].

Another C–T substitution +19 bp in the 3' UTR was therefore investigated. It was found in the tumors of four of five studied cancer patients and in none of the control placenta tissue but was suggested to be a polymorphism[48]. In addition, it was reported this 3' UTR is in strong linkage disequilibrium with the $(TTTA)_n$ polymorphism in intron 4 ($p < 0.001$)[54]. Accordingly, a significant difference in the distribution of genotypes between breast cancer patients and controls ($p = 0.007$), particularly among those presenting with high-stage disease ($p = 0.004$) and among patients with tumors larger than 5 cm

$(p = 0.001)^{55}$. However, it is not yet conclusively determined which of these polymorphisms is functional or if the function is determined by further polymorphisms in linkage disequilibrium. The C–T substitution in the 3′ UTR of CYP19 may influence the mRNA levels through mRNA stability. Indeed, a significant association between the presence of the T allele and mRNA levels $(p < 0.02)$ as well as a switch from the normally used adipose promoter to ovary promoter $(p < 0.01)^{55}$. So, the C–T substitution in the 3′ UTR of CYP19 may influence the mRNA levels through mRNA stability.

CYP1A1

CYP1A1 (mapping on 15q22–23) is a highly inducible member of the cytochrome P450 family[56]. CYP1A1 catalyzes the C-2, C-6α, and C-15α-hydroxylation of estradiol, but has been mostly studied as the principal enzyme activating cigarette-smoke constituents and other environmental pollutants such as polycyclic aromatic hydrocarbons, dioxin and derivatives, aromatic amines, polychlorinated biphenyls and nitrosamines, thus creating an enormous body of literature by itself[57]. The role of CYP1A1 in the metabolism of estradiol and its influence on human cancer risk has been shadowed by its role in the metabolism of these potent carcinogens. Several polymorphisms had been described in the human CYP1A1 gene. A MspI RFLP in the 3′ UTR[58], an adenine to guanine transition in the heme-binding domain of exon 7 (Ile[462]Val)[59], a promoter (TAAAA)$_n$ repeat polymorphism[56] and an African-American-specific RFLP in intron 7[60]. The first two have been found overrepresented among lung cancer patients in Japan[61], but reports in Caucasians are inconclusive[62]. Moreover, both have been related with a slightly elevated risk of colon and postmenopausal breast cancer[63–66]. In addition, the MspI polymorphism has been found associated with breast cancer in African-American women[67]. Esteller et al.[68] have found an enhanced endometrial cancer risk associated with the 3′ UTR and exon 7 CYP1A1 germ line polymorphisms. Finally, a new polymorphism in exon 7 of human CYP1A1 has been described resulting in a threonine to asparagine exchange in codon461 (Thr[461]Asn) in the heme-binding domain[69], showing a strong association with endometrial cancer risk with an OR of 6.36 (95% CI 1.99–26.5, $p < 0.001$)[70]. The significance of this variant is still unknown, although the exchange of the adjacent amino acid residues, isoleucine to valine, results in a change in enzyme activity[71].

CYP1B1

CYP1B1 (mapping on 2p21) is a dioxin-inducible member of the cytochrome P450 superfamily[72]. CYP1B1 catalyses the C4-hydroxylation of estradiol to 4OH-estradiol, as main product and also 2- and 16α-OH-metabolites[73]. The C4-hydroxylation activity of CYP1B1 has received particular attention because 4-OH-estrogens are carcinogenic in animal models[74,75]. Genetic polymorphism in the human CYP1B1 gene has recently been reported by Stoilov et al.[76], Bailey et al.[77] and Bejjani et al.[78] and results have suggested that there are at least six genetic polymorphisms in the CYP1B1 gene. Of these variants, amino acid replacements occur at exon 2 (Arg[48]-Gly and Ala[119]-Ser) and exon 3 (Val[432]-Leu and Asn[453]-Ser)[76,77]. These exon variants displayed 2.4- to 3.4-fold higher catalytic efficiencies than the wild type enzyme[73]. The data on CYP1B1 exon 3 polymorphisms are too preliminary or contradictory to evaluate possible association with breast or colon cancer risk[79–81], needing to be studied in larger and better-defined cohorts.

Recognition and signaling pathways of sex steroid molecules

Given the central role of sex steroids in female health, polymorphisms of genes encoding sex steroid receptors (ERs and PR) and their cofactor/repressor are certainly important candidates for the determination of postmenopause risk of disease.

Estrogen receptor (ERα and ERβ) polymorphisms

The known physiological actions of estrogens appear to be mediated on target cells primarily by two nuclear estrogen receptors (ERα and ERβ) which act as transcriptional factors[82,83].

Several polymorphisms about the *ERα* gene have been reported[84–88], but actually, the intron 1 *Pvu*II and *Xba*I restriction sites were the most studied variants. The presence of the restriction site for each endonuclease was conventionally indicated with lowercase letters (p or x, respectively for *Pvu*II and *Xba*I endonucleases), while uppercase letters (P or X) indicated the absence of the restriction site. In particular, in bone[89–93] and neurological disorders[94–96] where estrogens show protective effects, PP, XX or PPXX genotypes revealed a higher risk of onset of disease than opposite genotypes, with a dose-dependence for the p or x allele. Interestingly, Maruyama *et al.*[97] detected enhancer activity in intron 1 of the *ERα* gene and demonstrated that this enhancer activity differed among haplotypes of *Pvu*II and *Xba*I restriction sites. We recently located $(TA)_n$ repeat polymorphism[84] in the promoter region of *ERα* gene, and reported a high degree of linkage disequilibrium with *Pvu*II and *Xba*I polymorphic restriction sites[98]. Because of its position, between promoter A and B regions, it is possible to speculate that allelic variations due to different $(TA)_n$ dinucleotide repeat lengths might have physiological relevance, probably by affecting promoter usage. There was a strong linkage disequilibrium between intron 1 polymorphic sites and also between these sites and $(TA)_n$ repeats, with a high degree of coincidence of the short TA alleles and the presence of *Pvu*II and *Xba*I restriction sites. No significant relationship between *Pvu*II-*Xba*I polymorphisms and BMD was observed. A statistically significant correlation between $(TA)_n$ repeat allelic variants and lumbar BMD was observed ($p < 0.05$), with subjects with a low number of repeats (TA < 15) showing the lowest BMD values and increased incidence of vertebral

fracture[98]. Conversely, data of these *ERα* polymorphisms appear not conclusive with possible prevalence and severity of coronary artery disease[99,100]. What about reproductive tissues? Weel *et al.*[101] suggested that homozygous PP women had a 1.1 year ($p < 0.02$) earlier onset of menopause than opposite pp genotype, with a dose-dependence for the P allele corresponding to a 0.5 year ($p < 0.02$) earlier onset of menopause. Furthermore, PP genotype revealed a higher risk of surgical menopause because of hysterectomy due to menorrhagia and leiomyomas than women bearing the pp genotype[101], but we did not find any difference in leiomyoma onset risk between *Pvu*II-*Xba*I genotypes[102]. In a recent Swedish study[103], the *ERα* P and X, such as long $(TA)_n$ alleles appeared to confer a reduced risk for endometrial cancer. As for breast cancer susceptibility and prognostic markers, the presence of the *Xba*I restriction site was found more frequently in patients than in controls and p allele was associated with progesterone receptor negativity in primary tumors, as reported in larger series[104,105]. By contrast, no agreement was reached on different *ERα* polymorphism distribution both in ER protein expression and in age of cancer onset[104–107].

Rosenkranz *et al.*[108] detected a single polymorphism nucleotide exchange at nt 1730 (A–G) of the 3′ UTR of the *ERβ* gene. The 1730A–G polymorphism has presumably no functional implications, but its alleles might be in linkage disequilibrium to relevant mutations in the *ERβ* gene. Specific control-sequence of mRNA degradation pathway are located in the 3′ UTR region of *ERα* gene[109,110]. No comparable data are actually reported for *ERβ* gene. In our Caucasian population, we did not find any association between this 3′ UTR and $(CA)_n$ repeat polymorphisms[111] with lumbar BMD, contrasting with what previously was reported in a Japanese study[112].

Progesterone receptor (PR) polymorphism

Human progesterone receptor (*PR*) gene is located on chromosome 11q22–23 and belongs to the steroid–thyroid–retinoic acid receptor superfamily of transcriptional factors[113]. PR exists in two isoforms, PR_A and PR_B transcribed from the *PR* gene by alternative initiation. Several polymorphisms of *PR* are reported[114–116]. Rowe *et al.*[116] identified a variant of human *PR* gene, named *PROGINS*, containing a 306-bp *Alu* direct repeat insertion of the PV/HS-1 *Alu* subfamily in intron 7, which causes the previously reported additional *Taq*I restriction endonuclease site[117]. Furthermore, a consensus splice acceptor site $T_{(10)}TGAG$ was identified in the *Alu* insertion and a consensus splice branch site was located between nucleotides –53 and –47 relative to the consensus splice acceptor site[117]. This *Alu* insertion brings a consensus splice acceptor site into the proximity of an upstream consensus splice branch site, the combination of which potentially directs the encoding of a variant form of PR exon 8. The correct transcription of codons in this exon is essential to the function of the human PR. It has been demonstrated that encoding of an alternative exon 8 results in complete loss of both ligand binding and transcriptional activation in response to progesterone[118]. Thus, this insertion might result in expression of an aberrant splice form of PR with altered ligand and hormone-binding properties and hence hormonal regulation[119]. In addition, Kieback *et al.*[119] reported the polymorphic PR_A *PROGINS* allele to express an increased transcriptional activity and increased stability and,

thereby, PR_A *PROGINS* could repress estrogen receptor activation more efficiently. However, the functional role of the *PROGINS* allele is not known. Four hospital-based case–control studies have been published that analyzed the association between *PROGINS* polymorphism and breast or ovarian cancer risk in patient populations with different ethnic backgrounds without analyses regarding age and menopausal status[117,120–123]. It is unclear whether the *PROGINS* allele alters the risk for breast or ovarian cancer. However, Wang-Gohrke *et al.*[123] recently found a reduced risk of breast cancer in women by age of 50 years who carry at least one *PROGINS* allele and a statistically significant trend of decrease in risk with an increase in the number of *PROGINS* alleles, which is compatible with other previous observations of a decreased risk of breast cancer associated with the *PROGINS* allele[120,123].

Acknowledgements

Research performed within the frame of the Italian National Health System Project 'Human Exposure to Xenobiotics with Potential Endocrine Activities: Evaluation of the Risks for Reproduction and Development' and 'Environmental Risk of Postmenopausal Diseases' (2000); Cofin MURST 1999 and Telethon 1999–2000 to M.L.B.

References

1. World Health Organization. *Research on the Menopause in the 1990s. Report of a WHO Scientific Group*. WHO Technical Report Series. No. 866, 1996

2. Lindsay R, Hart DM, Clark DM. The minimum effective dose of estrogen for prevention of postmenopausal bone loss. *Obstet Gynecol* 1984; 63:759–63

3. Cummings SR, Kelsey JL, Nevitt MC, *et al.* Epidemiology of osteoporosis and osteoporotic fractures. *Epidemiol Rev* 1985;7:178–208

4. Lachance Y, Luu-The V, Labrie C, *et al.* Characterization of human 3 beta-hydroxysteroid dehydrogenase/delta 5-delta 4-isomerase gene and its expression in mammalian cells. *J Biol Chem* 1990;265:20469–75

5. Rheaume E, Lachance Y, Zhao HF, *et al.* Structure and expression of a new complementary DNA encoding the almost exclusive 3 beta-hydroxysteroid dehydrogenase/delta 5-delta 4-isomerase in human adrenals and gonads. *Mol Endocrinol* 1991;5:1147–57

6. Russell AJ, Wallace AM, Forest MG, *et al.* Mutation in the human gene for 3 beta-hydroxysteroid dehydrogenase type II leading to male pseudohermaphroditism without salt loss. *J Mol Endocrinol* 1994;12:225–37

7. Morissette J, Rheaume E, Leblanc JF, *et al.* Genetic linkage mapping of HSD3B1 and HSD3B2 encoding human types I and II 3 beta-hydroxysteroid dehydrogenase/delta 5-delta 4-isomerase close to D1S514 and the centromeric D1Z5 locus. *Cytogenet Cell Genet* 1995;69:59–62

8. Sutcliffe RG, Russell AJ, Edwards CR, *et al.* Human 3 beta-hydroxysteroid dehydrogenase: genes and phenotypes. *J Mol Endocrinol* 1996; 17:1–5

9. Lachance Y, Luu-The V, Verreault H, *et al.* Structure of the human type II 3 beta-hydroxysteroid dehydrogenase/delta 5-delta 4 isomerase (3 beta-HSD) gene: adrenal and gonadal specificity. *DNA Cell Biol* 1991;10: 701–11

10. Penning TM. Molecular endocrinology of hydroxysteroid dehydrogenases. *Endocr Rev* 1997;18:281–305

11. Lorence MC, Murry BA, Trant JM, *et al.* Human 3 beta-hydroxysteroid dehydrogenase/delta 5-4isomerase from placenta: expression in nonsteroidogenic cells of a protein that catalyzes the dehydrogenation/isomerization of C21 and C19 steroids. *Endocrinology* 1990;126:2493–8

12. Verreault H, Dufort I, Simard J, *et al.* Dinucleotide repeat polymorphisms in the HSD3B2 gene. *Hum Mol Genet* 1994;3:384

13. Devgan SA, Henderson BE, Yu MC, *et al.* Genetic variation of 3 beta-hydroxysteroid dehydrogenase type II in three racial/ethnic groups: implications for prostate cancer risk. *Prostate* 1997;33:9–12

14. Voutilainen R, Miller WL. Developmental expression of genes for the stereoidogenic enzymes P450scc (20,22-desmolase), P450c17 (17 alpha-hydroxylase/17,20-lyase), and P450c21 (21-hydroxylase) in the human fetus. *J Clin Endocrinol Metab* 1986;63:1145–50

15. Picado-Leonard J, Miller WL. Cloning and sequence of the human gene for P450c17 (steroid 17 alpha-hydroxylase/17,20 lyase): similarity with the gene for P450c21. *DNA* 1987;6:439–48

16. Carey AH, Chan KL, Short F, *et al.* Evidence for a single gene effect causing polycystic ovaries and male pattern baldness. *Clin Endocrinol* 1993;38:653–8

17. Feigelson HS, Coetzee GA, Kolonel LN, *et al.* A polymorphism in the CYP17 gene increases the risk of breast cancer. *Cancer Res* 1997;57: 1063–5

18. Feigelson HS, Shames LS, Pike MC, *et al.* Cytochrome P450c17alpha gene (CYP17) polymorphism is associated with serum estrogen and progesterone concentrations. *Cancer Res* 1998;58:585–7

19. Haiman CA, Hankinson SE, Spiegelman D, *et al.* The relationship between a polymorphism in CYP17 with plasma hormone levels and breast cancer. *Cancer Res* 1999;59:1015–20

20. Feigelson HS, McKean-Cowdin R, Pike MC, *et al.* Cytochrome P450c17alpha gene (CYP17) polymorphism predicts use of hormone replacement therapy. *Cancer Res* 1999;59: 3908–10

21. Kadonaga JT, Carner KR, Masiarz FR, *et al.* Isolation of cDNA encoding transcription factor Sp1 and functional analysis of the DNA binding domain. *Cell* 1987;51:1079–90

22. Nedelcheva Kristensen V, Haraldsen EK, Anderson KB, *et al.* CYP17 and breast cancer risk: the polymorphism in the 5′ flanking area of the gene does not influence binding to Sp-1. *Cancer Res* 1999;59:2825–8

23. Weston A, Pan CF, Bleiweiss IJ, *et al.* CYP17 genotype and breast cancer risk. *Cancer Epidemiol Biomarkers Prev* 1998;7:941–4

24. Helzlsouer KJ, Huang HY, Strickland PT, *et al.* Association between CYP17 polymorphisms and the development of breast cancer. *Cancer Epidemiol Biomarkers Prev* 1998;7:945–9

25. Dunning AM, Healey CS, Pharoah PD, *et al.* No association between a polymorphism in the steroid metabolism gene CYP17 and risk of breast cancer. *Br J Cancer* 1998;77:2045–7

26. Spurdle AB, Chen X, Abbazadegan M, *et al.* CYP17 promotor polymorphism and ovarian cancer risk. *Int J Cancer* 2000;86:436–9

27. Poutanen M, Miettinen M, Vihko R. Differential estrogen substrate specificities for transiently expressed human placental 17 beta-hydroxysteroid dehydrogenase and an endogenous enzyme expressed in cultured COS-m6 cells. *Endocrinology* 1993;133: 2639–44

28. Peltoketo H, Isomaa V, Maentausta O, *et al.* Complete amino acid sequence of human placental 17 beta-hydroxysteroid dehydrogenase

deduced from cDNA. *FEBS Lett.* 1988 Oct 24;239(1):73–7

29. Gast MJ, Sims HF, Murdock GL, *et al.* Isolation and sequencing of a complementary deoxyribonucleic acid clone encoding human placental 17 beta-estradiol dehydrogenase: identification of the putative cofactor binding site. *Am J Obstet Gynecol* 1989;161:1726–31

30. Andersson S, Geissler WM, Patel S, *et al.* The molecular biology of androgenic 17 beta-hydroxysteroid dehydrogenases. *J Steroid Biochem Mol Biol* 1995;53:37–9

31. Geissler WM, Davis DL, Wu L, *et al.* Male pseudohermaphroditism caused by mutations of testicular 17beta-hydroxysteroid dehydrogenase 3. *Nat Genet* 1994;7:34–9

32. Adamski J, Normand T, Leenders F, *et al.* Molecular cloning of a novel widely expressed human 80 kDa 17beta-hydroxysteroid dehydrogenase IV. *Biochem J* 1995;311:437–43

33. Luu The V, Labrie C, Zhao HF, *et al.* Characterization of cDNAs for human estradiol 17 beta-dehydrogenase and assignment of the gene to chromosome 17: evidence of two mRNA species with distinct 5′-termini in human placenta. *Mol Endocrinol* 1989;3:1301–9

34. Simard J, Feunteun J, Lenoir G, *et al.* Genetic mapping of the breast–ovarian cancer syndrome to a small interval on chromosome 17q12-21: exclusion of candidate genes EDH17B2 and RARA. *Hum Mol Genet* 1993; 2:1193–9

35. Normand T, Narod S, Labrie F, *et al.* Detection of polymorphisms in the estradiol 17 beta-hydroxysteroid dehydrogenase II gene at the EDH17B2 locus on 17q11-q21. *Hum Mol Genet* 1993;2:479–83

36. Mannermaa A, Peltoketo H, Winqvist R, *et al.* Human familial and sporadic breast cancer: analysis of the coding regions of the 17 beta-hydroxysteroid dehydrogenase 2 gene (EDH17B2) using a single-strand conformation polymorphism assay. *Hum Genet* 1994; 93:319–24

37. Puranen TJ, Poutanen MH, Peltoketo HE, *et al.* Site-directed mutagenesis of the putative active site of human 17 beta-hydroxysteroid dehydrogenase type 1. *Biochem J* 1994;304: 289–93

38. Friedman LS, Lynch ED, King MC. Two independent polymorphisms at the 17 beta-hydroxysteroid dehydrogenase (EDH17B) gene (17q21). *Hum Mol Genet* 1993;2:821

39. Peltoketo H, Isomaa V, Vihko R. Genomic organization and DNA sequences of human 17 beta-hydroxysteroid dehydrogenase genes and flanking regions. Localization of multiple Alu sequences and putative cis-acting elements. *Eur J Biochem* 1992;209:459–66

40. Means GD, Mahendroo MS, Corbin CJ, *et al.* Structural analysis of the gene encoding human aromatase cytochrome P-450, the enzyme responsible for estrogen biosynthesis. *J Biol Chem* 1989;264:19385–91

41. Hankinson SE, Willett WC, Manson JE, *et al.* Plasma sex steroid hormone levels and risk of breast cancer in postmenopausal women. *J Natl Cancer Inst* 1998;90:1292–9

42. Pike MC, Spicer DV, Dahmoush L, *et al.* Estrogens, progestogens, normal breast cell proliferation, and breast cancer risk. *Epidemiol Rev* 1993;15:17–35

43. Harada N, Ogawa H, Shozu M, *et al.* Genetic studies to characterize the origin of the mutation in placental aromatase deficiency. *Am J Hum Genet* 1992;51:666–72

44. Fisher CR, Graves KH, Parlow AF, *et al.* Characterization of mice deficient in aromatase (ArKO) because of targeted disruption of the cyp19 gene. *Proc Natl Acad Sci USA* 1998;95: 6965–70

45. Siegelmann-Danieli N, Buetow KH. Constitutional genetic variation at the human aromatase gene (Cyp19) and breast cancer risk. *Br J Cancer* 1999;79:456–63

46. Polymeropoulos MH, Xiao H, Rath DS, *et al.* Tetranucleotide repeat polymorphism at the human aromatase cytochrome P-450 gene (CYP19). *Nucleic Acids Res* 1991;19:195

47. Corbin CJ, Graham-Lorence S, McPhaul M, *et al.* Isolation of a full-length cDNA insert encoding human aromatase system cytochrome P-450 and its expression in nonsteroidogenic cells. *Proc Natl Acad Sci USA* 1988;85:8948–52

48. Sourdaine P, Parker MG, Telford J, *et al.* Analysis of the aromatase cytochrome P450 gene in human breast cancers. *J Mol Endocrinol* 1994; 13:331–7

49. Watanabe J, Harada N, Suemasu K, *et al.* Arginine-cysteine polymorphism at codon 264 of the human CYP19 gene does not affect aromatase activity. *Pharmacogenetics* 1997;7: 419–24

50. Kristensen VN, Andersen TI, Lindblom A, *et al.* A rare CYP19 (aromatase) variant may increase

the risk of breast cancer. *Pharmacogenetics* 1998;8:43–8

51. Haiman CA, Hankinson SE, Spiegelman D, *et al*. A tetranucleotide repeat polymorphism in CYP19 and breast cancer risk. *Int J Cancer* 2000;87:204–10

52. Healey CS, Dunning AM, Durocher F, *et al*. Polymorphisms in the human aromatase cytochrome P450 gene (CYP19) and breast cancer risk. *Carcinogenesis* 2000;21:189–93

53. Masi L, Becherini L, Gennari L, *et al*. Polymorphism of the aromatase gene in postmenopausal Italian women: distribution and correlation with bone and fracture risk. *J Clin Endocrinol Metab* 2001;86:in press

54. Kristensen T, Kristensen VN, Borresen-Dale AL. High-throughput screening for known mutations by automated analysis of single sequencing reactions. *Biotechniques* 1998;24:832–5

55. Kristensen VN, Borresen-Dale AL. Molecular epidemiology of breast cancer: genetic variation in steroid hormone metabolism. *Mutat Res* 2000;462:323–33

56. Durocher F, Morissette J, Simard J. Genetic linkage mapping of the CYP11A1 gene encoding the cholesterol side-chain cleavage P450scc close to the CYP1A1 gene and D15S204 in the chromosome 15q22.33-q23 region. *Pharmacogenetics* 1998;8:49–53

57. Nedelcheva V, Gut I. P450 in the rat and man: methods of investigation, substrate specificities and relevance to cancer. *Xenobiotica* 1994;24:1151–75

58. Kawajiri K, Nakachi K, Imai K, *et al*. Identification of genetically high risk individuals to lung cancer by DNA polymorphisms of the cytochrome P450IA1 gene. *FEBS Lett* 1990;263:131–3

59. Hayashi S, Watanabe J, Nakachi K, *et al*. Genetic linkage of lung cancer-associated MspI polymorphisms with amino acid replacement in the heme binding region of the human cytochrome P450IA1 gene. *J Biochem* 1991;110:407–11

60. Crofts F, Cosma GN, Currie D, *et al*. A novel CYP1A1 gene polymorphism in African-Americans. *Carcinogenesis* 1993;14:1729–31

61. Nakachi K, Imai K, Hayashi S, *et al*. Genetic susceptibility to squamous cell carcinoma of the lung in relation to cigarette smoking dose. *Cancer Res* 1991;51:5177–80

62. Raunio H, Husgafvel-Pursiainen K, Anttila S, *et al*. Diagnosis of polymorphisms in carcinogen-activating and inactivating enzymes and cancer susceptibility – a review. *Gene* 1995;159:113–21

63. Ambrosone CB, Freudenheim JL, Graham S, *et al*. Cytochrome P4501A1 and glutathione S-transferase (M1) genetic polymorphisms and postmenopausal breast cancer risk. *Cancer Res* 1995;55:3483–5

64. Sivaraman L, Leatham MP, Yee J, *et al*. CYP1A1 genetic polymorphisms and in situ colorectal cancer. *Cancer Res* 1994;54:3692–5

65. Rebbeck TR, Rosvold EA, Duggan DJ, *et al*. Genetics of CYP1A1: coamplification of specific alleles by polymerase chain reaction and association with breast cancer. *Cancer Epidemiol Biomarkers Prev* 1994;3:511–14

66. Kiss I, Sandor J, Pajkos G, *et al*. Colorectal cancer risk in relation to genetic polymorphism of cytochrome P450 1A1, 2E1, and glutathione-S-transferase M1 enzymes. *Anticancer Res* 2000;20:519–22

67. Taioli E, Trachman J, Chen X, *et al*. A CYP1A1 restriction fragment length polymorphism is associated with breast cancer in African-American women. *Cancer Res* 1995;55:3757–8

68. Esteller M, Garcia A, Martinez-Palones JM, *et al*. Susceptibility to endometrial cancer: influence of allelism at p53, glutathione S-transferase (GSTM1 and GSTT1) and cytochrome P-450 (CYP1A1) loci. *Br J Cancer* 1997;75:1385–8

69. Cascorbi I, Brockmoller J, Roots I. A C4887A polymorphism in exon 7 of human CYP1A1: population frequency, mutation linkages, and impact on lung cancer susceptibility. *Cancer Res* 1996;56:4965–9

70. Esteller M, Garcia A, Martinez-Palones JM, *et al*. Germ line polymorphisms in cytochrome-P450 1A1 (C4887 CYP1A1) and methylenetetrahydrofolate reductase (MTHFR) genes and endometrial cancer susceptibility. *Carcinogenesis* 1997;18:2307–11

71. Kawajiri K, Nakachi K, Imai K, *et al*. The CYP1A1 gene and cancer susceptibility. *Crit Rev Oncol Hematol* 1993;14:77–87

72. Tang YM, Wo YYP, Stewart J, *et al*. Isolation and characterization of the human cytochrome P450 CYP1B1 gene. *J Biol Chem* 1996;271:28324–30

73. Hanna IH, Dawling S, Roodi N, *et al.* Cytochrome P450 1B1 (CYP1B1) pharmacogenetics: association of polymorphisms with functional differences in estrogen hydroxylation activity. *Cancer Res* 2000;60:3440–4

74. Hayes CL, Spink DC, Spink BC, *et al.* 17 beta-estradiol hydroxylation catalyzed by human cytochrome P450 1B1. *Proc Natl Acad Sci USA* 1996;93:9776–81

75. Shimada T, Hayes CL, Yamazaki H, *et al.* Activation of chemically diverse procarcinogens by human cytochrome P-450 1B1. *Cancer Res* 1996;56:2979–84

76. Stoilov I, Akarsu AN, Alozie I, *et al.* Sequence analysis and homology modeling suggest that primary congenital glaucoma on 2p21 results from mutations disrupting either the hinge region or the conserved core structures of cytochrome P4501B1. *Am J Hum Genet* 1998; 62:573–84

77. Bailey LR, Roodi N, Dupont WD, *et al.* Association of cytochrome P450 1B1 (CYP1B1) polymorphism with steroid receptor status in breast cancer. *Cancer Res* 1998;58:5038–41

78. Bejjani BA, Lewis RA, Tomey KF, *et al.* Mutations in CYP1B1, the gene for cytochrome P4501B1, are the predominant cause of primary congenital glaucoma in Saudi Arabia. *Am J Hum Genet* 1998;62:325–33

79. Watanabe J, Shimada T, Gillam EM, *et al.* Association of CYP1B1 genetic polymorphism with incidence to breast and lung cancer. *Pharmacogenetics* 2000;10:25–33

80. Zheng W, Xie DW, Jin F, *et al.* Genetic polymorphism of cytochrome P450-1B1 and risk of breast cancer. *Cancer Epidemiol Biomarkers Prev* 2000;9:147–50

81. Fritsche E, Bruning T, Jonkmanns C, *et al.* Detection of cytochrome P450 1B1 Bfr I polymorphism: genotype distribution in healthy German individuals and in patients with colorectal carcinoma. *Pharmacogenetics* 1999;9: 405–8

82. Green S, Walter P, Greene G, *et al.* Cloning of the human oestrogen receptor cDNA. *J Steroid Biochem* 1986;24:77–83

83. Mosselman S, Polman J, Dijkema R. ER beta: identification and characterization of a novel human estrogen receptor. *FEBS Lett* 1996; 392:49–53

84. del Senno L, Aguiari GL, Piva R. Dinucleotide repeat polymorphism in the human estrogen receptor (ESR) gene. *Hum Mol Genet* 1992; 1:354

85. Schubert EL, Lee MK, Newman B, *et al.* Single nucleotide polymorphisms (SNPs) in the estrogen receptor gene and breast cancer susceptibility. *J Steroid Biochem Mol Biol* 1999;71:21–7

86. Iwase H, Greenman JM, Barnes DM, *et al.* Sequence variants of the estrogen receptor (ER) gene found in breast cancer patients with ER negative and progesterone receptor positive tumors. *Cancer Lett* 1996;108:179–84

87. Wang Y, Miksicek RJ. Characterization of estrogen receptor cDNAs from human uterus: identification of a novel PvuII polymorphism. *Mol Cell Endocrinol* 1994;101:101–10

88. Taylor JA, Li Y, You M, *et al.* B region variant of the estrogen receptor gene. *Nucleic Acids Res* 1992;20:2895

89. Kobayashi S, Inoue S, Hosoi T, *et al.* Association of bone mineral density with polymorphism of the estrogen receptor gene. *J Bone Miner Res* 1996;11:306–11

90. Gennari L, Becherini L, Masi L, *et al.* Vitamin D and estrogen receptor allelic variants in Italian postmenopausal women: evidence of multiple gene contribution to bone mineral density. *J Clin Endocrinol Metab* 1998;83:939–44

91. Carling T, Rastad J, Kindmark A, *et al.* Estrogen receptor gene polymorphism in postmenopausal primary hyperparathyroidism. *Surgery* 1997;122:1101–6

92. Kurabayashi T, Tomita M, Matsushita H, *et al.* Association of vitamin D and estrogen receptor gene polymorphism with the effect of hormone replacement therapy on bone mineral density in Japanese women. *Am J Obstet Gynecol* 1999;180:1115–20

93. Lorentzon M, Lorentzon R, Backstrom T, *et al.* Estrogen receptor gene polymorphisms, but not estradiol levels, is related to bone density in healthy adolescent boys: a cross-sectional and longitudinal study. *J Clin Endocrinol Metab* 1999;84:4597–601

94. Brandi ML, Becherini L, Gennari L, *et al.* Association of the estrogen receptor alpha gene polymorphisms with sporadic Alzheimer's disease. *Biochem Biophys Res Commun* 1999;265: 335–8

95. Isoe-Wada K, Maeda M, Yong J, *et al.* Positive association between an estrogen receptor gene polymorphism and Parkinson's disease with dementia. *Eur J Neurol* 1999;6:431–5

96. Isoe K, Ji Y, Urakami K, *et al*. Genetic association of estrogen receptor gene polymorphisms with Alzheimer's disease. *Alzheimer's Research* 1997;3:195–7

97. Maruyama H, Toji H, Harrington CR, *et al*. Lack of an association of estrogen receptor alpha gene polymorphisms and transcriptional activity with Alzheimer disease. *Arch Neurol* 2000;57:236–40

98. Becherini L, Gennari L, Masi L, *et al*. Evidence of a linkage disequilibrium between polymorphisms in the human estrogen receptor alpha gene and their relationship to bone mass variation in postmenopausal Italian women. *Hum Mol Genet* 2000;9: 2043–50

99. Matsubara Y, Murata M, Kawano K, *et al*. Genotype distribution of estrogen receptor polymorphisms in men and postmenopausal women from healthy and coronary populations and its relation to serum lipid levels. *Arterioscler Thromb Vasc Biol* 1997;17:3006–12

100. Kunnas TA, Laippala P, Penttila A, *et al*. Association of polymorphism of human alpha oestrogen receptor gene with coronary artery disease in men: a necropsy study. *BMJ* 2000; 321:273–4

101. Weel AE, Uitterlinden AG, Westendorp IC, *et al*. Estrogen receptor polymorphism predicts the onset of natural and surgical menopause. *J Clin Endocrinol Metab* 1999;84: 3146–50

102. Massart F, Becherini L, Gennari L, *et al*. Genotype distribution of estrogen receptor alpha gene polymorphisms in Italian women affected by surgical uterine leiomyomas. *Fertil Steril* 2001;75:567–70

103. Weiderpass E, Persson I, Melhus H, *et al*. Estrogen receptor alpha gene polymorphisms and endometrial cancer risk. *Carcinogenesis* 2000;21:623–7

104. Yaich L, Dupont WD, Cavener DR, *et al*. Analysis of the PvuII restriction fragment-length polymorphism and exon structure of the estrogen receptor gene in breast cancer and peripheral blood. *Cancer Res* 1992;52: 77–83

105. Andersen TI, Heimdal KR, Skrede M, *et al*. Oestrogen receptor (ESR) polymorphisms and breast cancer susceptibility. *Hum Genet* 1994;94:665–70

106. Hill SM, Fuqua SA, Chamness GC, *et al*. Estrogen receptor expression in human breast cancer associated with an estrogen receptor gene restriction fragment length polymorphism. *Cancer Res* 1989;49:145–8

107. Parl FF, Cavener DR, Dupont WD. Genomic DNA analysis of the estrogen receptor gene in breast cancer. *Breast Cancer Res Treat* 1989;14:57–64

108. Rosenkranz K, Hinney A, Ziegler A, *et al*. Systematic mutation screening of the estrogen receptor beta gene in probands of different weight extremes: identification of several genetic variants. *J Clin Endocrinol Metab* 1998; 83:4524–7

109. Kenealy MR, Flouriot G, Sonntag-Buck V, *et al*. The 3′-untranslated region of the human estrogen receptor alpha gene mediates rapid messenger ribonucleic acid turnover. *Endocrinology* 2000;141:2805–13

110. Keaveney M, Parker MG, Gannon F. Identification of a functional role for the 3′ region of the human oestrogen receptor gene. *J Mol Endocrinol* 1993;10:143–52

111. Tsukamoto K, Inoue S, Hosoi T, *et al*. Isolation and radiation hybrid mapping of dinucleotide repeat polymorphism at the human estrogen receptor beta locus. *J Hum Genet* 1998;43:73–4

112. Ogawa S, Hosoi T, Shiraki M, *et al*. Association of estrogen receptor beta gene polymorphism with bone mineral density. *Biochem Biophys Res Commun* 2000;269:537–41

113. Rousseau-Merck MF, Misrahi M, Loosfelt H, *et al*. Localization of the human progesterone receptor gene to chromosome 11q22-q23. *Hum Genet* 1987;77:280–2

114. Fuqua SA, Hill SM, Chamness GC, *et al*. Progesterone receptor gene restriction fragment length polymorphisms in human breast tumors. *J Natl Cancer Inst* 1991;83:1157–60

115. Tsukamoto K, Watanabe I, Shiba T, *et al*. Isolation of a polymorphic CA repeat sequence at the human progesterone receptor (PGR) locus. *J Hum Genet* 1998;43:287–8

116. Rowe SM, Coughlan SJ, McKenna NJ, *et al*. Ovarian carcinoma-associated TaqI restriction fragment length polymorphism in intron G of the progesterone receptor gene is due to an Alu sequence insertion. *Cancer Res* 1995; 55:2743–5

117. McKenna NJ, Kieback DG, Carney DN, *et al*. A germline TaqI restriction fragment length polymorphism in the progesterone receptor gene in ovarian carcinoma. *Br J Cancer* 1995;71:451–5

118. Vegeto E, Allan GF, Schrader WT, *et al*. The mechanism of RU486 antagonism is dependent on the conformation of the carboxy-terminal tail of the human progesterone receptor. *Cell* 1992;69:703–13

119. Kieback DG, Tong XW, Weigel NL, *et al*. A genetic mutation in the progesterone receptor (PROGINS) leads to an increased risk of non-familial breast and ovarian cancer causing inadequate control of estrogen receptor driven proliferation. *J Soc Gynecol Investig* 1998;5:40a

120. Lancaster JM, Berchuck A, Carney ME, *et al*. Progesterone receptor gene polymorphism and risk for breast and ovarian cancer. *Br J Cancer* 1998;78:277

121. Manolitsas TP, Englefield P, Eccles DM, *et al*. No association of a 306-bp insertion polymorphism in the progesterone receptor gene with ovarian and breast cancer. *Br J Cancer* 1997;75:1398–9

122. Garrett E, Rowe SM, Coughlan SJ, *et al*. Mendelian inheritance of a Taq I restriction fragment length polymorphism due to an insertion in the human progesterone receptor gene and its allelic imbalance in breast cancer. *Cancer Res Ther Control* 1995;4:217–2

123. Wang-Gohrke S, Chang-Claude J, Becher H, *et al*. Progesterone receptor gene polymorphism is associated with decreased risk for breast cancer by age 50. *Cancer Res* 2000;60:2348–50

Non-transcriptional mechanisms for estrogen receptors signaling

34

T. Simoncini, G. Varone, J. K. Liao and A. R. Genazzani

Non-transcriptional mechanisms for estrogen receptors signaling

Estrogen receptors (ER) have been characterized as transcription factors translating the signals from their relative ligands through transcriptional regulation of the expression of target genes[1,2]. According to this model, binding of estrogen to the specific ligand binding domain (LBD) induces a conformational modification of ER, leading to the separation of the receptor from cytoplasmic chaperone proteins such as heat shock protein 90 (HSP90) and to the exposure of nuclear localization sequences (NLS). This event favors nuclear translocation of the ligand-bound receptors, that are now able to dimerize with other ERs and to bind to estrogen response elements (ERE), i.e. nucleotide sequences specifically recognized by ERs, on the promoter regions of the target genes, thus regulating the expression of these genes by interfering with the transcription machinery[3].

However, observations of a series of effects elicited by steroid hormones that are too rapid to be compatible with the activation of the process of RNA and protein synthesis have prompted a search for alternative signaling mechanisms for these receptors. Different terms have been used in order to distinguish these non-conventional signaling mechanisms, the more popular of which are 'non-genomic' or 'non-nuclear'. In general, these mechanisms should be more properly indicated as 'non-transcriptional', so to underline that RNA synthesis is not required for the production of these effects. Actually, the classification of these effects is still quite fragmentary, due to poor knowledge of the real molecular basis explaining all the different phenomena that have been from time to time described as 'non-genomic' actions of steroid receptors. As practical rules, non-transcriptional effects can be indicated as: (1) actions that are too rapid to be compatible with RNA and protein synthesis, i.e. that ensue within seconds to minutes from the challenge with the hormone; (2) actions that steroid hormones induce in cells in which RNA and protein synthesis are nearly absent (such as spermatozoa); (3) actions that can be reproduced in the presence of inhibitors of RNA or protein synthesis; (4) actions that can be reproduced by using steroid hormones coupled to cell-membrane-impermeable molecules. It is therefore clear that a satisfactory understanding of the real nature of these mechanisms is still far from being accomplished, and up to now only a patchwork of descriptive information on different non-transcriptional effects of steroid hormones has been cumulated. However, there is growing evidence that many of these effects could be linked to the presence of functional and yet unidentified cell membrane steroid hormone receptors.

Regarding estrogen receptors, pioneering evidence of the existence of a distinct subpopulation of cell membrane receptors was provided at the end of the 1970s by the work of Pietras and Szego[4], who first described the presence of cell membrane binding sites for estradiol in endometrial cells. Since then, various observations on these receptors have been contributed (although there has never been an isolation or full characterization of this particular population of receptors), and evidence that these molecules mediate important cellular actions of estrogens has accumulated[5]. Indeed, plasma membrane estrogen receptors have been said to be involved in the regulation of cell membrane ion channels[6–8], of G-protein-coupled receptors[9] and of tyrosine kinases and mitogen-activated (MAP) kinases[10,11]. They have also been shown to activate adenylate cyclase production[12], as well as to trigger phospholipase C activation[13]. Little is yet known about the nature of these putative membrane estrogen receptors, but data from transfection studies suggest that both ERα and ERβ can localize to the cell membrane, although we have as yet no data on the possible structural differences of these particular subpopulations of receptors[14].

Estrogens and the cardiovascular system

In the past few years, the cardiovascular system has been demonstrated to be an important target for estrogens. Estrogen deficiency has been recently proposed to be a possible independent cardiovascular risk factor[15], and epidemiological studies have demonstrated that estrogen supplementation after menopause has significant beneficial effects on the cardiovascular system[16,17]. Together with these intriguing clinical data, we still face the problem of an insufficient knowledge of the mechanisms of action of sex steroid hormones on the vascular system, and thus on the possible different pathophysiological processes taking place in different patient populations or disease stages.

In this regard, non-transcriptional signaling represents a particularly important mechanism of action for estrogen receptors at the vascular wall level[18,19]. Female sex steroid hormones produce diverse effects on the vascular system, inducing rapid vasodilatation, blocking vessel wall response to injury, and decreasing the development of atherosclerosis[18,19]. All of these effects are the result of a multi-faceted series of actions on the various components of the vascular wall, from endothelial cells to smooth muscle cells, to macrophages and stromal vascular cells, and are the result of a complex interplay of estrogen receptor-mediated transcriptional as well as non-transcriptional actions.

Estrogen receptors and the vascular wall

Two subtypes of the human estrogen receptor (ER) have been identified, ERα[1] and ERβ[2]. ERα is expressed in human vasculature, both in endothelial[20] and in smooth muscle cells[21]. ERβ distribution in vascular tissues is less characterized, but human endothelial cells synthesize ERβ[22]. Blood vessels of non-human primates[23], mice and rats[24] also express this receptor subtype. The relative importance of the two receptor subtypes for estrogen's actions at the vascular level is still unclear. In fact, ERα-deficient mice are still protected by estrogen treatment from balloon vascular injury, like their wild-type controls[25], but also ERβ knock-out mice[26] are protected, suggesting that there may be an overlap between the actions of the two receptors, and that in the absence of one of the two, the other may provide a functional compensation. However, a male patient carrying a non-functional mutation of ERα showed impaired vascular function[27] as well as early atherosclerotic degeneration[28], suggesting that there may be distinct vascular functions for the estrogen receptor subtypes. This is suggested also by the recent finding of increased expression of ERβ, but not of ERα, after balloon vascular injury in male rats[24]. Additionally, recent studies show the presence of a cell membrane-specific estrogen receptor subpopulation in endothelial cells[29,30].

Estrogens and vascular tone regulation: 'transcriptional' and 'non-transcriptional' effects

A prototypical 'non-genomic' action of estrogen receptors is represented by vasodilatation induced by estrogen, which occurs in a matter of seconds to minutes[31]. This acute effect is

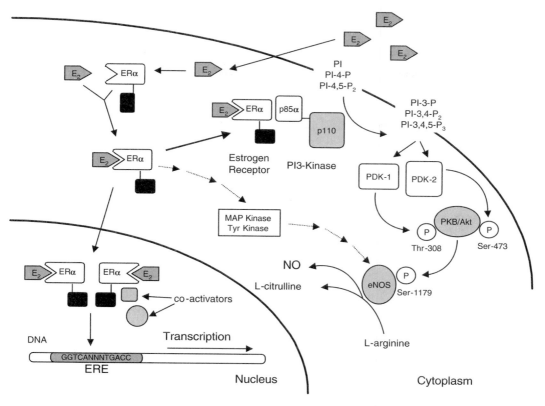

Figure 1 Estrogen and vascular tone regulation: 'genomic' and 'non-genomic' effects. Natural estrogen's regulation of vascular cell function through classic transcriptional ('genomic') mechanisms is mediated by binding of the engaged estrogen receptor to specific consensus DNA sequences (estrogen response elements, ERE) located in the promoter region of the target genes, with the contribution of other regulatory molecules (co-activators). This binding results in transcriptional regulation of the target gene (usually, but not always, induction of gene expression). Other mechanisms mediating the rapid vascular effects of estrogens have been identified, and since they are not dependent on gene transcription, they have been collectively indicated as non-transcriptional (or 'non-genomic'). There are probably very different types of 'non-genomic' effects, and some appear to be dependent on the estrogen receptor (ER). A typical example of estrogen-dependent non-transcriptional signaling mechanism is represented by rapid endothelial nitric oxide synthase (eNOS) activation upon treatment with estrogen, that has been shown to be elicited by a physical and functional coupling of ERα with PI3-kinase and with consequent activation of the PI3-kinase/Akt cascade, that leads to eNOS phosphorylation and enzymatic activation.

the result of a regulation of ionic fluxes as well as of vasoactive molecule release on endothelial and smooth muscle cells (Figure 1).

Regulation of nitric oxide (NO) synthesis and release is a major target of estrogen at the endothelial level. NO is a central controller of vascular function, acting as a potent vasodilator as well as an anti-inflammatory molecule[32]. Estrogen-induced endothelium-dependent vasodilatation *in vivo* is reliant on NO production[33], and estrogen has been shown to regulate NO release by several means. The principal mechanism is probably represented by the rapid activation of the endothelial isoform of nitric oxide synthase (eNOS)[34,35]. ERα is involved in the genesis of this phenomenon, which is independent from gene transcription and has been proposed to be in part due to the activation of MAP or tyrosine kinases-dependent pathways[36]. Another possible mechanism of regulation of eNOS by estrogen may involve the chaperone protein heat shock protein 90 (HSP90), which basally interacts with the estrogen receptor and dissociates from it upon binding with the ligand. In this regard, HSP90 has been recently demonstrated to interact with eNOS and to dynamically regulate its enzymatic activity[37].

We have recently demonstrated the existence of a novel, non-transcriptional mechanism of ERα signaling in endothelial cells potentially explaining estrogen's rapid effects on NO release[38]. Indeed, according to our data, ERα is able to interact with the lipid kinase phosphatidylinositol-3-kinase (PI3-kinase). The PI3-kinase is a heterodimeric phosphoinositide kinase composed of an 85 kD (p85α) adapter/regulatory subunit and a 110 kD (p110) catalytic subunit[39]. The PI3-kinase phosphorylates the D-3 position of the phosphatidylinositol ring, catalyzing the synthesis of lipid mediators that act as second messengers transferring the signaling cascade to intracellular protein kinases. One of the principal targets of this cascade is the serine–threonine protein kinase Akt. The activation of Akt mediates many of the downstream cellular effects of PI3-kinase including activation of cell survival pathways[40]. We have shown that upon binding with estradiol, ERα physically and functionally couples with the regulatory subunit of PI3-kinase, thus triggering an activation of the catalytic subunit and increasing intracellular production of phosphoinositides[38]. This association is strictly dependent on the concentration of estradiol, can be completely reversed by pure estrogen receptor antagonists, such as ICI 182,780, and is highly specific, since it is not elicited by the inactive estradiol stereoisomer 17α-estradiol. Moreover, this association follows in a time-delayed manner, being maximal after 20 minutes from estrogen treatment of endothelial cells in culture[38]. Endothelial cells treated with estradiol undergo a rapid increase in nitric oxide release due to an activation of eNOS, and the kinetics of this activation corresponds with the time course of the association with ERα and activation of PI3-kinase and with

the consequent production of lipid second messengers[38]. Moreover, eNOS activation by estrogen can be blocked by co-treatment of endothelial cells with a selective PI3-kinase inhibitor, wortmannin, as well as by the transfection of a negative dominant form of PI3-kinase, and can be reproduced in mouse fibroblasts lacking either eNOS, ERα or p85α subunit of PI3-kinase only after the molecular reconstitution of the cells by transfection of all the missing molecules, but not if any of the three is lacking[38]. Additional information is provided by the evidence that in order to get eNOS activation by estrogen treatment, the downstream PI3-kinase effector, Akt, necessarily has to be activated. Estrogen treatment of endothelial cells results in a time-consistent phosphorylation and enzymatic activation of Akt. Transfection of endothelial cells with negative dominant forms of Akt abolishes estrogen capacity to trigger increases in eNOS activity[38]. In agreement with our data, it has been recently shown that rapid eNOS activation can be accomplished by eNOS phosphorylation by Akt[41,42]. Additionally, we also showed that the activation of this signaling pathway by estrogen has significant pathophysiological implications *in vivo*, by demonstrating that estrogen-induced reduction in leukocyte adhesion to endothelium in vessels after ischemia/ reperfusion (evaluated by real-time intravital microscopy in pulsating cremaster muscle vessels) can be completely reversed by treatment with PI3-kinase as well as eNOS inhibitors[38].

Thus, by linking the estrogen receptor to PI3-kinase, a novel and potentially critical non-transcriptional action is described. In addition, the cellular effects of estrogen are considerably broadened since PI3-kinase is known to mediate various cellular functions[40,43]. As additional data, we have preliminary results suggesting that the interaction of PI3-kinase with ERα may occur via the co-localization of the two molecules at the cell membrane level, thus suggesting that estrogen-induced activation of PI3-kinase may be an additional and novel function

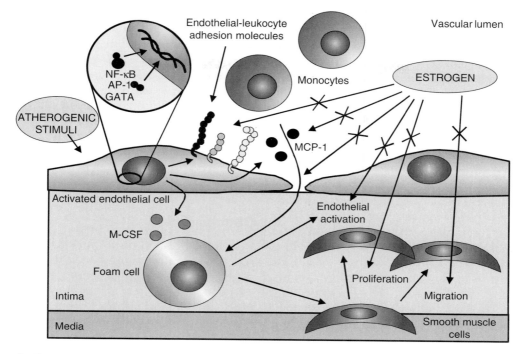

Figure 2 Estrogen receptor non-transcriptional signaling and atherosclerosis. Atherogenic stimuli have the common characteristic of inducing an inflammatory phenotype on endothelial cells (endothelial activation). This is dependent on the activation of inflammatory transcription factors (such as NF-κB and AP-1), which induce the expression of the genes encoding for endothelial leukocyte adhesion molecules (VCAM-1, ICAM-1, E-selectin), monocyte chemoattractants (MCP-1) and macrophage growth factors (M-CSF). This process leads to increased adherence of circulating monocytes to activated endothelial cells, and to their intimal accumulation. Here monocytes accumulate lipids and release inflammatory molecules, perpetrating the endothelial activation status and causing smooth muscle cell migration from the media to the intima and their proliferation, which are the earliest events in the development of atherosclerotic lesions. Estrogens produce a series of direct effects on several of these steps, thus potentially acting as a local anti-inflammatory and anti-atherogenic factor

of plasma membrane estrogen receptors (Simoncini *et al.* unpublished results).

Non-transcriptional estrogen receptor signaling and atherosclerosis

Estrogen regulates the structure of the vessel wall, controlling the proliferation, survival and migration of endothelium, smooth muscle, stromal cells and leukocytes[18,19]. Endothelial cell proliferation after injury is enhanced by estrogen both *in vitro*[44] and *in vivo*[44,45]. Endothelial cell apoptotic process is blocked by estrogen[46] as well, thus showing an endothelial protective effect which may be involved in estrogen's antiatherogenic properties and

important for the estrogen-induced improvement in functional recovery after vascular injury. Indeed, estrogen treatment is known to have antiatherogenic effects *in vivo*[47,48], and these effects are independent of cholesterol levels but tightly dependent on the state of arterial endothelium and on reduced endothelium–monocyte interactions[49].

Atherosclerosis is currently considered an inflammatory process[50], and vascular endothelium plays a pivotal role in its initiation and propagation[51]. Various atherogenic stimuli induce endothelial cell activation, defined as functional, and antigenic changes that promote monocyte adhesion and accumulation to the vessel wall[52] (Figure 2). In recent years, estrogen's antiatherogenic effects have been more and more associated with the anti-inflammatory effects exerted on vascular endothelium. Estrogen's cellular action on endothelial leukocyte adhesion molecules is mirrored by an inhibition of leukocyte adhesion to endothelial cells and transendothelial migration in vivo[53].

The inhibition of adhesion molecule expression is part of a general decrease in transcription of endothelial genes which are induced during endothelial activation, such as monocyte chemoattractant protein-1[54]. Several of these genes are transcriptionally induced by inflammatory transcription factors, such as nuclear factor-κB (NF-κB) and activator protein-1 (AP-1). This effect is due to binding of the activated factors on specific response elements located on the promoter region of these genes[55]. The genes encoding for leukocyte adhesion molecules have no known estrogen response elements[56], and estrogen's inhibitory action on adhesion molecule expression is actually mediated by functional interferences with the activation of these transcription factors[22]. Indeed, pretreatment of endothelial cells with estradiol prior to the induction of endothelial activation with an inflammatory cytokine is associated with a dramatic inhibition of the activation, nuclear translocation and DNA-binding activity of transcription factors NF-κB, AP-1 and GATA-binding proteins[22]. The effect on NF-κB is actually mediated by a non-transcriptional action of estrogen receptor, linked to the blockade of the cytokine-induced activation of the specific IκB kinase, IKKα, thus preventing the degradation of the NF-κB inhibitor IκBα and the nuclear translocation of NF-κB. This mechanism thus configures an additional, novel, non-transcriptional way of signal transduction of the estrogen receptor, with significant pathophysiological implications for the development of atherosclerotic lesions. Indeed, we have shown that different estrogen receptor agonists[57] and selective estrogen receptor modulators[58] can have differential effects on the expression of endothelial leukocyte adhesion molecules in cell culture, thus posing the question of the existence of potential differences in the efficacy of distinct treatments for postmenopausal women with regard to prevention of cardiovascular disease.

Conclusions

In summary, non-transcriptional estrogen receptor signaling represents a vast and still largely unknown array of actions triggered by estrogen through distinct molecular mechanisms in different tissues. There is growing evidence to suggest that part of these actions can be ascribed to estrogen receptors localized to the plasma membrane, although an isolation and characterization of this subpopulation of receptors is essential in order to confirm this hypothesis. Estrogen receptor non-transcriptional signaling mechanisms are particularly important at the vascular wall level, where estrogen can activate nitric oxide release via the interaction with the lipid kinase PI3-kinase, and can exert anti-inflammatory actions via the inhibition of transcription factors NF-κB, AP-1 and GATA-binding proteins, thus controlling vascular tone and exerting potent antiatherogenic effects. Understanding the molecular mechanisms through which these actions are exerted represents an important frontier, in order to have the key to engineer newer pharmacological tools for the prevention of cardiovascular disease in postmenopausal women.

References

1. Green S, Walter P, Kumar V, et al. Human oestrogen receptor cDNA: sequence, expression and homology to v-erb-A. Nature 1986; 320:134–9

2. Mosselman S, Polman J, Dijkema R. ER beta: identification and characterization of a novel human estrogen receptor. FEBS Lett 1996;392: 49–53

3. Truss M, Beato M. Steroid hormone receptors: interaction with deoxyribonucleic acid and transcription factors. *Endocr Rev* 1993;14: 459–79

4. Pietras RJ, Szego CM. Specific binding sites for oestrogen at the outer surfaces of isolated endometrial cells. *Nature* 1977;265:69–72

5. Levin ER. Cellular functions of the plasma membrane estrogen receptor. *Trends Endocrinol Metab* 1999;10:374–77

6. Tesarik J, Mendoza C. Nongenomic effects of 17 beta-estradiol on maturing human oocytes: relationship to oocyte developmental potential. *J Clin Endocrinol Metab* 1995;80: 1438–43

7. Nakajima T, Kitazawa T, Hamada E, *et al.* 17beta-estradiol inhibits the voltage-dependent L-type Ca^2+ currents in aortic smooth muscle cells. *Eur J Pharmacol* 1995;294:625–35

8. Valverde MA, Rojas P, Amigo J, *et al.* Acute activation of Maxi-K channels (hSlo) by estradiol binding to the beta subunit. *Science* 1999; 285:1929–31

9. Kelly MJ, Wagner EJ. Estrogen modulation of G-protein-coupled receptors. *Trends Endocrinol Metab* 1999;10:369–74

10. Migliaccio A, Di Domenico M, Castoria G, *et al.* Tyrosine kinase/p21ras/MAP-kinase pathway activation by estradiol-receptor complex in MCF-7 cells. *EMBO J* 1996;15:1292–300

11. Watters JJ, Campbell JS, Cunningham MJ, *et al.* Rapid membrane effects of steroids in neuroblastoma cells: effects of estrogen on mitogen activated protein kinase signalling cascade and c-fos immediate early gene transcription. *Endocrinology* 1997;138:4030–3

12. Aronica SM, Kraus WL, Katzenellenbogen BS. Estrogen action via the cAMP signaling pathway: stimulation of adenylate cyclase and cAMP-regulated gene transcription. *Proc Natl Acad Sci USA* 1994;91:8517–21

13. Le Mellay V, Grosse B, Lieberherr M. Phospholipase C beta and membrane action of calcitriol and estradiol. *J Biol Chem* 1997;272: 11902–7

14. Razandi M, Pedram A, Greene GL, *et al.* Cell membrane and nuclear estrogen receptors (ERs) originate from a single transcript: studies of ERalpha and ERbeta expressed in Chinese hamster ovary cells. *Mol Endocrinol* 1999;13:307–19

15. Braunwald E. Shattuck lecture – Cardiovascular medicine at the turn of the millennium: triumphs, concerns, and opportunities. *N Engl J Med* 1997;337:1360–9

16. Grodstein F, Stampfer M, Manson J, *et al.* Postmenopausal estrogen and progestin use and the risk of cardiovascular disease. *N Engl J Med* 1996;335:453–61

17. Grodstein F, Stampfer MJ, Colditz GA, *et al.* Postmenopausal hormone therapy and mortality. *N Engl J Med* 1997;336:1769–75

18. Mendelsohn ME, Karas RH. The protective effects of estrogen on the cardiovascular system. *N Engl J Med* 1999;340:1801–11

19. Simoncini T, Genazzani AR. Direct vascular effects of estrogens and selective estrogen receptor modulators. *Curr Opin Obstet Gynecol* 2000;12:181–7

20. Venkov CD, Rankin AB, Vaughan DE. Identification of authentic estrogen receptor in cultured endothelial cells. A potential mechanism for steroid hormone regulation of endothelial function. *Circulation* 1996;94: 727–33

21. Karas RH, Patterson BL, Mendelsohn ME. Human vascular smooth muscle cells contain functional estrogen receptor. *Circulation* 1994; 89:1943–50

22. Simoncini T, Maffei S, Basta G, *et al.* Estrogens and glucocorticoids inhibit endothelial vascular cell adhesion molecule-1 expression by different transcriptional mechanisms. *Circ Res* 2000;87:19–25

23. Register TC, Adams MR. Coronary artery and cultured aortic smooth muscle cells express mRNA for both the classical estrogen receptor and the newly described estrogen receptor beta. *J Steroid Biochem Mol Biol* 1998;64: 187–91

24. Lindner V, Kim SK, Karas RH, *et al.* Increased expression of estrogen receptor-beta mRNA in male blood vessels after vascular injury. *Circ Res* 1998;83:224–9

25. Iafrati MD, Karas RH, Aronovitz M, *et al.* Estrogen inhibits the vascular injury response in estrogen receptor alpha-deficient mice. *Nat Med* 1997;3:545–8

26. Karas RH, Hodgin JB, Kwoun M, *et al.* Estrogen inhibits the vascular injury response in estrogen receptor beta-deficient female mice. *Proc Natl Acad Sci USA* 1999;96:15133–6

27. Sudhir K, Chou TM, Messina LM, *et al.* Endothelial dysfunction in a man with disruptive mutation in oestrogen-receptor gene. *Lancet* 1997;349:1146–7

28. Sudhir K, Chou TM, Chatterjee K, *et al.* Premature coronary artery disease associated with a disruptive mutation in the estrogen receptor gene in a man. *Circulation* 1997;96: 3774–7

29. Russell KS, Haynes MP, Sinha D, *et al.* Human vascular endothelial cells contain membrane binding sites for estradiol, which mediate rapid intracellular signaling. *Proc Natl Acad Sci USA* 2000;97:5930–5

30. Stefano GB, Prevot V, Beauvillain JC, *et al.* Cell-surface estrogen receptors mediate calcium-dependent nitric oxide release in human endothelia. *Circulation* 2000;101: 1594–7

31. Gilligan DM, Quyyumi AA, Cannon RO 3rd. Effects of physiological levels of estrogen on coronary vasomotor function in postmenopausal women. *Circulation* 1994;89:2545–51

32. Liao JK. Endothelial nitric oxide and vascular inflammation. In Panza JA, Cannon ROI, eds. *Endothelium, Nitric Oxide and Atherosclerosis.* Armonk, NY: Futura, 1999:119–32

33. Guetta V, Quyyumi AA, Prasad A, *et al.* The role of nitric oxide in coronary vascular effects of estrogen in postmenopausal women. *Circulation* 1997;96:2795–801

34. Caulin-Glaser T, Garcia-Cardena G, Sarrel P, *et al.* 17 beta-estradiol regulation of human endothelial cell basal nitric oxide release, independent of cytosolic Ca2+ mobilization. *Circ Res* 1997;81:885–92

35. Lantin-Hermoso RL, Rosenfeld CR, Yuhanna IS, *et al.* Estrogen acutely stimulates nitric oxide synthase activity in fetal pulmonary artery endothelium. *Am J Physiol* 1997;273: L119–26

36. Chen Z, Yuhanna IS, Galcheva-Gargova Z, *et al.* Estrogen receptor alpha mediates the nongenomic activation of endothelial nitric oxide synthase by estrogen. *J Clin Invest* 1999; 103:401–6

37. Garcia-Cardena G, Fan R, Shah V, *et al.* Dynamic activation of endothelial nitric oxide synthase by Hsp90. *Nature* 1998;392:821–4

38. Simoncini T, Hafezi-Moghadam A, Brazil D, *et al.* Interaction of oestrogen receptor with the regulatory subunit of phosphatidylinositol-3-OH kinase. *Nature* 2000;407:538–541

39. Carpenter CL, Duckworth BC, Auger KR, *et al.* Purification and characterization of phosphoinositide 3-kinase from rat liver. *J Biol Chem* 1990;265:19704–11

40. Franke TF, Kaplan DR, Cantley LC. PI3K: downstream AKTion blocks apoptosis. *Cell* 1997;88:435–7

41. Dimmeler S, Fleming I, Fisslthaler B, *et al.* Activation of nitric oxide synthase in endothelial cells by Akt-dependent phosphorylation. *Nature* 1999;399:601–5

42. Fulton D, Gratton JP, McCabe TJ, *et al.* Regulation of endothelium-derived nitric oxide production by the protein kinase Akt. *Nature* 1999;399:597–601

43. Franke TF, Yang SI, Chan TO, *et al.* The protein kinase encoded by the Akt proto-oncogene is a target of the PDGF-activated phosphatidylinositol 3-kinase. *Cell* 1995;81:727–36

44. Morales DE, McGowan KA, Grant DS, *et al.* Estrogen promotes angiogenic activity in human umbilical vein endothelial cells *in vitro* and in a murine model. *Circulation* 1995;91: 755–63

45. Krasinski K, Spyridopoulos I, Asahara T, *et al.* Estradiol accelerates functional endothelial recovery after arterial injury. *Circulation* 1997; 95:1768–72

46. Spyridopoulos I, Sullivan AB, Kearney M, *et al.* Estrogen-receptor-mediated inhibition of human endothelial cell apoptosis. Estradiol as a survival factor. *Circulation* 1997;95:1505–14

47. Adams MR, Kaplan JR, Manuck SB, *et al.* Inhibition of coronary artery atherosclerosis by 17-beta estradiol in ovariectomized monkeys. Lack of an effect of added progesterone. *Arteriosclerosis* 1990;10:1051–7

48. Nascimento CA, Kauser K, Rubanyi GM. Effect of 17beta-estradiol in hypercholesterolemic rabbits with severe endothelial dysfunction. *Am J Physiol* 1999;276:H1788–94

49. Holm P, Andersen HL, Arroe G, *et al.* Gender gap in aortic cholesterol accumulation in cholesterol-clamped rabbits: role of the endothelium and mononuclear-endothelial cell interaction. *Circulation* 1998;98:2731–7

50. Ross R. Atherosclerosis – An inflammatory disease. *N Engl J Med* 1999;340:115–26

51. Gimbrone MA Jr. Vascular endothelium: an integrator of pathophysiologic stimuli in atherosclerosis. *Am J Cardiol* 1995;75:67B–70B

52. De Caterina R, Gimbrone MA Jr. Leukocyte-endothelial interactions and the pathogenesis of atherosclerosis. In Kristensen SD, Schmidt EB, De Caterina R, *et al.*, eds. *n-3 Fatty Acids – Prevention and Treatment in Vascular Disease.* London: Springer Verlag, 1995:9–24

53. Nathan L, Pervin S, Singh R, *et al*. Estradiol inhibits leukocyte adhesion and transendothelial migration in rabbits *in vivo*. Possible mechanisms for gender differences in atherosclerosis. *Circ Res* 1999;85:377–85

54. Simoncini T, Genazzani AR, De Caterina R. Towards a molecular understanding of the atheroprotective effects of estrogens: a review of estrogen effects on endothelial activation. *Ital Heart J* 2000;1:104–7

55. Collins T, Read MA, Neish AS, *et al*. Transcriptional regulation of endothelial cell adhesion molecules: NF-kappa B and cytokine-inducible enhancers. *FASEB J* 1995;9:899–909

56. Neish AS, Williams AJ, Palmer HJ, *et al*. Functional analysis of the human vascular cell adhesion molecule 1 promoter. *J Exp Med* 1992; 176:1583–93

57. Simoncini T, Genazzani AR. Tibolone inhibits leukocyte adhesion molecule expression in human endothelial cells. *Mol Cell Endocrinol* 2000;162:87–94

58. Simoncini T, De Caterina R, Genazzani AR. Selective estrogen receptor modulators: different actions on vascular cell adhesion molecule-1 (VCAM-1) expression in human endothelial cells. *J Clin Endocrinol Metab* 1999;84:815–18

Assessment of quality of life in the climacteric

35

H. P. G. Schneider

The first widely accepted attempt to measure the severity of menopausal complaints in women was the Kupperman Index. The main focus of this instrument is on symptomatic relief, assessed on the basis of the physician's summary of the severity of climacteric complaints and assisted by the index rather than by letting women respond independently. A new 'Menopause Rating Scale' (MRS) was validated in order to establish an instrument that can easily be filled in by patients. This scale was standardized and three important dimensions of the scale were characterized by cluster analysis: somatic, psychological and urogenital symptoms. The definition of the cluster 'somatic symptoms' such as hot flushes, vasomotor symptoms, insomnia and musculoskeletal disorders is quite apparent, the cluster 'psychological symptoms' includes depression, irritability, anxiety and mental exhaustion. Depression is the collective term that defines 'melancholia' according to Kupperman; it is a reactive process and often termed 'depressive mood' or 'moodiness'. Mental exhaustion is related to 'lack of energy' or 'tiredness' or terms such as 'weakness' and 'fatigue'. It also implies 'poor concentration' and 'forgetfulness'. Finally, 'urogenital symptoms' were defined as sexual dysfunction, urological complaints and vaginal atrophy. 'Sexual dysfunction' includes reduction in sexual desire, reduced sexual activity and/or satisfaction. Urological complaints include 'urgency', 'loss of urine' or 'incontinence'. Finally, vaginal atrophy is coincident with 'vaginal dryness' and 'dyspareunia'.

A comparative analysis with the Kupperman Index clearly demonstrated that both scales are measuring the same conditions. However, when the original degrees of severity of both the MRS and Kupperman Index are analyzed, the Kupperman Index classifies many more women of a population sample as so-called 'no/minor' as compared with the MRS. The MRS, standardized in a random population sample, has a different spread in its classification, and by looking at quartiles of both scales, the index categories of the MRS differentiate more appropriately in the higher and lower degrees of symptoms; also, the psychometric quality of the MRS in many ways is more elaborated than that of the Kupperman Index.

The results of our follow-up survey with the MRS demonstrate that the individual scores remain relatively stable unless intervening variables such as new diseases and treatments, or other conditions, occurred during the observational period. Multivariate analyses of the medical history including drug treatment, health status and contact with the healthcare system, besides age and a few social characteristics, give rise to a similar conclusion: the variation of scores and its direction are mainly influenced by co-morbidity such as cardiac failure, chest pain, chronic gastrointestinal problems, rheumatoid or joint-muscle complaints and others.

Our analyses very clearly demonstrate a striking correlation of the MRS classification of menopausal symptoms with the quality of life. The SF-36 profile is distinctly different among the four quartiles of the total MRS score. For both the somatic and psychological sum-scores, significant positive associations were found between MRS and short-form 36 (SF-36) scores, for example the MRS can be utilized as an age-condition-specific measure of quality of life. The MRS scores do not correlate equally well across all dimensions of the SF-36. The best differentiation was observed for scales which are known from clinical practice as particularly relevant for the menopausal transition: physical role functioning, bodily pain, vitality and emotional role functioning.

A well-defined menopausal complaint self-rating scale serves the purpose of a less troublesome, practical and less time-consuming instrument to address the impact of any therapy on various aspects of quality of life and at the same time avoid interpersonal bias of patients and health personnel. Introducing the MRS into the interaction between a women and her doctor would allow improved co-operation and a higher degree of long-term compliance and at the same time avoid wide-ranging batteries of questionnaires.

Hormone replacement therapy and lipid profile: effects of different routes of administration

36

N. O. Siseles, G. Berg, P. Gutierrez, M. S. Moggia and M. Prada

Introduction

The decrease in serum estrogen levels as a consequence of menopause is associated with an increase in different risk factors[1,2]. Among others, cardiovascular disease (CVD) is the most frequent cause of death for Western postmenopausal women[3,4].

Compared with premenopausal women, postmenopausal women have a larger plasma concentration of total cholesterol and LDL cholesterol[5,6]. There is also an increase in plasma triglycerides that is related to aging[4]. Other lipoproteins whose plasma concentrations increase in menopause are Lp(a)[7] and intermediate density lipoprotein (IDL)[6,8]. There is more controversy about the behavior of HDL cholesterol, which, according to some authors, decreases[9–11,13], whereas others do not observe changes after menopause has set in (Table 1)[8,14].

Both IDL and LDL are very heterogeneous lipoproteins, varying in size, density, molecular mass and chemical composition. Under normal conditions, these lipoproteins catabolize at the level of apoproteins B:E receptors, whose synthesis is stimulated by estrogens (Figure 1)[15]. During postmenopause, the low estrogen levels causes a decrease in the catabolism of these lipoproteins together with their concomitant increase in blood circulation[5,6]. This increase is independent of age[8,14].

The quality and plasma concentrations of IDL and LDL as well as the number of B:E receptors determine plasma residence time for these particles, and are directly related to their oxidability. LDL's most frequent alterations, such as a larger amount of triglycerides, glycosylation, or their turning into smaller, denser particles, are all factors that would accelerate LDL oxidability in the vessel wall[16].

These changes are related to an increased risk of cardiovascular disease. Estrogen therapy has proved to have beneficial effects regarding cardiovascular risk factors. A large body of epidemiological evidence shows 50% reduction of the risk of CVD in healthy estrogen users. Nevertheless, only 25–35% of the cardiovascular benefit of hormone replacement therapy (HRT) can be attributed to the alterations in lipid profile[17]. Some of these effects are related to estrogen's capacity to stimulate the synthesis of B:E receptors and to reverse deterioration of lipid profiles to premenopausal levels, though not all studies have yielded the same findings[18].

We should bear in mind additional factors that may alter therapeutic response to estrogen, for instance:

(1) quantity, dose and potency of the drug;

(2) quality, chemical structure of the drug;

(3) route of administration;

(4) duration of treatment;

(5) therapeutic strategies;

(6) basic hormonal and metabolic state of the recipient.

Table 1 Effect of menopause on lipids and lipoproteins

	Number	TC	TG	LDL	HDL	IDL
Matthews (1989)[11]	541	↑	↑	↑	↓	—
Jensen (1990)[9]	170	↑	↑	↑	↓	—
Razay (1992)[12]	394	↑	↑	—	↑	—
Stevenson (1993)[10]	542	↑	↑	↑	↓	—
Castelo-Branco (1993)[13]	95	↔	↔	↑	↓	—
Berg (2001)[8]	126	↑	↑	↑	↔	↑

↔, No change; ↑, increase; ↓, decrease. TC, total cholesterol; TG, triglycerides; LDL, low density lipoproteins; HDL, high density lipoproteins; IDL, intermediate density lipoproteins

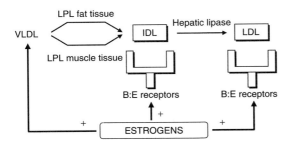

Figure 1 Effects of estrogens on plasma lipoproteins

Routes of administration

Hormone replacement in menopause may be performed by either oral or parenteral routes. Among the latter, the most usual are transdermal, by means of patches, or percutaneous, by means of gels[19]. A more recent development is the intranasal route as a new option[20]. These methods of administration have become more popular in the last few years because they do away with the hepatic first pass effect. This is the reason why it is possible to achieve more physiological concentrations of the estradiol (E2)/estrone (E1) index and less hepatic protein synthesis. Compared with oral treatments, which might produce side-effects like hypertension, hypercoagulation and gall bladder disease, non-oral therapy avoids these effects[19]. Accordingly, parenteral administration of estradiol by means of patches, gels or nasal spray is a valid option in HRT.

Oral therapy

Oral therapy has been the standard treatment both in the long and the short term. Hepatic first passage induces different enzymes to act on estrogen, producing metabolites with low or zero activity. Thus, it becomes necessary to obtain substances that can resist the action of such enzymes, or else to administer doses that surpass their clearance[21–23].

The use of high doses of estrogens determines their massive arrival at hepatic cells, causing intense enzyme activity and metabolic alterations such as the following:

(1) an increase in B:E receptors, with a concomitant decrease in atherogenic IDL and LDL lipoproteins[15];

(2) a decrease in Lp(a)[7];

(3) an increase in Apo A1[24];

(4) a decrease in hepatic lipase synthesis[24,25];

(5) a suppression of SR-B1 receptors[26].

The three last points entail a concomitant increase in HDL, mostly at the expense of HDL_2.

One of the observed unwanted effects is an increase in the synthesis of VLDL: if clearance capacity is surpassed by production, hypertriglyceridemia becomes evident[27–32].

Women with primary hypertriglyceridemia may develop severe hypertriglyceridemia on estrogen replacement therapy, and in such patients, estrogens should be used with caution and only after therapeutic reduction of triglyceride levels to less than 500 mg/dl[33].

The effects of oral estrogen therapy on lipid metabolism become manifest from the first month of treatment, and do not disappear for as long as the treatment lasts[34].

Non-oral therapies

Current alternatives to oral HRT represent a mixture of traditional drug delivery routes (vaginal gels, creams, pessaries and subcutaneous implants) and newer technologies (transdermal gels and patches, intrauterine devices, vaginal rings, intranasal sprays)[19,20].

In all cases, a more extended peripheral dilution is observed and, consequently, a relatively smaller hepatic concentration, with less E1 bioproduction; thus, the E2/E1 ratio is higher than 1, and is more physiological as it lies within the values observed in reproductive age women.

In the case of parenteral routes, effects on the lipid profile are weaker and can be detected after a longer time[13,35,36]. Walsh *et al.*[34] have observed no change in the short term with the transdermal route.

Some authors have reported a decrease of LDL, a decrease of Lp(a) and an increase of HDL; however, these findings are not conclusive[35-37]. By this route, intrahepatic estrogen levels are less than those required to reach an activity that could be compared to the one provided by enterohepatic circulation following oral administration. For this very reason, increase of triglycerides is not detected, for their alterations are dose-dependent; moreover, some authors have noted a decrease in triglycerides through some mechanism that cannot yet be explained[18,38].

Combination HRT

The addition of progestins, necessary for endometrial protection, may counteract some of the benefits provided by estrogens. In the case of natural progestins (micronized natural progestin) no significant changes of plasma lipoprotein levels were observed. On the other hand, synthetic progestins, particularly those with more androgenic activity (noretindrone, norgestrel) may have important metabolic effects[39].

The most frequently documented effects on lipid metabolism are the increase of hepatic lipase activity with a concomitant decrease of HDL (particularly HDL_2) and the decrease of triglyceride levels through some as yet unknown mechanism[26,40].

Levonorgestrel, which is used through an intrauterine device, has a lower impact on lipoprotein profile deterioration on account of the smaller systemic concentration it causes during the first uterine pass[41]. Levonorgestrel's metabolic effects appear favorable in terms of limited or no attenuation of beneficial estrogen effects at all doses, especially in the lower ones. We would like to consider separately tibolone, a synthetic substance of specific tissue action, since it offers estrogenic, progestogenic and androgenic properties depending on where it is operating[42]. We have conducted a study of this molecule on a group of postmenopausal women who were treated over a six-month period, and in whom we found total cholesterol levels had lowered (12%, $p < 0.025$), as had triglycerides (40%, $p < 0.02$), HDL cholesterol (29%, $p < 0.001$), VLDL cholesterol (40%, $p < 0.02$) and IDL cholesterol (34% NS). We did not find significant changes in LDL cholesterol[43]. The decrease of total cholesterol was partly ascribed to the decrease of HDL cholesterol and VLDL cholesterol. Moore has examined several studies of this molecule and found similar outcomes[42].

Summary of results from clinical studies

As can be seen from Table 2, most hormone combinations that were administered orally significantly reduced total cholesterol at the expense of LDL, with varying increase of HDL, as compared with basal values or placebo groups[44]. Unopposed estrogen administration proved to be more effective regarding increase of HDL and decrease of LDL[44]. Norethisterone acetate counteracted the expected effect of estrogens on HDL[45,46]; this was not the case with medroxyprogesterone acetate, which did not bring about the same increase as did estrogen by itself, but had beneficial effects on this lipoprotein. On the other hand, addition of progestin was not

Table 2 Clinical studies of effects of HRT on lipid profile: summary of results

Author	Therapies and regimen	Duration (months)	% Change from baseline TC	TG	HDL-C	LDL-C
Farish (1989)[45]	E₂ + NETA	12	1 ↓	↔	5.7 ↓	2.6 ↑
	E₂ + E₃ + NETA		4 ↓	7.7 ↓	9 ↓	1 ↓
PEPI Trial (1995)[44]	CEE + MPA	36	6 ↓	24 ↑	1.9–2.4 ↑	12–13 ↓
	CEE + MP		3.5 ↓	25 ↑	7 ↑	11 ↓
	CEE alone		3.5 ↓	23 ↑	9 ↑	10 ↓
	Placebo		↔	8 ↑	2 ↑	↔
Whitcroft et al. (1994)[46]	CEE + NOR	36	12 ↓	2.5 ↓	7.8 ↓	14.2 ↓
	TE₂ + NETA		8.4 ↓	16.4 ↑	10.7 ↑	6.6 ↑
	Reference		2.8 ↑	19.4 ↑	7 ↑	5.4 ↓
Hirvonen et al. (1997)[47]	E₂V + MPA	12	10 ↓	↔	11 ↑	ND
	E₂ gel + MPA		5 ↓	38 ↓	11 ↑	↔
Jensen et al. (1987)[35]	E₂ gel	24	5 ↓	5 ↑	10 ↑	10 ↓
	E₂ gel + MP		9 ↓	2.5 ↑	12 ↑	14 ↓
	Placebo		1.5 ↓	5 ↑	3 ↑	1 ↓
Berg et al. (1999)[48]	CEE + MPA	6	8 ↓	14 ↑	1 ↑	13 ↓
	TE₂ + MPA (RTS)		2 ↓	8 ↑	9 ↑	3 ↓
	TE₂ + MPA (MTS)		3 ↓	14 ↑	1 ↑	2 ↓
Mattsson et al. (2000)[20]	E₂ + DG	6	1.5 ↓	20.5 ↑	14.5 ↑	6.3 ↓
	E₂ nasal + DG		2.3 ↓	3.9 ↑	0.3 ↑	0.5 ↓

TC, total cholesterol; TG, triglycerides; CEE, conjugated equine estrogens; MPA, medroxyprogesterone acetate; MP, micronized progesterone; NETA, norethisterone acetate; E₂, 17β-estradiol; E₃, estriol; E₂V, estradiol valerate; NOR, DL-norgestrel; RTS, reservory transdermal system; MTS, matrix transdermal system; TE₂, transdermal estradiol; DG, desogestrel; ↓, decrease; ↔, no change; ↑, increase; ND, not determined significant regarding the effect of estrogen on LDL[20,35].

Micronized progesterone is practically inert on lipoprotein metabolism[35,44]. Transdermal estrogen administration shows a much lower response of HDL; very little variation is noted, and a considerable decrease is observed when gels are used[8,35,47,48].

While in search of correct therapeutic individualization, we believe suitable selection of progestogens and of the route of estrogen administration to be relevant to CVD prevention.

References

1. Wittemen J, Grobbee D, Kok F, et al. Increased risk of atherosclerosis in women after the menopause. *BMJ* 1989;298:642–4
2. Rosenberg L, Hennekens CH, Rosner B, et al. Early menopause and the risk of myocardial infarction. *Am J Obstet Gynecol* 1981;139:47–51
3. Mosca L, Manson J, Sutherland S, et al. Cardiovascular disease in women: a statement for healthcare professionals from the American Heart Association Writing Group. *Circulation* 1997;96:2468–82
4. Castelli WP. Cardiovascular disease in women. *Am J Obstet Gynecol* 1988;158:1553
5. Berg G, Halperín H, Siseles N, et al. Very low density lipoproteins and subclasses of intermediate density lipoproteins in postmenopausal women. *Medicina* 1996;56:479–86
6. Arca M, Lena Vega G, Grundy S. Hypercholesterolemia in postmenopausal women. *JAMA* 1994;271:453–9
7. Bruschi F, Meschia M, Soma M, et al. Lipoprotein (a) and other lipids after oophorectomy and estrogen replacement therapy. *Obstet Gynecol* 1996;88:950–4
8. Berg G, Siseles N, Gonzalez AI, et al. Increase in hepatic lipase activity in postmenopause. Relationship with atherogenic intermediate density and low density lipoproteins. *Menopause* 2001;8:51–7
9. Jensen J, Nilas L, Christiansen C. Influence of menopause on serum lipids and lipoproteins. *Maturitas* 1990;12:321–31
10. Stevenson J, Crook D, Godsland I. Influence of age and menopause on serum lipids and lipoproteins in healthy women. *Atherosclerosis* 1993;98:83–90
11. Matthews K, Meilahn E, Kuller L, et al. Menopause and risk factors for coronary heart disease. *N Engl J Med* 1989;321:641–6
12. Razay G, Heaton K, Bolton C. Coronary heart disease risk factors in relation to menopause. *QJ Med* 1992;85:307–8
13. Castelo-Branco C, Casals E, Sanllehy C, et al. Effect of oophorectomy and hormone replacement therapy on plasma lipids. *Maturitas* 1993;17:113–22
14. De Aloysio D, Gambacciani M, Meschia M, et al. The effect of menopause on blood lipid and lipoprotein levels. *Atherosclerosis* 1999;147:147–53
15. Ma PT, Yamamoto T, Goldstein J, et al. Increased mRNA for low density lipoproteins receptor in liver for rabbit treated with 17-a-ethinyl estradiol. *Proc Natl Acad Sci USA* 1986;83:792–6
16. Steimberg D. Low density lipoprotein oxidation and its pathobiological significance. *J Biol Chem* 1997;272:20963–6
17. Mijatovic V, van der Mooren M, Stehouwer A, et al. Postmenopausal hormone replacement, risk estimators for coronary artery disease and cardiovascular protection. *Gynecol Endocrinol* 1999;13:130–44
18. Krauss R. Lipid and lipoproteins and effects of hormone replacement. In Lobo R, ed. *Treatment of the Postmenopausal Woman: Basic and Clinical Aspects*, 2nd edn. Philadelphia: Lippincott Williams & Wilkins, 1999;32:369–76
19. Crook D. The metabolic consequences of treating postmenopausal women with non-oral hormone replacement therapy. *Br J Obstet Gynaecol* 1997;104:(Suppl. 16)4–13
20. Mattsson LA, Christiansen C, Colau J-C, et al. Clinical equivalence of intranasal and oral 17 β-estradiol for postmenopausal symptoms. *Am J Obstet Gynecol* 2000;182:545–52
21. De Lignieres B, Basdevant A, Thomas G, et al. Biological effects of estradiol-17 beta in postmenopausal women: oral versus percutaneous administration. *J Clin Endocrinol Metab* 1986;62:536–41
22. Elkik F, Gomfiel A, Mercier-Bodard C, et al. Effects of percutaneous estradiol and conjugated estrogens on the level of plasma proteins

and triglycerides in postmenopausal women. *Am J Obstet Gynecol* 1982;143:888–92

23. Elkin F, Gomfield A, Mercier-Bodard C, *et al*. Effects of percutaneus estradiol and conjugated estrogens on the level of plasma proteins and triglycerides in post menopausal women. *Am J Obstet Gynecol* 1982;143:888–92

24. Brinton EA. Oral estrogen replacement therapy in postmenopausal women selectively raises levels and production rates of lipoprotein A-I and lowers hepatic lipase activity without lowering the fractional catabolic rate. *Arterioscler Thromb Vasc Biol* 1996;16:431–40

25. Tikkanen MJ, Nikkila EA, Kuusi T, *et al*. Effects of oestradiol and levonorgestrel on lipoprotein lipids and post-heparin plasma lipase activities in normolipoproteinemic women. *Acta Endocrinol* 1982;99:630–5

26. Landschulz KT, Pathak RK, Rigotti A, *et al*. Regulation of scavenger receptor class B, type I, a high density lipoprotein receptor, in liver and steroidogenic tissues of the rat. *J Clin Invest* 1996;98:984–95

27. Farish E, Fletcher C, Hart D, *et al*. Effects of bilateral oophorectomy on lipoprotein metabolism. *Br J Obstet Gynaecol* 1990;97:78–82

28. Punnonen R, Rauramo L. Effect of bilateral oophorectomy and peroral estradiol valerate on serum lipids. *Int J Gynaecol Obstet* 1976;14:13–16

29. Punnonen R, Rauramo L. Effect of castration and estrogen therapy on serum high-density lipoprotein cholesterol. *Int J Gynaecol Obstet* 1980;17:434–6

30. Pansini F, Bergamini C, Bettochi S, *et al*. Short-term effect of oophorectomy on lipoprotein metabolism. *Gynecol Obstet Invest* 1984;18:134–9

31. Montgomery J, Crook D, Godsland I, *et al*. Plasma lipid risk factors in oophorectomized women. *Br J Obstet Gynaecol* 1989;96:1236–8

32. Higano M, Cohen W, Robinson R. Effect of sex steroids on lipids. *Ann NY Acad Sci* 1959;72:979–84

33. Glueck C, Scheel D, Fishback J, *et al*. Estrogen-induced pancreatitis in patients with previously covert familiar type V hyperlipoproteinemia. *Metabolism* 1972;21:657–66

34. Walsh BW, Schiff I, Rosner B, *et al*. Effects of postmenopausal estrogen replacement on the concentrations and metabolism of plasma lipoproteins. *N Engl J Med* 1991;325:1196–204

35. Jensen J, Riis B, Ström V, *et al*. Long-term effects of percutaneous estrogens and oral progesterone on serum lipoprotein in postmenopausal women. *Am J Obstet Gynecol* 1987;156:66–71

36. Castelo-Branco C. Valoración clínica y metabólica del 17 beta estradiol por vía percutánea en el tratamiento hormonal sustitutivo. Zaragoza: *Libro de ponencias III Congreso Nacional de la Asociación Española para el Estudio de la Menopausia* 1994

37. Taskinen MR, Puolakka J, Pyorala T, *et al*. Hormone replacement therapy lowers plasma Lp(a) concentration. Comparision of cyclic transdermal and continuos estrogen-progestin regimens. *Arterioscler Thromb Vasc Biol* 1996;16:1215–21

38. Crook D. Hormone replacement therapy choices for women with hypertriglyceridemia. In Whitehead M, ed. *The Prescriber's Guide to Hormone Replacement Therapy*. Carnforth, UK: Parthenon Publishing, 1998;183–91

39. Lobo RA. Effects of hormonal replacement on lipids and lipoproteins in post menopausal women. Clinical review 27. *J Clin Endocrinol Metab* 1991;73:925–7

40. Tikkanen MJ, Nikkila EA, Kuusi T, *et al*. High density lipoprotein-2 and hepatic lipase: reciprocal changes produced by estrogen and norgestrel. *J Clin Endocrinol Metab* 1982;54:1113–7

41. Riphagen F. Intrauterine application of progestins in hormone replacement therapy: a review. *Climacteric* 2000;3:199–211

42. Moore RA. Livial: a review of clinical studies. *Br J Obstet Gynaecol* 1999;106(Suppl. 19):1–21.

43. Siseles NO, Halperin H, Benencia HJ, *et al*. A comparative study with two hormone replacement therapy regimens on safety and efficacy variables. *Maturitas* 1995;21:201–10

44. Postmenopausal Estrogen/Progestin Interventions Trial. Effects of estrogen or estrogen/progestin regimens on heart disease risk factors in postmenopausal women. *JAMA* 1995;273:199–208

45. Farish E, Fletcher CD, Dagen MM, *et al*. Lipoprotein and apolipoprotein levels in postmenopausal women on continuous oestrogen/progestogen therapy. *Br J Obstet Gynaecol* 1989;96:358–64

46. Whitcroft SI, Crook D, Godsland IF, *et al*. Long-term effects of oral and transdermal

hormone replacement therapies on serum lipid and lipoprotein concentrations. *Obstet Gynecol* 1994;84:222–6

47. Hirvonen E, Cacciatore B, Wahlström T, *et al.* Effects of transdermal oestrogen therapy in postmenopausal women: a comparative study of an oestradiol gel and an oestradiol delivering patch. *Br J Obstet Gynaecol* 1997;104 (Suppl. 16):26–31

48. Berg G, Aisemberg L, Siseles N, *et al.* Comparision of the effect of the orally and transdermally administered hormone replacement therapy (HRT) on the lipid and lipoprotein profile. *Gynecol Endocrinol* 1999;13:168

Effect of DHEA on carbohydrate and lipid metabolism in postmenopausal women

37

A. Milewicz, D. Jędrzejuk and A. Bohdanowicz-Pawlak

Introduction

Dehydroepiandrosterone (DHEA) is a 'juvenile' hormone, revealing its serum peak at the period of adrenarche, and subsequently declining from approximately 25 years of age. A major reason for this decline is a progressive reduction in the activity of the fundamental adrenal steroidogenesis enzyme 17,20-desmolase.

On the basis of isotope investigations in humans, it was concluded that both DHEA and its derivative dehydroepiandrosterone sulfate (DHEAS), which are weak androgens, are peripherally converted into estrogens (estrone and estradiol), as well as potent androgens, specifically testosterone and androstendione, though the extent of these transformations are determined by sex[1]. In relation to the above, an indirect effect of DHEA as a prehormone for estrogens and androgens on estrogen and androgen receptors in target tissues both in women and men was suggested. Significant influence on cytokine levels, i.e. interleukin-2 (II-2) and II-6 was also proposed[2]. Beneficial effects of exogenous DHEA in animal models on carbohydrate and lipid metabolism led to the investigation of its action in humans. Evidence for the efficacy of exogenous DHEA in humans is contentious, and many studies were not placebo-controlled trials.

The aim of the present study was to investigate whether the concentration of endogenous DHEAS affects anthropometric parameters, and lipid and carbohydrate metabolism, and if this influence is age related.

The effect of exogenous DHEA on the above parameters was also studied.

Subjects and methods

Seventy-seven volunteers, including 53 postmenopausal women aged 56.02 ± 3.12 years with body mass index (BMI) 27.2 ± 4.35 kg/m^2 and 24 men aged 58.22 ± 5.61 years with BMI 26.1 ± 2.98 kg/m^2 were recruited to the study. All subjects were non-smokers. They were administered DHEA p.o. at 50 mg/day for 3 months. The study was approved by the medical ethics committee.

Anthropometrical parameters were measured to calculate BMI and waist to hip ratio (WHR). Measurements of percent adipose tissue and calculation of android/gynoid fat deposit ratios (percent fat content in measured area to the total fat) were performed using the dual energy X-ray absorptiometry densitometer (DEXA) technique (DPX (+), Lunar, USA).

Blood was drawn from the cubical vein after a 12 h fast. Serum hormone concentrations (growth hormone (GH), estradiol, testosterone, DHEAS, leptin, insulin, insulin-like growth factor-1 (IGF-1)) were estimated with commercially available radioimmunoassay (RIA) kits (DPC, Germany). Blood lipid measurements (total cholesterol, HDL-cholesterol, triglycerides) and glucose were carried out with kits supplied by Boehringer Mannheim. LDL-cholesterol was calculated by the Friedewald formula.

Table 1 Effect of endogenous dehydroepiandrosterone sulphate (DHEAS) levels on body mass index (BMI), waist to hip ratio (WHR), insulin/glucose ratio and testosterone in healthy female volunteers

	DHEAS concentration (Mean ± SD)		
	< 1000 (ng/ml)	> 1000 (ng/ml)	p value
BMI (kg/m^2)	26.08 ± 3.126	28.32 ± 5.12	0.031
WHR	0.8 ± 0.04	0.83 ± 0.07	0.031
Insulin/glucose ratio (mIU/ml/mg %)	0.1065 ± 0.036	0.1363 ± 0.081	0.045
Testosterone (ng/ml)	0.252 ± 0.12	0.432 ± 0.35	0.009

Table 2 Effect of low (< 1000) endogenous dehydroepiandrosterone sulphate (DHEAS) levels on various metabolic parameters in male and female volunteers

	DHEAS concentration < 1000 ng/ml		
	Women Mean ± SD	Men Mean ± SD	p value
WHR	0.8 ± 0.04	0.92 ± 0.05	0.00001
Adipose tissue (%)	38.44 ± 4.687	22.41 ± 2.21	0.00001
Android fat deposit	9.28 ± 1.43	13.92 ± 1.72	0.00001
Total cholesterol (mg/dl)	224.45 ± 40.5	195 ± 21.61	0.015
HDL-cholesterol (mg/dl)	61.75 ± 12.77	46.38 ± 11.95	0.0008
Glucose (mg/dl)	81.91 ± 9.27	87.88 ± 8.66	0.038
Estradiol (pg/ml)	2.99 ± 4.22	15.95 ± 8.69	0.00001
Testosterone (ng/ml)	0.252 ± 0.12	4.52 ± 1.93	0.00001
Estradiol/testosterone ratio (pg/ml:ng/ml)	7.657 ± 7.94	3.5824 ± 1.732	0.00001

The total group of women was divided into two subgroups: I ($n = 26$) with reduced endogenous DHEAS (< 1000 ng/ml), II ($n = 27$) with normal DHEAS concentration (> 1000 ng/ml).

Results

Comparative analysis of anthropometrical parameters, lipid and carbohydrate metabolism, apart from BMI, WHR, insulin/glucose ratio and testosterone levels (Table 1), did not vary statistically. Data obtained showed a positive relationship between BMI, WHR, insulin/glucose ratio and testosterone and endogenous DHEAS concentrations in women, which may be responsible for an increased cardiovascular disease risk. Women with decreased DHEAS levels (< 1000 ng/ml) ($n = 26$) were compared to the group of men with decreased DHEAS levels ($n = 11$) see Table 2. Statistically significant differences between the women ($n = 27$) and men ($n = 13$) with normal DHEAS concentrations (> 1000 ng/ml) are shown in Table 3.

In women with decreased endogenous DHEAS levels, lower glucose and estradiol/testosterone ratio, and higher total cholesterol and percentage adipose tissue than in men were observed. Women with higher (> 1000 ng/ml) DHEAS concentrations showed higher BMI, percentage adipose tissue and HDL-cholesterol concentration than men with DHEAS levels > 1000 ng/ml. It can be concluded that the effect of endogenous

Table 3 Effect of normal (> 1000 ng/ml) endogenous dehydroepiandrosterone sulphate (DHEAS) levels on various metabolic parameters in male and female volunteers

| | DHEAS concentration > 1000 (ng/ml) | | |
	Women Mean ± SD	Men Mean ± SD	p value
BMI (kg/m^2)	28.31 ± 5.12	25.44 ± 3.12	0.035
Adipose tissue (%)	39.51 ± 5.51	21.88 ± 4.03	0.00001
Android fat deposit	9.88 ± 1.576	14.16 ± 2.33	0.00001
Estradiol (pg/ml)	3.83 ± 5.49	21.4 ± 8.15	0.00001
Testosterone (ng/ml)	0.43 ± 0.35	4.31 ± 1.15	0.00001

DHEA on lipid and carbohydrate metabolism is influenced by sex.

After 3-month oral DHEAS administration at 50 mg/day in women with initially decreased DHEAS level (< 1000 ng/ml) ($n = 26$), significant increases in estradiol levels (from 1.27 ± 1.21 pg/ml to 14.32 ± 9.65 pg/ml; $p = 0.0003$) and DHEAS levels (784.0 ± 168.96 to 2748 ± 1718.88 ng/ml, $p = 0.0016$) were accomplished. In women with initially normal DHEAS (> 1000) ($n = 27$), a decline in GH concentrations (2.4 ± 0.3 mIU/ml to 1.92 ± 0.2 mIU/ml, $p = 0.007$) and an increase in DHEAS levels (1465 ± 350.3 to 2944 ± 795.8 ng/ml, $p = 0.0001$) was observed. No other significant differences in anthropometrical parameters, carbohydrate or lipid metabolism were revealed.

Conclusions

After 3 months of 50 mg/day DHEA oral administration we have not observed significant differences in estimated anthropometric and biochemical parameters in the treated women, except for the increase in serum estradiol and DHEAS levels, and decrease of serum GH levels, which are dependant on the initial serum DHEAS levels. Our results do not support the observations of Labrie[3] and Genazzani[4], which may be due to different times of treatment and for route of administration.

References

1. Legrain S, Massien CH, Lahlou N, *et al*. Dehydroepiandrosterone replacement administration: pharmacokinetic and pharmacodynamic studies in healthy elderly subjects. *J Clin Endocrinol Metab* 2000;85:3208–17
2. Arlt W, Callies F, Van Vlijmen C, *et al*. Dehydroepiandrosterone replacement in women with adreal insufficiency. *N Engl J Med* 1999;341: 1013–20
3. Labrie F. DHEA replacement therapy as source of androgens and estrogens at menopause. *Gynecol Endocrinol* 2000;14(Suppl. 2):5
4. Genazzani AR, Stomati M, Genazzani AD, *et al*. Central and peripheral effects of DHEAS relacement therapy in early and late postmenopausal women. *Gynecol Endocrinol* 2000; 14(Suppl. 2):18

DHEA replacement therapy as a source of androgens and estrogens at menopause

38

F. Labrie, A. Bélanger, V. Luu-the, J. Simard and C. Labrie

Introduction

There is no medical problem related to women's health with a higher negative impact on morbidity (and frequently mortality) than the menopause, a condition closely associated with declining sex steroid availability. The most important problems associated with the menopause are osteoporosis and atherosclerosis. It seems appropriate to mention that in Canada alone, osteoporosis affects more than 2 million people, while this already serious problem grows with the increasing life expectancy of the population. Osteoporosis results in approximately 30 000 hip fractures annually in Canada with an annual increase of 1000 to 2000 due to aging of the population. More than 50% of hip fracture patients loose their social independence permanently. Moreover, between 12 and 20% of hip fracture patients die within one year from fracture complications.

The most widely recognized fact concerning the menopause is that there is a progressive decrease and finally an arrest of estrogen secretion by the ovaries. The cessation of ovarian estrogen secretion is illustrated by the marked decline in circulating 17β-estradiol levels. This easily measurable change in circulating 17β-estradiol levels coupled with the demonstrated beneficial effects of estrogens on menopausal symptoms and bone resorption[1] has concentrated most of the efforts of hormone replacement therapy (HRT) on various forms of estrogen, alone or in combination with progestin in order to avoid the potentially harmful stimulatory effects of estrogen on the endometrium. It should be mentioned that convincing data indicate that progestins have a negative impact on breast cancer[2–4], with clinical reports indicating an increased risk of this cancer[5–7].

Despite the well-known beneficial effects of estrogen therapy on menopausal symptoms[8–10] and their role in reducing bone loss and coronary heart disease[11–16], compliance is low. Most women decide not to take estrogens or stop treatment early because of the fear of breast and uterine cancer[10] and of symptoms associated with this therapy, namely uterine bleeding, breast tenderness and fluid retention.

Intracrinology

An important finding in the field of sex steroids is that a large proportion of androgens and estrogens in men and women are synthesized locally in peripheral target tissues from the inactive adrenal precursors dehydroepiandrosterone (DHEA), DHEA sulfate (DHEAS), and androstenedione (Figure 1). In fact, in postmenopausal women, almost 100% of sex steroids are synthesized in peripheral tissues from DHEA and DHEAS of adrenal origin, except for a small contribution from ovarian and/or adrenal testosterone and androstenedione. Thus, in postmenopausal women, almost all active sex steroids are made in target tissues by an intracrine mechanism.

The secretion of DHEA and DHEAS by the adrenals increases during the adrenarche in

249

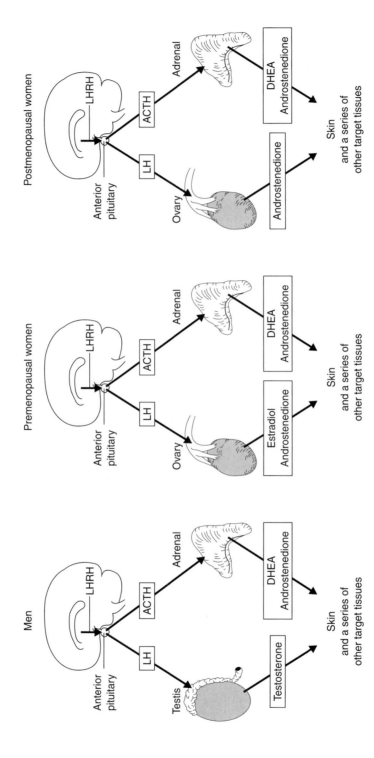

Figure 1 Schematic representation of the role of gonadal (testicular and ovarian) and adrenal sources of sex steroids in men and women. After menopause, the secretion of estradiol by the ovaries ceases and almost 100% of sex steroids are made locally in peripheral target intracrine tissues. LH, luteinizing hormone; ACTH, adrenocorticotropic hormone; DHEA, dehydroepiandrosterone

children at the age of 6–8 years and elevated values of circulating DHEA and DHEAS are maintained throughout adulthood, thus providing the high level of substrates required for conversion into potent androgens and estrogens in peripheral tissues. In fact, plasma DHEAS levels in adult men and women are 100–500 times higher than those of testosterone and 1000 to 10 000 times higher than those of estradiol, thus providing a large reservoir of substrate for conversion into androgens and/or estrogens in peripheral intracrine tissues.

This local formation of sex steroids provides autonomous control to target tissues which are thus able to adjust the formation and metabolism of sex steroids according to local needs[17]. The situation of a high secretion rate of adrenal precursor sex steroids in men and women is completely different from the animal models used in the laboratory, namely the rat, mouse, guinea pig and all others (except monkeys), where the secretion of sex steroids takes place exclusively in the gonads[18–22]. In these lower animal species, no significant amounts of androgens or estrogens are made outside the testes or ovaries and there is no sex steroid production after castration.

The term intracrinology was coined in 1988[23] to focus our attention on the synthesis of active steroids in peripheral tissues where the active steroids exert their action in the same cells where synthesis takes place without release in the extracellular space and in the general circulation[17] (Figure 2). The rate of formation of each sex steroid thus depends upon the level of expression of each of the specific androgen- and estrogen-synthesizing enzymes in each cell of each tissue[17,18,24–26] (Figure 3).

As mentioned above, transformation of the adrenal precursor steroids DHEAS and DHEA into androgens and/or estrogens in peripheral target tissues depends upon the level of expression of the various steroidogenic and metabolizing enzymes in each of these tissues. Knowledge in this area has recently made rapid progress with the elucidation of the structure of most of the tissue-specific genes that encode the steroidogenic enzymes responsible for the transformation of DHEAS and DHEA into androgens and/or estrogens in peripheral tissues[21,26–29] (Figure 3). The particular importance of DHEA and DHEAS is illustrated by the finding that approximately 50% of total androgens in the prostate of adult men derive from these adrenal precursor steroids[18,30,31]. As mentioned above, our best estimate of the intracrine formation of estrogens in peripheral tissues in women is in the order of 75% before menopause and close to 100% after menopause[17].

Because the molecular structure of most of the key non-P450-dependent enzymes required for sex steroid formation had not been elucidated and knowing that local formation of sex steroids is most likely to play a major role in both normal and tumoral hormone-sensitive tissues, an important proportion of our research program and that of other groups has been devoted to this exciting and therapeutically promising area[21,26,32–35].

Age-related decline in DHEA levels

To gain a better knowledge of the role of DHEA and DHEAS transformation in both men and women, we analyzed the serum levels of 18 conjugated C21- and C19-steroids[36]. We thereby wanted to assess precisely the changes occurring in the serum concentration of these steroids over a range of ages from the peak adrenal secretion of DHEA and DHEAS (20–30 years) to the lowest values found at 70–80 years.

The data obtained show a dramatic decline in the circulating levels of DHEA, DHEAS, androst-5-ene-3β,17β-diol/(androstenediol), androstenediol sulfate, androstenediol fatty acid esters, and androstenedione in both men and women between the ages of 20 and 80 years. In the 50- to 60-year-old group, serum DHEA has already decreased by 74% and 70% from its 20–30-year-old peak values in men and women, respectively (Figure 4). The serum concentrations of the conjugated metabolites of dihydrotestosterone, namely

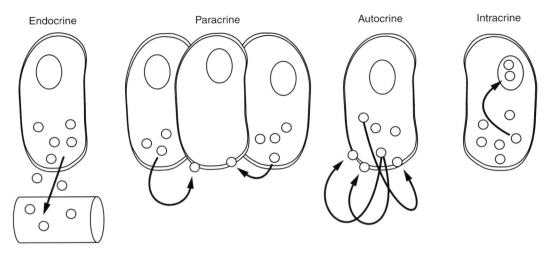

Figure 2 Schematic representation of endocrine, paracrine, autocrine and intracrine secretion. Classically, endocrine activity includes the hormones secreted in specialized glands called the endocrine glands. These hormones are released in the general circulation and are transported to distant target cells. On the other hand, hormones released from one cell can influence neighboring cells (paracrine activity) or can exert a positive or negative action on the cell of origin (autocrine activity). Intracrine activity describes the formation of active hormones which exert their action in the same cells where synthesis took place without release into the pericellular compartment

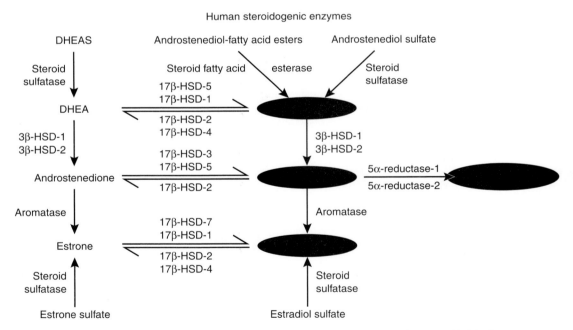

Figure 3 Human steroidogenic enzymes in peripheral intracrine tissues. HSD, hydroxysteroid dehydrogenase

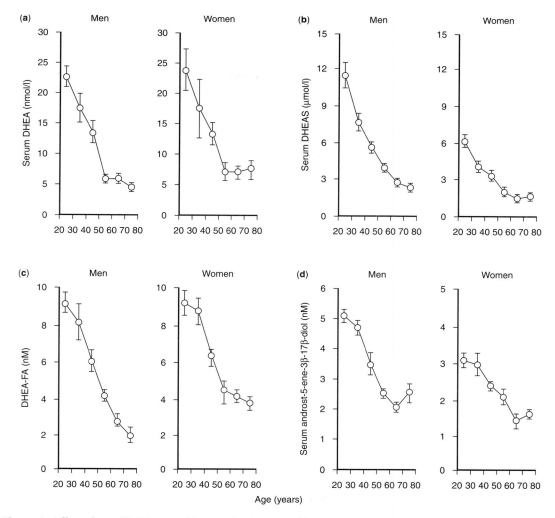

Figure 4 Effect of age (20–30-years-old versus 70–80-years-old) on serum concentration of (a) DHEA, (b) DHEAS, (c) DHEA-fatty acid esters (DHEA-FA) and (d) androstenediol in men and women (reproduced with permission from reference 36)

androsterone glucuronide, androstane-3α, androstane-3β,17β-diolglucuronide and androsterone sulfate are the most reliable parameters of the total androgen pool in both men and women while serum testosterone and dihydrotestosterone can only be used as markers of testicular secretion in men and interstitial ovarian secretion in women. The serum concentration of these various conjugated androgen metabolites decreased by 40.8% to 72.8% from the 20–30 to the 70–80 age groups in men and women, thus suggesting a parallel decrease in the total androgen

pool with age. As estimated by measurement of the circulating levels of these conjugated metabolites of dihydrotestosterone, it is noteworthy that androgen levels in women are approximately 66% of the levels found in men: in women, most of these androgens originate from the transformation of DHEA and DHEAS into testosterone and dihydrotestosterone in peripheral intracrine tissues while in men, the testes and DHEA plus DHEAS provide approximately equal amounts of androgens at the age of 50 to 60 years. An additional potentially highly significant

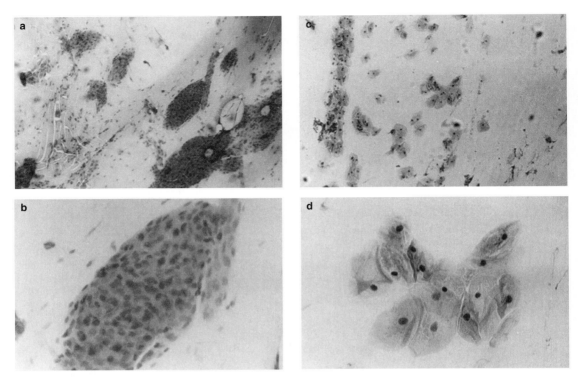

Figure 5 (a) Atrophic vaginal smear with numerous parabasal cells in a 65-year-old woman before starting treatment with DHEA (X100); (b) Atrophic vaginal smear with numerous parabasal cells in a 65-year-old woman before starting treatment with DHEA at larger magnification (X400); (c) Vaginal smear from the same patient as Figure 4a after 12 months of DHEA treatment showing superficial pyknotic cells (X100); (d) Vaginal smear from the same patient as Figure 4b after 12 months of DHEA administration showing superficial pyknotic cells at larger magnification (X400) [41]

observation is that the majority of the marked decline in circulating adrenal C19 steroids and in their resulting androgen metabolites takes place between the age groups of 20–30 years and 50–60 years with smaller changes observed after the age of 60 years[36] (Figure 4).

Role of androgens in bone physiology

In order to assess the relative role of the androgenic and/or estrogenic components of DHEA action, we have studied the effect of 12-month administration of DHEA, alone or in combination with the pure antiandrogen flutamide or the antiestrogen EM-800 on bone mineral content (BMC) and density (BMD), on bone histomorphometry as well as on other parameters of bone formation and turnover

in the rat. Treatment with DHEA not only completely reversed the inhibitory effect of ovariectomy but led to femoral BMC and BMD values 26% and 8% above those found in intact animals. Simultaneous treatment with the pure antiandrogen flutamide reversed by 76% the stimulatory effect of DHEA on both femoral BMC and BMD, while treatment with the pure antiestrogen EM-800 had no statistically significant effect on the stimulation by DHEA of femoral BMC and BMD[37].

This study by Martel *et al.*[37] also showed that the DHEA-induced stimulation of femoral, lumbar spine and total body BMD and BMC are accompanied by an increase in serum alkaline phosphatase concentration, a marker of bone formation, and a decrease in urinary hydroxyproline excretion, a marker of bone resorption. These data clearly suggest

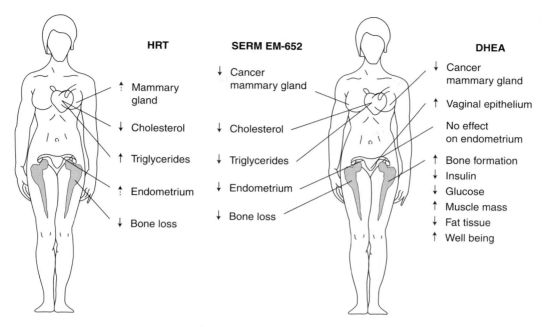

Figure 6 Comparison of the potential benefits of combining DHEA with EM-652.HCl, a selective estrogen receptor modulator (SERM) having pure antiestrogenic activity in the mammary gland and endometrium compared with standard HRT. Plain arrow, benefits; dotted arrow, negative effects from available evidence. There are no negative effects expected from the combination EM-652.HCl plus DHEA, while potential stimulation of breast and endometrial cancers are the risks associated with estrogen therapy. The combination EM-652.HCl plus DHEA has a series of potential benefits not achievable with standard ERT

the potential of a new approach using DHEA to prevent and treat problems associated with menopause, especially osteoporosis.

Inhibition of growth of breast cancer xenografts in nude mice

Since androgens inhibit breast cancer[38,39], we have studied the possibility that DHEA could inhibit the growth of the human breast cancer ZR-75-1 cell line *in vivo* in nude mice. In order to avoid the inhibitory effects of DHEA on gonadotropin secretion, and be able to assess the direct effects of DHEA-derived steroids on breast cancer growth, we have used ovariectomized animals supplemented with estrone.

Estrone by itself caused a 9.4-fold increase in ZR-75-1 tumor area after 9.5 months of treatment whereas the daily oral administration of 15, 50 or 1000 µg of EM-800 in estrone-supplemented mice led to inhibitions of 88%,

93% and 94%, respectively. DHEA, at doses of 0.30 mg, 1.0 mg and 3.0 mg, inhibited tumor weight by 67%, 82% and 85%, respectively[40]. Combination of a daily 15 µg oral dose of EM-800 with the three doses of topical DHEA produced 84 to 94% inhibitions of estrone-stimulated ZR-75-1 tumor growth, these values being not significantly different from the 88% inhibition achieved by EM-800 alone.

Effects of DHEA in postmenopausal women

Total hip BMD increased significantly from 0.744 ± 0.021 g/cm^2 to 0.753 ± 0.023 g/cm^2 (1.2%) after 6 months of treatment ($p < 0.05$) and to 0.759 ± 0.025 g/cm^2 (2.0%) after 12 months of DHEA administration ($p < 0.05$). On the other hand, after the 12 months of DHEA treatment, the femoral Ward's triangle BMD increased from 0.486 ± 0.026 g/cm^2 to 0.494 ± 0.026 g/cm^2 (1.6%) while the lumbar spine BMD increased from 0.829 ± 0.030 g/cm^2 to 0.839 ± 0.033 g/cm^2 (1.2%), although these changes did not reach the level of statistical significance[41].

The serum concentration of osteocalcin, a marker of bone formation, increased from 1.16 ± 0.30 µg/l at pretreatment to 1.95 ± 0.59 µg/l (NS), 2.28 ± 0.53 µg/l ($p < 0.05$), 2.49 ± 0.58 µg/l ($p < 0.01$, 115% over control), and 2.44 ± 0.47 ($p < 0.01$, 110% over control) after 3, 6, 9 and 12 months of treatment, respectively.

Vaginal cytology was examined as a specific parameter of the estrogenic action of DHEA. Before treatment, ten women had a completely atrophic vaginal smear exclusively composed of parabasal cells (Figures 5a and 5b). In eight of these ten women on DHEA treatment, the vaginal cytology was converted into a pattern typical of normal cycling women showing mainly the presence of superficial pyknotic cells (Figures 5c and 5d, as example)[41].

Considering the major concern related to the stimulatory effect of estrogens on endometrial proliferation with the related risk of endometrial carcinoma[42,43], an endometrial biopsy was performed before starting treatment and after 12 months of DHEA administration. The endometrial atrophy seen in all women at start of treatment remained unaffected by 12 months of DHEA administration[41].

Combination with a pure SERM (EM-652)

The inhibitory effect of DHEA on the growth of human breast cancer xenografts supports the use of DHEA as hormone replacement therapy in women. Moreover, since the administration of DHEA does not interfere with the inhibitory effect of EM-800 on ZR-75-1 tumor growth, combined treatment with DHEA and EM-800 (or EM-652) could possibly be a more beneficial chemopreventive and therapeutic approach in breast cancer.

EM-652 is a fourth generation selective estrogen receptor modulator (SERM), having pure and potent antiestrogenic activity in the mammary gland and endometrium while decreasing serum cholesterol and triglyceride levels and preventing bone loss[44]. The potential benefits of such combination can be seen in Figure 6. Most importantly, such a combination appears to possess the ideal characteristics for prevention of breast and uterine cancer while preventing bone loss, cardiovascular risks and a series of other problems associated with menopause.

References

1. Christiansen C, Christensen MS, Larsen NE, et al. Pathophysiological mechanisms of estrogen effect on bone metabolism. Dose–response relationships in early postmenopausal women. *J Clin Endocrinol Metab* 1982;55:1124–30
2. Horwitz KB. The molecular biology of RU486. Is there a role for antiprogestins in the treatment of breast cancer? *Endocr Rev* 1992;13: 146–63
3. Musgrove ES, Lee CS, Sutherland RL. Progestins both stimulate and inhibit breast cancer cell cycle progression while increasing expression of transforming growth factor alpha, epidermal growth factor receptor, c-fos, and c-myc genes. *Mol Cell Biol* 1991;11:5032–43
4. Clarke CL, Sutherland RL. Progestin regulation of cellular proliferation. *Endocr Rev* 1990;11: 266–301
5. Colditz GA, Hankinson SE, Hunter DJ, et al. The use of estrogens and progestins and the risk of breast cancer in postmenopausal women. *N Engl J Med* 1995;332:1589–93
6. Ross RK, Paganini-Hill A, Wan PC, et al. Effect of hormone replacement therapy on breast cancer risk: estrogen versus estrogen plus progestin. *J Natl Cancer Inst* 2000;92:328–32
7. Magnusson C, Baron JA, Correia N, et al. Breast-cancer risk following long-term oestrogen- and oestrogen–progestin-replacement therapy. *Int J Cancer* 1999;81:339–44

8. Lomax P, Schonbaum E. Postmenopausal hot flushes and their management. *Pharmacol Ther* 1993;57:347–58

9. Greendale GA, Judd HL. The menopause: health implications and clinical management. *J Am Geriatr Soc* 1993;41:426–36

10. Grady D, Rubin SM, Petitti DB, *et al*. Hormone therapy to prevent disease and prolong life in postmenopausal women. *Ann Intern Med* 1992;117:1016–37

11. Lobo RA. Clinical review 27: Effects of hormonal replacement on lipids and lipoproteins in postmenopausal women. *J Clin Endocrinol Metab* 1991;73:925–30

12. Harris ST, Genant HK, Baylink DJ, *et al*. The effects of estrone (Ogen) on spinal bone density of postmenopausal women. *Arch Intern Med* 1991;151:1980–4

13. Stampfer MJ, Colditz GA, Willett WC, *et al*. Postmenopausal estrogen therapy and cardiovascular disease. Ten year follow up from the Nurses' Health Study [see comments]. *N Engl J Med* 1991;325:756–62

14. Barrett-Connor E, Bush TL. Estrogen and coronary heart disease in women [see comments]. *JAMA* 1991;265:1861–7

15. Lindsay R. Hormone replacement therapy for prevention and treatment of osteoporosis. *Am J Med* 1993;95:37s–39s

16. Field CS, Ory SJ, Wahner HW, *et al*. Preventive effects of transdermal 17 beta estradiol on osteoporotic changes after surgical menopause: a two year placebo controlled trial. *Am J Obstet Gynecol* 1993;168(1 Pt 1):114–21

17. Labrie F. Intracrinology. *Mol Cell Endocrinol* 1991;78:C113–18

18. Labrie F, Dupont A, Bélanger A. Complete androgen blockade for the treatment of prostate cancer. In de Vita VT, Hellman S, Rosenberg SA, eds. *Important Advances in Oncology*. Philadelphia: JB Lippincott, 1985:193–217

19. Labrie F. Intracrinology: its impact on prostate cancer. *Curr Opin Urol* 1993;3:381–7

20. Cutler Jr GB, Glenn M, Bush M, *et al*. Adrenarche: a survey of rodents, domestic animals and primates. *Endocrinology* 1978;103:2112–18

21. Labrie F, Simard J, Luu-The V, *et al*. Structure, function and tissue-specific gene expression of 3β-hydroxysteroid dehydrogenase/5-ene-4-ene isomerase enzymes in classical and peripheral intracrine steroidogenic tissues. *J Steroid Biochem Mol Biol* 1992;43:805–26

22. Bélanger B, Bélanger A, Labrie F, *et al*. Comparison of residual C-19 steroids in plasma and prostatic tissue of human, rat and guinea pig after castration: unique importance of extratesticular androgens in men. *J Steroid Biochem* 1989;32:695–8

23. Labrie C, Bélanger A, Labrie F. Androgenic activity of dehydroepiandrosterone and androstenedione in the rat ventral prostate. *Endocrinology* 1988;123:1412–7

24. Hobkirk R. Steroid sulfation: current concepts. *Trends Endocrinol Metab* 1993;4:69–74

25. Stewart PM, Sheppard MC. Novel aspects of hormone action: intracellular ligand supply and its control by a series of tissue-specific enzymes. *Mol Cell Endocrinol* 1992;83:C13–C18

26. Labrie F, Luu-The V, Lin S-X, *et al*. Intracrinology: role of the family of 17β-hydroxysteroid dehydrogenases in human physiology and disease. *J Mol Endocrinol* 2000;25:1–16

27. Labrie F, Sugimoto Y, Luu-The V, *et al*. Structure of human type II 5α-reductase. *Endocrinology* 1992;131:1571–3

28. Luu-The V, Zhang Y, Poirier D, *et al*. Characteristics of human types 1, 2 and 3 17β-hydroxysteroid dehydrogenase activities: oxidation–reduction and inhibition. *J Steroid Biochem Molec Biol* 1995;55:581–7

29. Labrie Y, Durocher F, Lachance Y, *et al*. The human type II 17β-hydroxysteroid dehydrogenase gene encodes two alternatively-spliced messenger RNA species. *DNA Cell Biol* 1995;14:849–61

30. Bélanger A, Brochu M, Cliche J. Levels of plasma steroid glucuronides in intact and castrated men with prostatic cancer. *J Clin Endocrinol Metab* 1986;62:812–15

31. Labrie F, Bélanger A, Dupont A, *et al*. Science behind total androgen blockade: from gene to combination therapy. *Clin Invest Med* 1993;16:475–92

32. Labrie F, Simard J, Luu-The V, *et al*. Structure, regulation and role of 3β-hydroxysteroid dehydrogenase, 17β-hydroxysteroid dehydrogenase and aromatase enzymes in formation of sex steroids in classical and peripheral intracrine tissues. In Sheppard MC, Stewart PM, eds. *Hormone, Enzymes and Receptors*. London: Baillière Tindall, 1994:451–74

33. Pelletier G, Dupont E, Simard J, *et al*. Ontogeny and subcellular localization of 3β-hydroxysteroid dehydrogenase (3β-HSD) in

the human and rat adrenal, ovary and testis. *J Steroid Biochem Mol Biol* 1992;43:451–67

34. Labrie F, Simard J, Luu-The V, *et al.* The 3β-hydroxysteroid dehydrogenase/isomerase gene family: lessons from type II 3β-HSD congenital deficiency. In Hansson V, Levy FO, Taskén K, eds. *Signal Transduction in Testicular Cells Ernst Schering Research Foundation Workshop.* Berlin, Heidelberg, New York: Springer-Verlag, 1996:185–218

35. Labrie F, Luu-The V, Lin SX, *et al.* The key role of 17β-HSDs in sex steroid biology. *Steroids* 1997;62:148–58

36. Labrie F, Bélanger A, Cusan L, *et al.* Marked decline in serum concentrations of adrenal C19 sex steroid precursors and conjugated androgen metabolites during aging. *J Clin Endocrinol Metab* 1997;82:2396–402

37. Martel C, Sourla A, Pelletier G, *et al.* Predominant androgenic component in the stimulatory effect of dehydroepiandrosterone on bone mineral density in the rat. *J Endocrinol* 1998; 157:433–42

38. Dauvois S, Geng CS, Lévesque C, *et al.* Additive inhibitory effects of an androgen and the antiestrogen EM-170 on estradiol-stimulated growth of human ZR-75-1 breast tumors in athymic mice. *Cancer Res* 1991;51:3131–5

39. Kennedy BJ. Fluxymesterone therapy in treatment of advanced breast cancer. *New Engl J Med* 1958;259:673–5

40. Couillard S, Gutman M, Labrie C, *et al.* Comparison of the effects of the antiestrogens EM-800 and tamoxifen on the growth of human breast ZR-75-1 cancer xenografts in nude mice. *Cancer Res* 1998;58:60–4

41. Labrie F, Diamond P, Cusan L, *et al.* Effect of 12-month DHEA replacement therapy on bone, vaginum, and endometrium in postmenopausal women. *J Clin Endocrinol Metab* 1997;82:3498–505

42. Franceschi S. The epidemiology of endometrial cancer. *Gynecol Oncol* 1991;41:1–16

43. Friedl A, Jordan VC. What do we know and what don't we know about tamoxifen in the human uterus. *Breast Cancer Res Treat* 1994;31: 27–39

44. Labrie F, Labrie C, Bélanger A, *et al.* EM-652 (SCH 57068), a third generation SERM acting as pure antiestrogen in the mammary gland and endometrium. *J Steroid Biochem Mol Biol* 1999;69:51–84

Long-term testosterone replacement therapy with slow-release silastic implants

39

E. M. Coutinho, C. Erdens Teixeira, A. Maltez and H. Maia, Jr

Introduction

In healthy women the level of ovarian secretion of estradiol drops from 40–80 µg/day during reproductive years to less than 20 µg/day during menopause. Ovarian secretion of estrone drops from 20–50 µg/day to less than 10 µg/day[1]. Unlike estrogen, androgen levels do not drop as markedly at the menopause. However, their decline with increasing age is greater than that of estrogen[2]. Total circulatory levels in women in their forties are approximately 50% of those of women in their twenties. In addition, reduction of ovarian secretion rates of androgens also occurs and, although not as marked as that of the estrogens, it is also significant. Testosterone drops from 50–70 µg/day to 40–50 µg/day, whereas androstenedione declines from 1.0–1.5 mg/day to 0.3–0.6 mg/day[3]. The physiologic decrease in the estrogen–androgen ratio is the cause of the increased facial hair growth that occurs in some women postmenopausally. Replacement therapy with estrogen corrects the estrogen deficiency but increases the estrogen–androgen ratio in favor of estrogen, creating a relative androgen deficiency in which loss of libido and sexual satisfaction becomes one of the most disturbing consequences. In addition, lowered testosterone levels contribute to increased risk of invertebral crush fractures[4].

Methods

For the past twenty years we have been providing testosterone supplementation as replacement therapy to women with low testosterone blood levels. We have also offered hormone replacement therapy (HRT) with estrogen and testosterone using silastic implants to both oophorectomized and menopausal women who were unhappy with their estrogen–alone or estrogen–progestogen HRT. The silastic implants were made with segments of silastic tubing (Technical Products Inc., Decatur, Georgia), measuring 4 cm in length and filled with 50 mg of testosterone-17β-ol or 50 mg 17β-estradiol. The implants were sterilized with either steam or ethylene oxide. Insertion was made in the gluteal region following local anesthesia with procaine 2%. The standard dose consisted of 6–8 capsules of estradiol, totalling 300–400 mg, and 2–4 capsules of testosterone, totalling 100–200 mg. The set of estradiol implants provided blood levels of estradiol of 35–50 pg/ml of estradiol whereas the two implants of testosterone provided 50–80 ng/dl of testosterone. The release rate of estradiol was in the range of 0.8–1.09 mg/day, whereas that of testosterone was 0.2–0.8 mg/day over one year[5].

Implants containing levonorgestrel (Norplant®) or other progestins such as nomegestrol acetate (Uniplant®) were available for those women whose endometrial thickness surpassed 10 mm for a period of two months or longer.

The women included in these studies were: (1) women with intact ovaries but low testosterone blood levels; (2) young, oophorectomized women; and (3) menopausal women.

The third group included both those with intact ovaries and oophorectomized women.

Most women had been treated previously with estrogen, alone or in combination with progestin, and considered the previous treatment unsatisfactory because they felt depressed, lacked energy and enthusiasm, and suffered loss of libido. Some of them complained of memory loss.

Testosterone treatment in intact, cycling women

Eighty-eight intact, cycling women complaining solely of loss of libido and presenting total testosterone levels below 80 ng/dl (normal levels 50–180 ng/dl) were inserted with two capsules of testosterone. Blood levels of the hormone measured during implant use were higher than 80 ng/dl but never higher than the physiological limit of 180 ng/dl. Following insertion of the implants, these women were evaluated for effects on libido. In this group of 88 women the effect of the hormone on libido on a scale of 0–10 was rated 8 by 36 women (41%). Twenty-eight women (32%) rated the response between 5 and 7, and the remaining 24 (27%) rated it below 5. Half of these latter women (12) had no change in libido at all (Table 1).

No virilizing effects, such as hoarseness, hirsutism and acne, were observed at the 100 mg (two implants) dose level. In women who reported no effect or a response well below that which was desired, an additional capsule or set of two capsules was offered with the warning that the higher blood levels resulting from this additional dosage could result in side-effects. All 12 women who had no response and ten of those who had rated the response below 5 opted for a supplement. Of the 22 women receiving a supplement, 20 received one more capsule and only two received two additional capsules. After three months these women were re-evaluated. Of the 20 women who were now bearing three capsules, eight women rated the response superior to that attained with two capsules,

Table 1 Effects of testosterone implants on the libido of intact, cycling women

Number	%	Rating
36	41	8–10
28	32	5–7
24	27	0–5

i.e. above 5 but below 8. Three women rated the response above 8. One of these women considered the effect exaggerated and requested removal of the extra capsule. This subject reported the development of an unwelcome desire for other women. The remaining nine women reported no improvement with the extra implant.

One of the two women who received two additional capsules rated the response between 5 and 7 but the other remained unresponsive. Both developed hoarseness, seborrhea and acne. In over 50% of all women receiving these implants a line of very soft, downy hair grew over the skin covering the implant. In some women (15%), a slight depression at the site of the implant developed, indicating loss of fat.

Testosterone replacement therapy in young, oophorectomized women

In women who had been oophorectomized for various reasons, which included endometriosis, abscesses, benign cysts and malignant disease, testosterone replacement therapy with implants was carried out in conjunction with estrogen replacement therapy. The combined set consisted of 6–8 implants containing 50 mg each (total of 300–400 mg) and 2–4 implants of testosterone containing 50 mg each (total of 100–200 mg). The sets provided enough hormones to maintain blood levels of estrogen in the range of 40–80 pg/ml and testosterone in the range of 50–80 ng/dl.

Forty-eight oophorectomized women, aged 15–45, were inserted with either 6 or 8 implants of estradiol and 2–4 implants of testosterone, depending on body weight, and were followed up for 1–5 years. (Women with ovarian agenesis were not included in this group). Twenty-eight of these women who had an intact uterus (subgroup A) were offered two alternative regimens of progesterone therapy: (1) oral administration of medroxyprogesterone 5 mg for two weeks followed by two weeks off; or (2) an implant of nomegestrol acetate containing 50 mg of the progestin inserted from the outset. The second alternative was the choice of 19 women (68%). Nine women (32%) opted for cyclic withdrawal bleeding.

Testosterone replacement therapy provided the necessary support for normal sexual receptivity and libido according to the subject's own evaluation at six months, one year and every successive year in over 50% of the women in both subgroups. Twenty-one out of 28 women who had intact uteri (subgroup A) reported a satisfactory response to masturbation. Over half of this group had no sexual partner, which made evaluation of sexual receptivity, sex drive and orgasm during coitus impossible. In the 20 women who had no uterus and who received no progestin supplementation (subgroup B), the response to sexual stimulation was reported as satisfactory in 17/20 subjects (85%). Only two subjects reported no orgasm when masturbating.

Testosterone replacement therapy in menopausal women

The use of subdermal implants with testosterone in menopausal women has the advantage of providing natural testosterone in physiological dosage over a long period of time. In clinics at both the Federal University of Bahia's Climério de Oliveira Maternity Hospital and at CEPARH (Centro de Pesquisa e Assistência em Reprodução Humana) in Salvador, Bahia, Brazil, we have been providing our menopausal patients with hormone replacement therapy, including testosterone implants, for over twenty years. Although several thousand women over the last ten years have received a small supplement of subdermal testosterone to maintain a physiological level

of the hormone, we are reporting here on only 153 women who opted for that form of therapy and who have been followed up for 1–5 years (mean 3.5 years). The women were aged 42–72 years. The standard procedure was to offer all the women a set of implants containing 4–6 capsules of estradiol and 1–3 capsules of testosterone. In intact women whose blood levels of both estrogen and testosterone, albeit low, remained within the physiological range, the combination set contained four capsules of estradiol and one to two capsules of testosterone. Whenever the blood levels of these hormones were below the physiological range, the higher dose was prescribed. Of the 153 women, 108 were intact women who required monitoring of the uterus by ultrasound at 6-monthly intervals for evaluation of endometrial thickness. The other 45 women had been hysterectomized prior to admission to this study for reasons which included leiomyomata, endometrial hyperplasia and/or excessive bleeding. In addition to sonographic monitoring, all the women were evaluated on a yearly basis with a mammography and breast ultrasound, as well as blood analysis which included cholesterol, high-density lipoprotein (HDL), low-density lipoprotein (LDL), triglycerides, testosterone, estradiol, thyroid-stimulating hormone (TSH), follicle-stimulating hormone (FSH), luteinizing hormone (LH) and prolactin. Bone densitometry was also carried out on a yearly basis.

A total of 634 woman-years of use of the estradiol–testosterone implant combination was analyzed. Except in the case of smokers, the symptomatology associated with the menopause, which included hot flushes, sweating and tachycardia, was maintained under control during implant use with the standard dose for a full year following implant insertion. The control of depression and headaches was likewise complete in over 72% of those who presented with these symptoms.

A total of 426 woman-years of use were completed by women with an intact uterus and the remaining 208 woman-years of use were from women hysterectomized before initiation of therapy.

At the end of the first week following implant insertion, most women (84%) who had complained of hot flushes, tachycardia and sweating at admission reported complete relief from these symptoms. By the end of the second month of use, 72% of implant users reported relief from depression and a moderate (32%) to marked (56%) improvement in their sexuality. Smokers in both intact and oophorectomized groups were those who felt that the standard dose was insufficient to control their symptoms. In these women, blood levels of both estrogen and testosterone were lower than in non-smokers. Moreover, the steroid supply from the implant needed replacement much earlier (3–6 months) in the smokers, never reaching the one year they lasted in non-smokers.

Weight changes at one year were moderate (mean 1.5 kg). Thirty-eight per cent of women presented no change or a reduction in body weight. Thirty-three per cent presented an increase of 0.5–3.0 kg. The remaining women (29%) presented increases greater than 3 kg. Two women, both with hypothyroidism, had increases in body weight above 8 kg and one subject, who had type II diabetes, gained 12 kg during the first year of use but lost 8 kg during the second year with proper dieting and medication. There were no complaints of hoarseness or other voice changes.

Thirty-two women (21.3%) complained of body and facial hair growth but none of them found the effect serious enough to discontinue use of the implant. Only one woman complained of clitoral hypertrophy. Discontinuation at one year was only 7.8% (12/153 women). The reasons for discontinuation were known in only three cases, where subjects felt the implantation procedure to be painful or unpleasant (2) or felt that the treatment was below expectations (1). The other nine women dropped out because they moved away from Salvador or because they had been advised to discontinue HRT. Of the 153 women admitted to the study, 141 wanted to be reinserted for the second year (92.2%). At the end of the second year, 14 women dropped out (9.2%). One hundred and twenty-seven

Table 2 Discontinuations and continuation rate over five years of implant use

Year	Number of patients	Continuation rate from previous year	Woman-years of study
1	153	–	153
2	141	92.2%	294
3	127	90.1%	421
4	111	85.8%	532
5	102	91.9%	634

remained for a third year. Reasons for dropout at the end of the second year were similar to those given at the end of the first year: moving away from the area or lack of motivation for continuation.

At the end of the third year, 16 women dropped out (10.5%). Some gave as a reason being too old (over 60) to carry on, others the loss of their husband. In no case were side-effects presented as a reason for discontinuation. One hundred and eleven women opted for continuation for a fourth year. At the end of the fourth year, only nine women (8.1%) dropped out, leaving 102 from the original group of 153, who felt they should continue with the therapy. Continuation rate at five years is therefore 2/3 (66%) of the original group (Table 2).

Twenty-six out of 108 women who had an intact uterus developed endometrial thickness above the 10 mm limit, which did not regress following shedding after a course of levonorgestrel (Nortrel®) or medroxyprogesterone acetate (Provera®) daily for ten days. These women were submitted to hysteroscopy and/or endometrial ablation. Five of these opted for hysterectomy. Endometrial changes detected by hysteroscopy were diagnosed as hyperplasia of the glandular epithelium or endometrial polyp. In none of these cases was malignant change detected.

No adverse changes were detected which could be correlated with the therapy in blood levels of cholesterol, HDL, LDL, triglycerides or total lipids. Elevated blood pressure developing during treatment in seven women, one of them diabetic, did not seem to be associated with the therapy according to their cardiologists' comments. No abnormal bone loss occurred during treatment as documented by bone densitometry carried out at yearly intervals in all patients.

Study conclusions

These observations of the use of subdermal silastic implants, which release physiological doses of testosterone, show that the hormone should be included in HRT whenever possible because of its remarkable benefits on mood, memory and sexuality of women with low blood levels of the hormone. That the users feel better when on testosterone than when without the hormone is indicated by the high continuation rates, which show two-thirds of the subjects remaining faithful to the therapy at 5 years. It is possible that other benefits of the implant method, which include liberating the woman from the need to apply or take medication for a full year, make this method more attractive. The relative lack of side-effects associated with the use of progestins, such as lowered libido and depression, is another attractive feature of this method.

There is a strong association between the menopause and a marked decrease in coital frequency and sexual interest, which is independent of age and seems to be more associated with testosterone than estrogen decrease[6]. The response to testosterone included an increase in sexual desire, sex drive, receptivity, skin sensitivity, particularly at the nipples and clitoris, better lubrication and enhanced response at orgasm. In addition to the benefits to psychosexual function, testosterone plays an important role in the development and maintenance of bone mass, reducing bone loss and the risk of fractures. This is supported in our studies by normal bone densitometry showing normal densities over the duration of the study.

The studies also show that the association of testosterone and estrogen at physiological doses reduces the need to use progesterone in order to protect the endometrium. It has been shown recently that androgens,

particularly androstenedione, can inhibit human endometrial epithelial cell growth and secretory activity *in vitro*. No significant effects of the two most potent androgens, testosterone and dihydrotestosterone, were shown in these studies, probably because the binding of the two steroids to proteins of the calf serum in the *in-vitro* system used reduced bioavailability[7].

Studies in our own laboratory confirm the existence, previously reported, of androgen receptors in the endometrium. The effects of testosterone on the endometrium are complex. The androgen receptor in the endometrium is located mainly in the stroma with very few detected in the glandular epithelium[8]. This predominantly stromal distribution of receptors is observed in various benign endometrial pathologies such as polyps and non-atypical hyperplasia. This indicates that most of the effects of testosterone on the normal endometrium are exerted through the stroma, where it stimulates, for instance, prolactin production[9]. This effect of testosterone on prolactin is similar to the one observed with progestins. In fact, several studies have shown that high and prolonged doses of androgens can induce endometrial atrophy. This has been observed to occur in women with gender dysphoria, who had used androgens for at least a year[10]. Androgens, when used to treat endometriosis, are also effective in causing endometrial atrophy despite the presence of normal circulating levels of estrogens[11]. Estrogens can induce the synthesis of androgen receptors in the endometrium in the same way as they do for progesterone receptors[12]. Testosterone, like progesterone, is also known to affect predominantly cellular differentiation and not proliferation in the endometrium[13]. These findings suggest that testosterone may exert an antiproliferative effect on the normal endometrium when a proper ratio with estrogen can be achieved. In fact, in postmenopausal patients using estradiol and testosterone implants, the endometrium remains atrophic throughout the treatment with very few signs of endometrial proliferation.

When these patients develop an abnormal thickening of the endometrium, this is due in most cases to the growth of endometrial polyps[14]. The growth of polyps in the uterine cavity seems to be unabated by testosterone. Similarly, endometrial polyps also seem to be insensitive to the antiproliferative effects of progesterone, growing in response to estrogen and displaying various grades of hyperplasia in their glandular epithelium[15]. The reasons for the insensitivity of endometrial polyps to both testosterone and progestins are still far from being understood. We have recently found that approximately 50% of endometrial polyps show amplification for the c-erbB2 oncoprotein and this is related to higher proliferation rates[16]. However, the association between c-erbB2 amplification and unresponsiveness to testosterone or progestins has not yet been established. Recent studies, on the other hand, have suggested that epidermal growth factor receptor could activate the estrogen receptor in the absence of estrogens by means of a chemical signal originating at the plasma membrane. This chemical signal would probably involve the phosphorylation of estrogen receptors and their subsequent activation[17]. Because c-erbB2 protein is a membrane glycoprotein growth factor receptor, which shares molecular homology with the EGF receptor, its overexpression in endometrial polyps may therefore permanently activate the estrogen receptor, markedly increasing the proliferative

response to estrogens and possibly blocking the differentiating effect of testosterone. Although an association between c-erbB2 overexpression and testosterone resistance in endometrial polyps is purely speculative at present, such an association might explain the development of endometrial polyps in postmenopausal patients using implants of testosterone and estradiol and the low incidence of diffuse endometrial hyperplasia as the cause of endometrial thickness and abnormal uterine bleeding in these patients.

Summary

Testosterone supplementation with slow-releasing subdermal silastic implants was provided to women with low testosterone blood levels. The women included in these studies were women with intact ovaries but testosterone blood levels below 80 ng/dl, young oophorectomized women and menopausal women. In all three groups of women, testosterone replacement therapy provided the necessary support for normal sexual receptivity and libido, according to the subjects' own evaluation at 6 months, one year and every successive year in over 50% of the women. The use of subdermal implants with testosterone and estrogen in menopausal women has the advantage of providing natural hormones in physiological dosages over a long period of time.

References

1. Judd HL. Hormonal dynamics associated with the menopause. *Clin Obstet Gynecol* 1976;19: 775–88
2. Judd HL, Yen SSC. Serum androstenedione and testosterone levels during the menstrual cycle. *J Clin Endocrinol Metab* 1973;36:481
3. Muschayandebvu T, Castracane DV, Gimpel T, *et al*. Evidence for diminished midcycle ovarian androgen production in older reproductive aged women. *Fertil Steril* 1996;65:721–3
4. Longscope C, Baker RS, Hui SL, *et al*. Androgen and estrogen dynamics in women with

vertebral crush fractures. *Maturitas* 1984;6: 309–18
5. Coutinho EM. Clinical experience with implant contraception. *Contraception* 1978;18:411–27
6. Montgomery M, Coutinho EM. Androgens, sexuality and menopause. In Coutinho EM, Spinola P, eds. *Current Knowledge in Reproductive Medicine* 2000. Excerpta Medica International Congress Series 1206. Amsterdam. Elsevier Science BV, 2000;409–13
7. Tuckerman EM, Okon MA, Tin-Chiu Li Ana, Laird SM. Do androgens have a direct effect on

endometrial function? An *in vitro* study. *Fertil Steril* 2000;74:771–9

8. Maia H Jr, Maltez A, Fahel P, *et al*. Detection of testosterone and estrogen receptors in post-menopausal endometrium. *Maturitas* 2000; in press

9. Narukawas S, Kanzaki H, Inoue T. Androgens induce prolactin production by human endometrial stromal cells *in vitro*. *J Clin Endocrinol Metab* 1994;78:165–8

10. Miller N, Bedard YC, Cooter NB, *et al*. Histological changes in the genital tract in transsexual women following androgen therapy. *Histopathology* 1986;10:661–9

11. Rose GL, Dowsett M, Mudge JE, *et al*. The inhibitory effects of danazol, danazol metabolites, gestrinone and testosterone on the growth of human endometrial cells *in vitro*. *Fertil Steril* 1998;49:224–8

12. Adesanya-Famuyiwa OO, Zhou J, Wu G, *et al*. Localization and sex steroid regulation of androgen receptor gene expression in rhesus monkey uterus. *Obstet Gynecol* 1999;93:265–70

13. Neulen J, Wagner B, Runge M, *et al*. Effect of progestins, androgens, estrogens and anti-estrogens on 3H-thymidine uptake by human endometrial and endosalpinx cells *in vitro*. *Arch Gynecol Obstet* 1987;240:225–32

14. Maia H Jr, Maltez A, Fahel P, *et al*. Hysteroscopic findings in postmenopausal patients with a thick endometrium after using implants of estradiol and testosterone. *Gynaecol Endoscopy* 2000;9:259–65

15. Maia H Jr, Maltez A, Calmon LC, *et al*. Histopathology and steroid receptors in endometrial polyps of postmenopausal patients under hormone replacement therapy. *Gynaecol Endoscopy* 1998;7:267–72

16. Maia H Jr, Maltez A, Fahel P, *et al*. Histochemical detection of c-erbB2 over-expression in endometrial polyps removed by hysteroscopy. *Gynaecol Endoscopy* 2000;9:253–8

17. Speroff L. The estrogen receptor: changing concepts. Clinical lessons from molecular biology. In Coutinho EM Spinola P, eds. *Reproductive Medicine: A Millennium Review*. Carnforth, UK: Parthenon Publishing, 1999;155–61

Delta 5-androgen replacement therapy in postmenopausal women   40

A. R. Genazzani, B. Quirici, M. Stomati and M. Luisi

Introduction

In women, climacteric and postmenopause are characterized by several endocrine, neuro-endocrine and metabolic modifications, producing short-term and long-term effects on sex steroid-sensitive tissues. The short-term effects are vasomotor symptoms (hot flushes and sweats), mood and neurogenic disturbances (depression, anxiety, migraine/headaches, insomnia), skin collagen loss and dyslipidemia. Long-term consequences are atrophic vaginitis, dispareunia, decrease of libido, urinary disturbances (stress incontinence, nocturnal enuresis), osteoporosis and increased risk of cardiovascular diseases. Estrogen–progestin replacement therapy is considered the principal approach to ameliorate these symptoms.

Experimental studies have shown direct and indirect effects of sex steroids on the brain. Estrogen administration directly increases total cerebral and cerebellar blood flow by 30% and augments cerebral glucose utilization[1]. Moreover, the central effects of gonadal steroids depend on their action on neuroactive transmitters and neuropeptides that regulate the function of specific brain areas. The positive effect of estrogens on mood depends on their action on different central neurotransmitters. In fact, they increase serotonin (5-HT) synthesis and levels of its main metabolite 5-hydroxyindoleacetic acid (5-HIAA). Estrogen administration improves cognitive functions[2,3], in particular by exerting a positive effect on memory and reaction time tests[4,5]. Estrogen modulates the cholinergic system by increasing choline acetyltransferase activity, the enzyme responsible for acetylcholine synthesis[6]. Acetylcholine is a key neurotransmitter in learning and memory and a disturbance of the cholinergic system is the most significant neurochemical defect of Alzheimer's disease. The onset of vasomotor disturbances coincides with neuroendocrine impairment: noradrenergic, opiatergic and dopaminergic systems play a key role in the physiopathology of these symptoms[7,8]. The decrease in plasma β-endorphin levels has also been shown to be related to the pathogenesis of mood, behavior and nociceptive disturbances of the postmenopausal period[9,10]. The positive effect of hormone-replacement therapy (HRT) on vasomotor and subjective psychobehavioral symptoms may be mediated through the opiatergic pathway. In fact, oral estrogen replacement therapy subsequent to spontaneous or surgically-induced menopause is followed by a significant increase in circulating β-endorphin levels[11,12].

Only a few studies have focused attention on androgen replacement therapy and in particular on those symptoms directly related to androgens deficiency, such as sexual disorders, reduction in well-being and energy, mood disorders, neuroendocrine dysfunction, metabolic and bone mass effects. The androgen activity in normal female physiology and the consequences of deficiency have not been clarified because these steroids are normally considered to be male hormones. However, androgens are normally produced in large amounts by the ovaries and the adrenals and play a relevant role in women from fetal life to adrenopause.

Androstenedione, testosterone and dehydro-epiandrosterone (DHEA) are produced in women by the ovaries and the adrenals. The adrenals also produce DHEA sulfate (DHEAS)[13]. DHEAS is synthesized by the conversion of free DHEA, which is secreted in large amounts (70–80%) by the adrenals and in lower amounts by the ovaries (20%). The Δ5-androgens DHEA and DHEAS (DHEA(S)) are the major circulating products of the adrenal cortex[14,15]. Both Δ5-androgens are peripherally converted to androstenedione, testosterone, dehydro-testosterone (DHT) and estrogens.

The decline of circulating androgens results from ovarian failure and age-related decline in adrenal androgen synthesis. The relative androgen deficiency in postmeno-pausal women provokes impairment of sexual function, lessened well-being, loss of energy and negative effects on bone mass. However, the decline in circulating testosterone, androstenedione and in particular DHEA(S) levels starts in the decades that precede the menopause and sometimes the above mentioned symptoms could occur in the pre-menopausal years. In some reports, the clinical symptoms related to androgen deficiency have been described as related to the adrenopause. For this reason, as menopause is characterized by the decline in gonadal function, it is possible to associate the adrenopause with the age-related decrease in Δ5-adrenal pathway biosynthesis.

The present chapter focuses on the Δ5-androgens and in particular on the endocrine, neuroendocrine and peripheral effects of DHEA(S) in postmenopausal women.

Δ5 androgens: basic and clinical trials

In humans, the synthesis and release of DHEA(S) in adrenal reticular zone cells declines linearly with age[14–16], starting from the third decade of life, and is independent of menopausal transition. After 70 years of age,

DHEA(S) levels are maintained at 20% or less of the maximum plasma concentrations, while cortisol levels remain unchanged[17]. The decrease in adrenal DHEA(S) secretion is not related to cortisol changes, and studies performed in postmenopausal women suggest that reduction in 17,20-desmolase activity, the enzyme that governs the biosynthesis of the Δ5-adrenal pathway, may provoke modifications in DHEA(S) synthesis[18–23] (Figure 1). Some authors have reported an overlap of values between sexes, showing 10–25% lower DHEA(S) levels in women than in men. In particular, postmenopausal women showed markedly reduced DHEA ultradian and circadian rhythms, which results in a further decline in Δ5-androgen production[23].

Other factors that may modify circulating levels of DHEA(S) are body mass index (BMI) and insulin/glucose balance. Obesity has been shown to be associated with an increased adrenal activity in both adults and children. In fact, in obese prepubertal and pubertal girls, circulating Δ5-androgen levels are significantly higher than in those of normal weight age-matched girls[24,25].

Epidemiological studies have also focused the attention on the relationship between the progressive decrease in circulating DHEA(S) levels and the increase in cardiovascular morbidity in men[26] and breast cancer in women[27,28], and the decline of immune competence in both sexes[29].

The evidence that DHEA(S) administration reduces some of the problems related to age-ing[30,31] has opened new perspectives for clinical research[30,32–35]. Morales and colleagues[36] administered 50 mg DHEA/day, orally, for 2 months to normal men and women. In both men and women, circulating levels of DHEA and DHEAS increased two- to three-fold. Thus, in both men and women, approximately 70–75% of the administered DHEA appeared in the circulation as DHEAS and only 7–10% as DHEA. In women, the circulating levels of androstenedione, testosterone and DHT all increased two- to three-fold. No modifications in serum estrone or estradiol were observed in

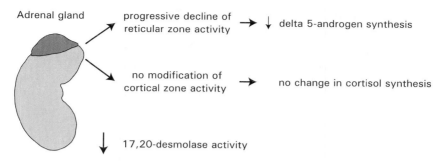

Figure 1 Modification of adrenal cortex activity with aging in men and women

both sexes. Other studies have shown that low doses of DHEA or DHEAS (50–100 mg/day) produce an improvement in psychological and physical well-being and ameliorate immune system function and bone mineral density in both sexes[31,37–40]. Moreover, other trials have shown that DHEA administration increases sex hormone circulating levels (DHEAS, testosterone and estrogens) to young adult values (with no steroid accumulation during the treatment), improves libido and exerts an anti-depressant role (30–90 mg/day for 4 weeks) in middle-aged and elderly patients with major depression and low basal DHEA(S) levels, without modification of cardiovascular parameters[41,42].

Effects of DHEA(S) in postmenopausal women

Neuroendocrine systems

Few studies have investigated the role of DHEA(S) on the CNS in humans, but several *in vitro* and *in vivo* experiments have tried to study the modulating effects of Δ5-androgens on human neuroendocrine systems. DHEA and DHEAS are considered to be neurosteroids because they are produced in the CNS and may directly affects CNS functions. In fact, DHEA(S) concentrations in the CNS are 5–10 times greater than plasma levels. At present, the origin of DHEA in the brain is unknown because the adult rat brain does not have 17β-hydroxylase activity and cannot convert

pregnenolone or progesterone to hydroxylated compounds, nor C21 to C19 steroids[43]. However, the DHEA(S) concentrations in rat brain remain unchanged for a long time after the removal of gonads and adrenals, thus the synthesis of classical neurosteroids, including DHEA, probably proceeds through different pathways to those of adrenals or gonads. Glial cells contain additional steroid metabolizing enzymes that transform classical steroid hormones into a variety of compounds[43–45].

Experimental evidence suggests that the effects of DHEA and DHEAS on the CNS occur directly through a specific binding to the γ-aminobutyric acid$_A$ (GABA$_A$) receptor, thus blocking GABA-induced chloride transport or current in synaptoneurosomes and neurons in a dose-dependent manner, with an increase in neuronal excitability[46]. Moreover, a potentiating effect of DHEA on N-methyl-D-aspartate (NMDA) and sigma receptors has been reported in rat brain[43] (Figure 2).

In order to clarify the effects of DHEA(S) on neuroendocrine functions, our group has investigated the effects of DHEA(S) supplementation on the opiatergic tonus in postmenopausal women. In particular, the attention was focused on β-endorphin, the most important and biologically active endogenous opioid peptide, having behavioral, analgesic, thermoregulatory and neuroendocrine properties[46,47].

In postmenopausal women, sex steroid hormone withdrawal modifies neuroendocrine equilibrium and produces a

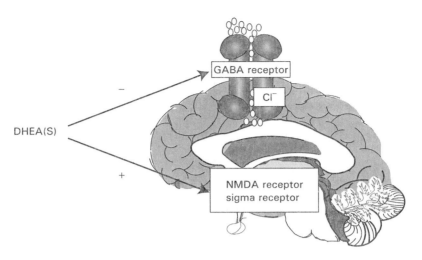

Figure 2 Dehydroepiandrosterone (DHEA) and dehydroepiandrosterone sulfate (DHEAS) regulation of the GABA$_A$ receptor and NMDA receptor in the CNS

decrease in plasma β-endorphin levels acting on the opiatergic system[48]. Neuroactive transmitters such as noradrenaline, dopamine, serotonin, acetylcholine, GABA and corticotrophin-releasing factor (CRF), modulate β-endorphin synthesis and release[49]. A typical example of the neuroendocrine modifications occurring postmenopausally is the response of an opioid peptide to a bolus injection of naloxone, an opioid receptor antagonist, and clonidine, an α_2-presynaptic receptor agonist. In fertile subjects, both clonidine and naloxone increase β-endorphin levels. In postmenopausal subjects the β-endorphin response to clonidine and to naloxone is completely absent, while HRT restores basal plasma β-endorphin levels to those present in fertile women as well as the β-endorphin response to clonidine and naloxone[49,50].

To further investigate this evidence, in a preliminary trial, postmenopausal women received oral DHEA (100 mg/day) (Rottapharm, Milan, Italy) for 7 days. Women underwent a clonidine test (0.150 mg i.v.), before and after 7 days of treatment. After treatment, a significant increase in plasma β-endorphin levels was observed as response of the adrenergic activation with clonidine[51]. Further data have been obtained in

postmenopausal women with a normal BMI and basal plasma DHEA levels < 4 ng/ml. Women received DHEAS (50 mg orally/day) (Rottapharm, Milan, Italy), 17β-estradiol alone (50 μg/patch) or DHEAS plus 17β-estradiol. Subjects were observed monthly during the 3 months of therapy for the determination of steroid hormone and β-endorphin levels. Before and after 3 months of therapy, β-endorphin levels were evaluated in response to three neuroendocrine tests: clonidine (0.150 mg), naloxone (4 mg i.v.) and fluoxetine (30 mg orally). Androgens and estrogens (DHEA, DHEAS, androstenedione, testosterone, estrone and estradiol) and β-endorphin levels significantly increased after each month of DHEAS treatment, while the group receiving 17β-estradiol alone showed an increase in estrogens (estrone and estradiol) and β-endorphin. Sex hormone-binding globulin (SHBG), cortisol, and 17-OH progesterone levels did not show significant variations in the three groups[52]. While no response to the three tests was observed before treatment in each group of subjects, a significant increase in plasma β-endorphin levels was shown after 3 months in response to clonidine and naloxone tests, with no differences between the three kinds of therapies.

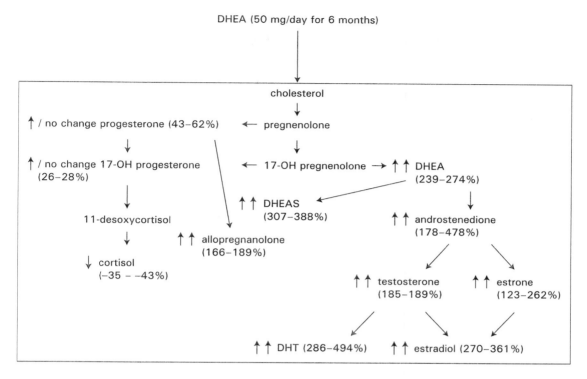

Figure 3 Six-month oral dehydroepiandrosterone (DHEA) supplementation in postmenopausal women: modification of circulating levels of androgen and estrogen DHEAS, dehydroepiandrosterone sulfate; DHT, dihydrotestosterone

These findings suggest that DHEAS restores the neuroendocrine control of α_2-adrenergic, opioidergic and serotonin receptors in terms of anterior pituitary β-endorphin secretion with the same potency as 17β-estradiol. Neuroendocrine pathway modulation after DHEAS supplementation may be mediated by a specific estrogenic action of DHEAS metabolites or, alternatively, by a similar receptor specificity of DHEAS and estrogen–progestin compounds on opiatergic and adrenergic neurons[52].

In conclusion, in postmenopausal women a restoration of the circulating steroid levels to values similar to those present in young subjects has been observed and the neuroendocrine response of β-endorphin to specific stimuli can be restored, suggesting that DHEAS, and/or its active metabolites, modulate the neuroendocrine control of pituitary β-endorphin secretion.

Circulating steroids, gonadotropins, SHBG, β-endorphin and adrenal function

In a recent study we aimed to investigate the effects of a 6-month DHEA supplementation (50 mg/day) in early and late postmenopausal women, with different BMIs, on circulating steroid, SHBG, β-endorphin and gonadotropin levels, and on the adrenal gland response to dexamethasone suppression and adrenocorticotropic hormone (ACTH) stimulation[53].

Early and late postmenopausal women both of normal weight (BMI 20–24) and overweight (BMI 26–30), were treated with oral DHEA (50 mg orally/day) (Rottapharm, Milan, Italy) for 6 months.

Circulating DHEA, DHEAS, 17-OH pregnenolone, progesterone, 17-OH progesterone, allopregnanolone, androstenedione, testosterone, DHT, estrone, estradiol, SHBG,

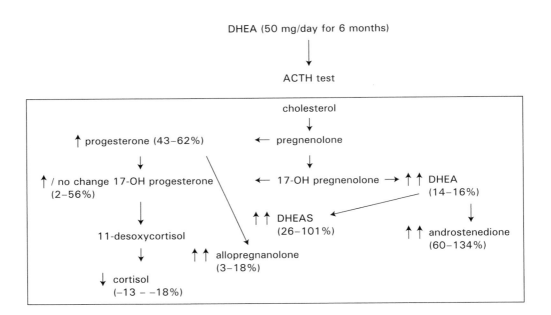

Figure 4 Six-month oral dehydroepiandrosterone (DHEA) supplementation in postmenopausal women: modification fo the response of the adrenal steroids to the adrenocorticotropic hormone (ACTH) test DHEAS, dehydroepiandrosterone sulfate

cortisol, luteinizing hormone (LH), follicle-stimulating hormone (FSH) and β-endorphin levels were evaluated monthly. Before and after 3 and 6 months of therapy, each woman underwent an ACTH stimulation test after dexamethasone (0.5 mg orally) suppression. Before and after each month of therapy, a Kupperman questionnaire was completed. It included complaints such as subjective vaso-motor and psychological symptoms.

DHEA, DHEAS, androstenedione, testosterone, DHT, estrone, estradiol, 17-OH progesterone, allopregnanolone and β-endorphin levels increased during the 6 months of treatment. Progesterone and 17-OH pregnenolone remained constant. SHBG levels significantly decreased only in overweight late postmenopausal women while cortisol and gonadotropin levels progressively decreased in all groups[53] (Figure 3). In basal conditions, dexamethasone significantly suppressed all the adrenal steroids and this suppression was greater after 3 and 6 months of treatment in terms of DHEA, DHEAS and allopregnanolone, while it remained unchanged for

other steroids. ACTH stimulation induced a significant increase in all parameters and, after treatment, it prompted a greater increase in Δ5- and Δ4-androgens, progesterone and 17-OH progesterone, while cortisol responded less both in younger and older normal weight subjects[53] (Figure 4). The endometrial thickness did not vary during the treatment. The Kupperman score improved in all groups, with major effects on the vasomotor symptoms in early postmenopausal subjects[53].

Conclusion

The present findings confirm that DHEA supplementation produces physiological and supraphysiological modifications in steroid milieu in both men and women. The beneficial effects of DHEA on the quality of life and in reverting the ageing processes, described in the literature, may be related to changes in the release of adrenal products and/or peripheral steroids, with an increase in anxiolytic (allo-pregnanolone), anabolic (androstenedione, testosterone, DHT) and estrogenic (estrone, estradiol) molecules, a beneficial decrease in cortisol and an increase in pituitary β-endorphin production[53]. We believe that the Δ5-androgens DHEA and DHEAS are active as pre-hormones because they produce active metabolites that induce positive modifications in the physiology of women, which may counteract the negative phenomena related to menopause and ageing. Consequently, DHEA should be considered a medication, not simply a 'dietary supplement' or an anti-ageing compound, and should, therefore, not be freely accessible to the public as it is now. More extensive studies are required to confirm the lack of effects on the endometrium and the breast, and to evaluate any alterations in metabolic parameters as well as the efficacy of lower doses of the drug.

References

1. Ohkura T, Teshima Y, Isse K. Estrogen increases cerebral and cerebellar blood flows in postmenopausal women. *Menopause* 1995;2:13–18

2. Furuhjelm M, Feder-Freybergh P. The influence of estrogens on the psyche in climacteric and postmenopausal women. In: van Keep PA, Albeaux M, Greenblatt R, eds. *Consensus on Menopause Research*. Baltimore: University Press, 1976:84–93

3. Caldwell BM, Watson RI. Evaluation of psychological effects of sex hormone administration in aged women: results of therapy after 6 months. *J Gerontol* 1952;7:228–44

4. Hackman BW, Galbraith D. Six month study of oestrogen therapy with piperazine oestrone sulphate and its effect on memory. *Curr Med Res Opin* 1977;4(Suppl):21–7

5. Fedor-Freybergh P. The influence of oestrogen on well being and mental performance in climacteric and postmenopausal women. *Acta Obstet Gynaecol Scand* 1977;64(Suppl):5–69

6. Lawrence AD, Sahakian BJ. Alzheimer disease, attention, and the cholinergic system. *Alzheimer Dis Assoc Disord* 1995;9(2):43–9

7. Genazzani AR, Petraglia F, Facchinetti F, *et al.* Increase of proopiomelanocortin-related peptides during subjective menopausal flushes. *Am J Obstet Gynecol* 1984;149:775–9

8. Linghtman SL, Jacobs HS, Maguire AK, *et al.* Climacteric flushing: clinical and endocrine response to infusion of naloxone. *Br J Obstet Gynaecol* 1981;88:919–24

9. Adler MW. Minireview: opioid peptides. *Life Sci* 1980;26,496–510

10. O'Donohue TL, Dorse DM. The opiomelanotropinergic neuronal and endocrine system. *Peptides* 1982;3:383–95

11. Genazzani AR, Petraglia F, Facchinetti F, *et al.* Steroid replacement increases beta-endorphin and beta-lipotropin plasma levels in postmenopausal women. *Gynecol Obstet Invest* 1988;26:153–9

12. Genazzani AR, Petraglia F, Cleva M, *et al.* Norgestimate increases pituitary and hypothalamic concentrations of immunoreactive beta-endorphin. *Contraception* 1989;5:605–13

13. Judd HL, Bardin CW. Serum androstenedione and testosterone levels during the menstrual cycle. *J Clin Endocrinol Metab* 1973;36:475–81

14. Parker LN, Odell WD. Control of adrenal androgen secretion. *Endocr Rev* 1980;4:392–410

15. Yamaji T, Ibayashi H. Serum deydroepiandrosterone sulphate in normal and pathological conditions. *J Clin Endocrinol Metab* 1969;29:273–8

16. Sherwin BB, Gelfand MM, Brender W. Androgen enhances sexual motivation in females: a prospective, crossover study of sex steroid administration in surgical menopause. *Psychosom Med* 1985;47:339–51

17. Davis SR, Burger HG. Androgens and the postmenopausal woman. *J Clin Endocrinol Metab* 1996;81:2759–63

18. Parker L, Gral T, Perrigo V, Skowksy R. Decreased adrenal androgen sensitivity to ACTH during aging. *Metabolism* 1981;30:601–4

19. Dorgan JF, Reichman ME, Judd JT, *et al.* Relationship of age and reproductive characteristics with plasma estrogens and androgens in premenopausal women. *Cancer Epidemiol Biomarkers Prev* 1995;4:381–6

20. Liu CH, Laughlin GA, Fisher UG, Yen SS. Marked attenuation of ultradian and circadin rhythms of dehydroepiandrosterone in post-menopausal women: evidence for a reduced 17,20 desmolase enzymatic activity. *J Clin Endocrinol Metab* 1990;71:900–6

21. Utian WH. The true clinical features of post-menopausal oophorectomy and their response to estrogens replacement therapy. *S Afr Med J* 1972;46:732–7

22. Campbell S, Whitehead M. Oestrogen therapy and the menopausal syndrome. *Clin Obstet Gynecol* 1977;4:31–47

23. Burger HG, Hailes J, Menelaus M. The management of persistent symptoms with estradiol-testosterone implants: clinical, lipid and hormonal results. *Maturitas* 1984;6:351–8

24. Genazzani AR, Pintor C, Corda R. Plasma levels of gonadotropins, prolactin, thyroxine, and adrenal and gonadal steroids in obese prepubertal girls. *J Clin Endocrinol Metab* 1978;47(5):974–9

25. Azziz R, Zacur HA, Parker Jr CR, *et al*. Effects of obesity on the response to acute adrenocorticotropin stimulation in eumenorrheic women. *Fertil Steril* 1991;56:427–33

26. Barret-Connor E, Khaw K, Yen SSC. A prospective study of DS mortality and cardiovascular disease. *N Engl J Med* 1986;315:1519–24

27. Helzlsouer KJ, Gordon GB, Alberg A, *et al*. Relationship of prediagnostic serum levels of DHEA and DS to the risk of developing pre-menopausal breast cancer. *Cancer Res* 1992;52:1–4

28. Bulbrook RD, Hayward JL, Spicer CC. Relation between urinary androgen and corticoid secretion excretion and subsequent breast cancer. *Lancet* 1975;2:395–8

29. Thoman ML, Weigle WO. The cellular and subcellular bases of immunosenescence. *Adv Immunol* 1989;46:221–61

30. Von Eckardstein S, Nieschlag E. Pharmacology, pharmacokinetics and effects/side-effects of different androgen preparations. *Aging Male* 1998;1:28–34

31. Wolf OT, Neumenn O, Helhammer DH, *et al*. Effects of a two-week physiological dehydroepiandrosterone substitution on cognitive performance and well-being in healthy elderly women and men. *J Clin Endocrinol Metab* 1997;82:2363–41

32. Davis SR, Mc Cloud P, Srauss BJC, *et al*. Testosterone enhances estradiol's effects on postmenopausal bone density and sexuality. *Maturitas* 1995;21:227–36

33. Berr C, Lafont S, Debuire B, *et al*. Relationships of dehydroepiandrosterone sulphate in elderly with functional, physiological, mental status and short term mortality: a French community-based study. *Proc Natl Acad Sci USA* 1996;93:13410–15

34. Ravaglia G, Forti P, Maioli F, *et al*. The relationship of dehydroiepiandrosterone sulphate (DHEAS) to endocrine-metabolic parameters and functional status in the oldest-old. Results from an Italian study on healthy free-living over ninety-years-old. *J Clin Endocrinol Metab* 1996;81:1173–8

35. Baulieu EE. Dehydroepiandrosterone (DHEA): a fountain of youth? *J Clin Endocrinol Metab* 1996;81:3147–52

36. Morales AJ, Nolan JJ, Nelson JC, Yen SS. Effects of replacement dose of dehydroepiandrosterone in men and women of advancing age. *J Clin Endocrinol Metab* 1994;78:1360–7

37. Blauer KI, Rogers WM, Benton EW. Dehydroepiandrosterone antagonizes the suppressive effects of glucocorticoids on lymphocyte proliferation. Presented at *Proc of the 71st Annual Meet of The Endocrine Soc*, 1989

38. Rogers WM, Blauer KL, Bernton W. Dehydroepiandrosterone protection against dexamethasone induced thymus involution: flow cytometric and mechanism studies. Presented at *Proc of the 71st Annual Meet of The Endocrine Soc*, 1989

39. Taelman P, Kayman JM, Janssens X, *et al*. Persistence of increased bone-resumption and possible role of dehydroepiandrosterone as a bone metabolism determinant in osteoporotic women in late menopause. *Maturitas* 1989;11:65–73

40. Nordin BEC, Robertson A, Seamark RF. The relation between calcium absorption, serum DHEA and vertebral mineral density in postmenopausal women. *J Clin Endocrinol Metab* 1985;60:651–7

41. Wolkowitz OM, Reus VI, Roberts E, *et al*. Dehydroepiandrosterone (DHEA) treatment of depression. *Biol Psychiatry* 1997;41:311–18

42. Baulieu EE, Thomas G, Legraln S, *et al*. Dehydroepiandrosterone (DHEA), DHEA sulphate and ageing: contribution of the DHEAge study to a sociobiomedical issue. *Proc Natl Acad Sci* 2000;97:3–8

43. Mellon SH. Neurosteroids: biochemistry, modes of action, and clinical relevance. *J Clin Endocrinol Metab* 1994;78:1003–8

44. Majewska MD. Neurosteroids: endogenous bimodal modulators of the GABA-A receptor. Mechanism of action and physiological significance. *Progress in Neurobiol* 1992;38: 379–95

45. Corpechot C, Young J, Calvel M, *et al.* Neurosteroids: 3α-hydroxy-5α-pregnan-20-one and its precursors in the brain, plasma, and steroidogenic glands of male and female rats. *Endocrinology* 1993;133:1003–9

46. Majewska MD, Demirgoren S, Spivak CE, *et al.* The neurosteroid DHEA is an allosteric antagonist of the GABA A receptor. *Brain Res* 1990; 526:143–6

47. Genazzani AR, Petraglia F, Mercuri N, *et al.* Effect of steroid hormones and antihormones on hypothalamic beta-endorphin concentrations in intact and castrated female rats. *J Endocrinol Invest* 1990;13:91–6

48. Petraglia F, Comitini G, Genazzani AR, *et al.* β-Endorphin in human reproduction. In: Herz A. *Opiods II.* Springer-Berlin: Verlag, 1993:763–80

49. Stomati M, Bersi C, Rubino S, *et al.* Neuroendocrine effects of different oestradiol–progestin regimens in postmenopausal women. *Maturitas,* 1997:28;127–35

50. Schneider HPG, Genazzani AR. A new approach in the treatment of climacteric disorders. *De Gruiter* 1992;134–54

51. Rubino S, Stomati M, Bersi C, *et al.* Neuroendocrine effect of a short-term treatment with DHEA in postmenopausal women. *Maturitas* 1998;28:251–7

52. Stomati M, Rubino S, Spinetti A, *et al.* Endocrine, neuroendocrine and behavioral effects of oral dehydroepiandrosterone sulfate supplementation in postmenopausal women. *Gynecol Endocrinol* 1999;13:15–25

53. Stomati M, Monteleone P, Quirici B, *et al.* Six month oral dehydroepiandrosterone supplementation in early and late postmenopause. *Gynecol Endocrinol* 2000;14:342–63

Hormone therapy in uterine bleeding disorders and menorrhagia

41

A. E. Schindler

Introduction

Uterine bleeding disorders and menorrhagia are one of the most disturbing symptoms for women[1,2]. Bleeding disorders present clinically in different ways such as: polymenorrhea, oligomenorrhea, hypermenorrhea; pre- and postmenstrual bleeding; metrorrhagia (irregular bleeding episodes); menorrhagia (excessive bleeding); and epimenorrhagia (inter-menstrual bleeding). The etiology of uterine bleeding disturbances and menorrhagia contains a broad spectrum of organic lesions and functional disturbances such as anovulation which can result in organic tissue changes such as endometrial hyperplasia. Some of the main organic causes are listed in Table 1.

Uterine bleeding disorders increase during the reproductive years, starting from about 8% in young women between 15 and 19 years of age, and rising to nearly 50% in women between 40 and 49 years of age[3,4]. Therefore, heavy menstrual bleeding is a significant factor of ill health in women. It accounts for 12% of all gynecological referrals in the UK[5]. Eighty per cent of women with heavy menstrual bleeding have no anatomical pathology. Therefore, medical therapy is indicated[5]. Each year about £7 million are spent in primary care prescribing for menorrhagia in the UK, and it is felt that medical therapy is indicated when there is no obvious pelvic abnormality and the woman wishes to retain her fertility[6].

Medical treatment

Although there is clearly a place for surgery, medical therapy, however, has an enormous

Table 1 Organic causes of uterine bleeding disorders

Pregnancy related
Spontaneous abortion
Incomplete or threatened abortion
Ectopic pregnancy
Placental detachment
Gestational trophoblastic disease
Genital tract infection
Vaginitis
Cervicitis
Endometritis
Premalignant and malignant genital tract changes
Cervical dysplasia/carcinoma
Cervical polyp
Endometrial polyp
Endometrial hyperplasia/carcinoma
Uterine leiomyomata (particularly submucous myoma)
Uterine adenomyosis
Fallopian tube carcinoma
Ovarian estrogen-producing tumor
Systemic illnesses
Thrombocytopenia
von Willebrand's disease
Fanconi's anemia
Thyroid disease
Liver disease

potential for most women with uterine bleeding disorders, especially those with dysfunctional uterine bleeding[7]. Treatment options for uterine bleeding disorders and menorrhagia are:

(1) Surgical (D&C, endometrial ablation, hysterectomy); and

(2) Medical.

The medical treatment options are:

(1) Progestins including natural progesterone;

(2) Estrogen/progestin combinations;

Table 2 Classification of progestins

Progestin	Example
Natural progesterone	
Progesterone derivatives	medrogestone
Retroprogesterone derivatives	dydrogesterone
17-Hydroxyprogesterone derivatives	medroxyprogesterone acetate, megastrol acetate, chlormadinone acetate, cyproterone acetate
19-Norprogesterone derivatives	demegestone, promegestone
17-Hydroxy-19-norprogesterone derivatives	nomegestrol acetate
Testosterone derivatives	ethisterone
19-Nortestosterone derivatives	norethisterone acetate, lynestrenol, levonorgestrel, gestodene, desogestrel, norgestimate, dienogest
Spirolactone derivatives	drospirenone

(3) Danazol/gestrinone;

(4) gonadotropin-releasing hormone (GnRH) analogs; and

(5) Conjugated estrogens.

Estrogens

For acute heavy uterine bleeding with no obvious malignant organic change, 20 mg intravenous equine conjugated estrogen can be used effectively[8]. This can be repeated every 4 hours for a total of six doses. A progestin should be added concomitantly followed by hormonal oral contraceptive pills with or without progestin added[9]. An alternative is the oral use of an estrogen/progestin preparation 3 times daily for 10 to 20 days. Oral contraceptives by virtue of their high progestin activity reduce the blood loss by 50%[9].

Progestins

For clinical use there are various groups of progestins available. The classification of the progestins is summarized in Table 2. These progestins include compounds with different partial effects as shown in Table 3. An example of the variation in biological effects of these compounds on the endometrium is shown in Table 4.

Progestin can be used for therapeutic purposes in various forms: tablet, depot injection, implant, patch, gel and vaginal suppository. Therefore, the route of application can be: oral, parenteral (intramuscular, subdermal), transdermal and vaginal.

Cyclic treatment with progestins At first, cyclic progestins can be used for 10 to 15 days in the second half of the cycle using 5 to 15 mg of a progestin per day[6,7]. Progesterone needs to be used in higher doses (100 mg 2 to 3 times per day)[11]. Over 50% of these women experience successful regulation of their bleeding problems[7]. Reduction of blood loss can be influenced by the length of the cyclic progestin therapy. Treatment between days 5 and 26 has a more profound effect than treatment from days 19 to 26[6].

Continuous treatment with progestins Progestin can be applied continuously by:

(1) Oral tablets;

(2) Long acting intramuscular injections;

(3) Progestin-containing intra-uterine devices; and

(4) Subdermal implants.

Continuous administration of progestins may be more effective in treating uterine bleeding disorders than cyclic doses since amenorrhea is the goal of a continuous systemic progestin application[7].

Table 3 Mechanism of action of progestins (modified according to Neumann and Düsterberg[10])

Progestin	Endometrium effect	Anti-gonadotropic effect	Anti-estrogenic effect	Estrogenic effect	Anabolic effect	Anti-androgenic effect	Gluco-corticoid effect	Anti-mineralocorticoid effect
Progesterone	+	+	+	−	−	±	+	+
Dydrogesterone	+	−	+	−	−	±	−	±
Hydroxy-progesterone derivatives								
Medrogestone	+	+	+	−	−	±	−	−
Chlormadione acetate	+	+	+	−	−	+	−	−
Cyproterone acetate	+	+	+	−	−	+	−	−
Megestrol acetate	+	+	+	−	−	+	−	−
Medroxy-progesterone acetate	+	+	+	−	±	−	+	−
Spirolactone derivative								
Drospirenone	+	+	+	−	−	+	−	+
19-Nortestosterone derivatives								
Norethisterone	+	+	+	+	+	−	−	−
Lynestrenol	+	+	+	+	+	−	−	−
Norethinodrel	±	+	±	+	±	−	−	−
Levonorgestrel	+	+	+	−	+	−	−	−
Norgestimate	+	+	+	−	+	−	−	−
3-Keto-desogestrel	+	+	+	−	+	−	?	−
Gestodene	+	+	+	−	+	−	+	+
Dienogest	+	+	−	−	−	+	−	−

Table 4 Biological effects of progesterone and progestins (modified according to Neumann and Düsterberg[10])

Progestin	Dose of ovulation inhibition (mg/day p.o.)	Transformation dose (mg/cycle p.o.)
Progesterone	> 100	200 (i.m.)
Medrogestone	10	60
Dydrogesterone	> 30	140
Norethisterone	0.5	100–150
Norethisterone acetate	0.5	30–60
Lynestrenol	2	70
Norgestimate	0.2	7
Levonorgestrel	0.05	6
Desogestrel	0.06	2
Gestodene	0.03	3
Dienogest	1	6
Chlormadione acetate	1.5–2	20–30
Cyproterone acetate	1	20
Medroxyprogesterone acetate	10	80
Drospirenone	2	40–80

In recent years many clinical data have been gathered on the use of levonorgestrel-intrauterine devices (IUD). Recurrent hypermenorrhea refractory to oral treatment can be effectively treated by the levonorgestrel-IUD. On the one hand the device is particularly advantageous for younger patients, who might wish to have their conception potential preserved. On the other hand the levonorgestrel-IUD treatment can be used in place of approximately 75% of endometrial ablations[12]. The clinical effect increases with time; a maximum appears to be reached after 12 months[13,14]. The amount of menstrual blood loss (MBL) with a levonorgestrel-IUD after 3 months was 81.6%, after 6 months 88% and after 12 months 95.8%[14]. This positive effect seems to be achieved in different races. For example, Chinese women who had menorrhagia without organic cause and suffered from anemia had a 54%, 87%, and 95% reduction in menstrual blood loss at the first, third and sixth month of treatment, respectively. These reductions were statistically significant with p values of 0.004, 0.03 and 0.008, respectively[15]. In a randomized comparative trial of levonorgestrel-IUD and norethisterone for the treatment of idiopathic menorrhagia the levonorgestrel-IUD reduced blood loss by 94% and oral norethisterone (3×5 mg/day

from days 5 to 26 for three cycles) by 87%[16]. Both the levonorgestrel-IUD and oral norethisterone are effective in menorrhagia in terms of reducing menstrual blood loss to within normal limits. The levonorgestrel-IUD was associated with higher rates of satisfaction and continuation with treatment[16].

Therefore, the levonorgestrel-IUD appears to be an effective nonsurgical treatment modality for the management of menorrhagia and dysmenorrhea. The device has additional benefits as a contraceptive and for relieving premenstrual symptoms[17]. In addition, it should be noted that a marked and safe relief from adenomyosis-associated menorrhagia can be obtained with the use of the levonorgestrel-IUD[18].

Similar control of uterine bleeding disorders can be obtained with progestin implants[19]. Recent studies have indicated a continuous induction of plasminogen activator inhibitor-1 (PAI-1), which may contribute to the therapeutic effect on menorrhagia[20].

GnRH analogs

GnRH analogs can be used to effectively reduce blood loss by pituitary down-regulation and subsequent inhibition of ovarian function, in most cases causing amenorrhea. Because of the estrogen withdrawal symptoms, add-back therapy might be considered either with progestin, estrogen/progestin combination or tibolone.

Danazol

Studies have shown that the MBL can be reduced by between 50 and 85% by treatment with danazol. For the induction of amenorrhea 400–600 mg orally per day are necessary. Clinical use, however, is limited by its androgenic side-effects and long-term metabolic effects[6].

Gestrinone

With 2.5 mg oral gestrinone twice weekly, about 50% of women become amenorrheic and a marked reduction of MBL is observed in 40%. Androgenic side-effects have to be considered[21].

Periovulatory bleeding

A short treatment with estrogens can suffice to cope with the problem. The suggested dose is 2 mg estradiol valerate orally per day from days 12 to 16 of the menstrual cycle[22].

Polymenorrhea with shortened luteal phase

Oral synthetic progestins should be used from days 15/16 to 24/25; also progesterone gel (8%) can be applied. In cases where conception is desired, follicular stimulation with an antiestrogen (e.g. clomifen, tamoxifen) or gonadotropins is indicated[22].

Polymenorrhea with shortened follicular phase

The therapeutic aim is to retard follicular growth. This can be achieved with oral estrogens such as estradiol valerate 2 mg orally from days 3 to 7 of the cycle or with ethinylestradiol 0.02 mg from days 3 to 7 of the cycle[22].

Postmenstrual bleeding

One approach is to use estradiol valerate 2 mg orally from days 3 to 6 of the menstrual cycle; on the other hand progestin from days 15 to 24 can be used[22].

References

1. Kaufert PA. The perimenopausal woman and her use of the health service. *Maturitas* 1980;2: 197–205
2. Coulter A. Definition and epidemiology of menorrhagia. In Cameron IT, Fraser IS, Smith SK, eds. *Clinical Disorders of the Endometrium and Menstrual Cycle*. Oxford: Oxford University Press, 1998:89–104
3. Cameron IT, Fraser IS, Smith SK. *Clinical Disorders of the Endometrium and Menstrual Cycle*. Oxford: Oxford University Press, 1998
4. Ballinger CB, Browing NC, Smith AHW. Hormonal profiles and psychological symptoms in perimenopausal women. *Maturitas* 1987;9: 235–51
5. Lathaly A, Irome G, Camerone I. Cyclical progestins for heavy menstrual bleeding. *Cochrane-Data. The Data-Base-Syst-Rev.* 2000; 2:CD001016
6. Rees MCP. The medical management of menorrhagia. In Cameron IT, Fraser IS, Smith SK, eds. *Clinical Disorders of the Endometrium and Menstrual Cycle*. Oxford: Oxford University Press, 1998:155–66
7. Munro MG. Medical management of abnormal uterine bleeding. *Obstet Gynecol Clin North Am* 2000;27:287–304
8. DeVore GR, Ovens O, Kasi N. Use of intravenous premarin in the treatment of dysfunctional uterine bleeding – a double blind randomised controlled study. *Obstet Gynecol* 1982;59:285–91
9. Rubins JC, Liu J. Alternatives to hysterectomy for the treatment of excessive uterine bleeding. *Int J Clin Pract* 2000;54:233–7
10. Neumann F, Düsterberg B. Entwicklung auf dem Gebiet der Gestagene. *Reproduktionsmedizin* 1998;14:257–64

11. Saarikoski S, Yliskowski M, Penttila I. Sequential use of norethisterone and natural progesterone in premenopausal bleeding. *Maturitas* 1990;12:89–97

12. Römer TH. Prospective comparison study of levonorgesterol IUD versus Roller-Ball endometrial ablation in the management of refractory recurrent hypermenorrhea. *Europ J Obstet Gynecol Reprod Biol* 2000;90:27–9

13. Andersson JK, Rybo G. Levonorgestrel releasing intrauterine device in the treatment of menorrhagia. *Br J Obstet Gynaecol* 1999;97:690–4

14. Milso I, Andersson K, Andersch B, Rybo G. A comparison of flurbiprofen, tranexamic acid, and a levonorgestrel-releasing intrauterine contraceptive device in the treatment of idiopathic menorrhagia. *Am J Obstet Gynecol* 1991; 164:879–83

15. Tang GWK, Lo SST. Levonorgestrel intrauterine device in the treatment of menorrhagia in Chinese women: efficacy versus acceptability. *Contraception* 1995;51:231–5

16. Irvine GA, Campbell-Brown MB, Lumsden MA, *et al*. Randomised comparative trial of the levonorgestrel intrauterine system and norethisterone for treatment of idiopathic menorrhagia. *Br J Obstet Gynaecol* 1998;105:592–8

17. Barrington JW, Bowen-Simpkins P. The levonorgestrel intrauterine system in the management of menorrhagia. *Br J Obstet Gynaecol* 1997;104:614–16

18. Fedele L, Portuese A, Bianchi S, *et al*. Treatment of adenomyosis-associated menorrhagia with a levonorgestrel-releasing intrauterine device. *Fertil Steril* 1997;68:426–9

19. Affandi B. Eine integrierte Analyse des Vaginalblutungsverhaltens in klinischen Studien über Implanon®. *Contraception* 1998;58:99–107

20. Rutanen EM, Hurskainen R, Finne P, Nokelainen K. Induction of endometrial plasminogen activator-inhibitor 1: a possible mechanism contributing to the effect of intrauterine levonorgestrel in the treatment of menorrhagia. *Fertil Steril* 2000;73:1020–4

21. Turnbull AC, Rees MCP. Gestrinone in the treatment of menorrhagia. *Br J Obstet Gynaecol* 1990;97:713–15

22. Schubert J, Distler W. Hormonelle Behandlung von benignen Blutungsstörungen in den verschiedenen Lebensphasen der Frau. *Gynäkologe* 2000;33:652–8

Soy and the treatment of menopause 42

M. M. Seibel

Introduction

Over the next decade, the number of women entering menopause will expand at an extraordinary rate. Roughly 4000 women daily turn 50, adding to the 40 million menopausal and postmenopausal women currently in the USA. However, as a result of fear that taking estrogen will either lead to an increased risk of developing breast and uterine cancer or result in unpleasant side-effects such as continuing menstrual periods, depression and mood swings, as many as 85% of postmenopausal women cannot or will not take estrogen. In one study of 2500 postmenopausal women, 20–30% never collected their initial estrogen prescription, 10% of those who used estrogen did so only intermittently, and an additional 20% discontinued their therapy within eight months[1].

Despite the fears associated with taking estrogen, menopause is associated with certain health issues that might benefit from estrogen replacement therapy, such as hot flashes, heart disease, osteoporosis and an increased risk of certain cancers. This paper will discuss how soy may serve as an alternative to estrogen in accomplishing these goals.

Isoflavones and the Asian diet

It has been known for more than 60 years that soybeans contain 100–300 mg/100 g of the glycosides (inactive form) of the two isoflavones daidzin and genistin. Intestinal microflora cleave the glycoside from the 7 position of the A ring to form the major respective aglycones (unconjugated or active forms) daidzein (4',7-dihydroxy-isoflavone) and genistein (4',5,7-trihydroxyisoflavone)[2]. Soybeans also contain much lower concentrations of glycitein (7,4'-dihydroxy-6-methoxy-isoflavone) and its glycoside, glycitin[3]. Cleavage of the oligosaccharide side chain is an essential step in isoflavone absorption. Once cleaved, these oligosaccharides pass into the large intestine because the human intestinal mucosa contains no alpha-galactosidase to digest them. There they are metabolized by bacteria forming large amounts of carbon dioxide, hydrogen and methane[4]. As a practical note, the resulting flatulence can be substantially reduced if the water in which beans are boiled is changed at least once[5].

The isoflavonoid phytoestrogens are heterocyclic phenols that are structurally similar to estrogens (Figure 1). The position of the benzenoid B ring is the basis for dividing the flavonoid class into flavonoids (2-position) and isoflavonoids (3-position). Although isoflavones occur in numerous plants, the soybean is, for practical purposes, the only nutritionally relevant source of these compounds[6]. Dr Herman Adlercreutz, one of the pioneers in researching the benefits of soy, studied the urinary excretion of soy isoflavonoid phytoestrogens in Japanese or oriental women and compared his findings with urinary levels found in American and Finnish omnivorous women[7]. The excretion of the isoflavonoids in the urine of the Japanese women was associated with intake of soy products and much higher than in the American and Finnish women, and as high in children as in middle-aged and old people. Soy consumption has been associated with a number of epidemiological benefits attributed to the Asian diet.

Isoflavones possess between 1×10^{-4} and 1×10^{-3} the activity of 17β-estradiol[8]. Although their potency is low, their serum

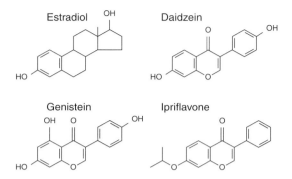

Figure 1   The isoflavonoid phytoestrogens

concentrations can reach levels that are several orders of magnitude higher than those of physiologic estrogens. It is generally believed that isoflavones act as a selective estrogen receptor modulator, exerting antiestrogenic effects in the high-estrogen environment of premenopause and estrogenic effects in the low-estrogen environment of postmenopause. For example, ovariectomized mice fed soy and not given exogenous estrogen had increased uterine weight compared with control animals, whereas ovariectomized mice fed soy and given exogenous estrogen had decreased uterine weight compared with controls[9]. Soy protein (60 g containing 45 mg isoflavones) given daily for one month to pre-menopausal women with regular ovulatory cycles significantly increased follicular phase length and/or delayed menstruation[10]. Soy consumption also significantly suppressed midcycle surges of luteinizing hormone (LH) and follicle-stimulating hormone (FSH) while significantly increasing plasma estradiol concentrations in the follicular phase. While these findings have not been found in every study, this potentially dichotomous biological effect of soy must be appreciated to anticipate some of soy's activity.

Soy and hot flashes

Despite an increased risk of heart disease, osteoporosis and breast cancer, relief from hot flashes is the single most common reason menopausal women seek medical intervention

during the climacteric. Because Asian women report a much lower incidence of hot flashes than Western women[11] and possess higher levels of isoflavones in their diets[7], a great interest has developed in using soy for the treatment of hot flashes.

Murkies *et al.* studied 58 menopausal women suffering from hot flashes and supplemented their diets with 45 g soy flour daily. A comparison group received the same amount of bleached wheat, which contains virtually no isoflavones[12]. By twelve weeks, the women who received soy flour had 40% fewer hot flashes daily compared with the control group, who experienced 25% fewer hot flashes.

Another study of 145 menopausal women[13] supplemented phytoestrogens (mostly soy but some flaxseed) as one fourth of the diet in half of the subjects, while the other half avoided phytoestrogens altogether. As in the first study, both groups reported some improvement in their menopausal symptoms, but the women consuming phytoestrogens improved significantly more.

Albertazzi *et al.* provided 51 women aged 48–61 with a daily dose of 60 g soy protein while 53 similarly-aged women took a placebo. The women taking soy experienced a 26% reduction by three weeks, a 33% reduction by week 4 and a 45% reduction in the mean number of hot flashes by the end of the 12th week compared with a 30% reduction with placebo[14].

Soy isoflavone supplements have also been used to treat hot flashes. In one study[15], participants in the control group were given placebo while the treatment group received 50 mg/day of isoflavones. After six weeks of treatment, the soy group had a significant reduction (45%) in hot flashes and night sweats compared with the placebo group (25%). More recently, 50 mg of isoflavones administered in a double-blind, randomized, placebo-controlled study in 177 patients confirmed the benefits of soy supplements on hot flashes[16] (Figure 2). Soy isoflavone extract was effective in reducing frequency and severity of hot flashes and did not stimulate the endometrium.

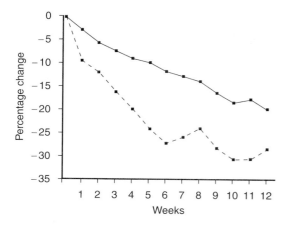

Figure 2 Mean percentage change in daily hot flush severity score per week ——, placebo; - - -, soy ($p = 0.01$)

Although one report of 177 breast cancer survivors given either 150 mg/day of soy isoflavones or a placebo for four weeks found a comparable decline in hot flashes in both groups of 24% and 30% respectively, both groups did experience some improvement in this very short study[17]. Because there is a placebo effect on hot flashes and because soy or soy supplements are typically 15–20% better than placebo, skeptics have suggested that the difference is statistically significant but not meaningful. Such thinking is inaccurate. Peri- and postmenopausal women who have hot flashes tend to have lower sleep efficiencies and longer rapid eye movement (REM) latencies than women who do not experience hot flashes[18]. The reduction in hot flashes provided by soy and soy supplements allows women to have less sleep disruption through the night. This improvement may allow them to achieve a sufficiently improved quality of life so that they can elect not to take HRT.

Soy and cancer

There are numerous studies linking diet and cancer[19,20]. The fact that certain cancers are less prevalent in the Asian population than in Western culture has led a number of investigators to investigate whether soy is responsible for those differences[21,22]. Soybeans contain five anticarcinogenic compounds: isoflavones,

saponins, phytates, protease inhibitors and phytosterols[23]. Isoflavones are by far the best-studied. High concentrations of the isoflavone genistein inhibit most types of cancer cells and may even inhibit metastases[24].

Breast cancer

One of the most important questions surrounding soy and isoflavones is their potential impact on breast cancer. Does soy as a phytoestrogen pose an increased protection or an increased risk for women developing breast cancer?

The basis for this consideration lies in epidemiological studies showing that Asian women whose diets are high in phytoestrogens have lower rates of breast cancer[25,26]. When Japanese women immigrate to North America, their incidence of breast cancer is higher than their Japanese counterparts, and dietary change is implicated as a risk factor for breast cancer[27]. In addition, premenopausal Singaporean women with high soy consumption[28] and Chinese women with high urinary excretion of total isoflavones[29] have been associated with reduced breast cancer risk. Not every study has shown that high intake of various soy products protects against breast cancer[30]. However, among women in Western society, the lowest phytoestrogen levels have been found in women with breast cancer[31]. Similarly, low urinary levels of daidzein and genistein have been associated with a higher incidence of breast cancer in non-Asian Australian women, again suggesting a protective effect from phytoestrogens on breast cancer risk[32]. Another case-controlled study from Australia found a significant reduction in breast cancer risk among both premenopausal and postmenopausal women with increased excretion of the lignan enterolactone and the isoflavone equol[33].

Animal data suggest that soy consumption begun prepubertally may be even more protective[34]. Some[10] though not all[35] studies have also shown soy capable of prolonging menstrual cycle length and suppressing mid-cycle surges of LH and FSH. Should these findings be borne out, they may be important, as menstrual cycle length is inversely related to breast cancer risk[36,37]. Soy has also been shown to prevent cancer in some breast cancer models[38] and genistein alone has prevented breast cancer in animal models[39]. In contrast, HRT is feared as potentially increasing the risk of breast cancer, especially if taken with progesterone[40].

With so much positive information, why doesn't every menopausal woman choose soy over HRT? There is a handful of reports that have added some caution to the answer. One animal study administered low levels (10–100 nM) of genistein to ovariectomized athymic mice implanted with estrogen-dependent human breast cancer (MCF-7) cells and found that the genistein enhanced tumor cell growth, though not nearly as much as 17β-estradiol. Equally important, however, > 20 μM inhibited cancer cell growth[41]. Other investigators have also found that phytoestrogens enhance estrogen-induced DNA synthesis in estrogen receptor (ER)-positive human breast cancer cell lines at low concentrations, but inhibit ER-positive and ER-negative breast cancer cell growth in higher concentrations, demonstrating anticarcinogenic effects[42]. One human study of 48 women undergoing mastectomy for benign and malignant disease showed increased markers of breast lobular epithelium proliferation after 14 days of receiving 60 g soy supplement containing 45 mg isoflavones[43]. However, a subsequent study in 84 premenopausal women taking identical amounts of soy for the same duration of time found no effect on breast epithelial cell proliferation, estrogen and progesterone receptor status, apoptosis or mitosis, suggesting that the proliferation markers the earlier study used may not equal proliferation[44]. These final studies require that a definitive statement on soy's impact on the breast undergo further investigation, despite a large body of evidence about soy's benefits on the breast[45]. Studies on the effect of soy and soy isoflavones under way at the University of North Carolina in women with advanced breast cancer, and at the University

of California at Los Angeles in patients with bilateral cancer recurrence who have had a mastectomy, may further shed light on this question.

Endometrial cancer

As with breast cancer, there is a low incidence of endometrial cancer in countries where large amounts of isoflavones are consumed[46,47]. Animal studies have shown that in ovariectomized models, soy extract does not increase uterine weight or increase endometrial proliferation[48,49]. Furthermore, when soy isoflavones were added to estradiol-treated animals, endometrial proliferation was no longer significantly different from control[50].

Similar findings in human studies have been produced. A recent report using soy extract corresponding to 50 mg daily of isoflavones reported no estrogenic activity on the reproductive tract, demonstrated by the lack of changes in vaginal and endometrial cytology and pulsatility index using transvaginal color Doppler sonography. These findings held true when conjugated equine estrogen was added to the soy isoflavones, suggesting a protective role for soy in the presence of estrogen[51]. Even a dose of 144 mg/day of soy extract had no effect on the increase in uterine weight observed with the equivalent of 0.5 mg or 2 mg estradiol, and a significant inhibition of the response to the 1 mg dose was observed. Other human studies have also shown that soy does not exert an estrogenic role on the endometrium[52,53]. Taken together, soy foods or extracts not only appear safe for the endometrium, but also may blunt the effects of estradiol.

Soy and bone health

Osteoporosis affects 28 million Americans, eighty per cent of whom are women. Because estrogen is effective in both preventing and treating osteoporosis, there is great excitement that the structural similarity between estrogen and isoflavones will promote bone health[54]. This is particularly true since Asian women have a lower incidence of hip fracture than American women[55], although the same is not true for vertebral fractures[56].

In animals, low doses of genistein have bone-conserving properties when administered to ovariectomized lactating rats consuming a low-calcium diet[57,58]. Another study demonstrated that either daidzin or genistin blunted bone loss in ovariectomized rats[59]. Similar findings were observed when soy protein was used in place of casein in the diet of estradiol-treated ovariectomized rats. Soy inhibited bone loss, though slightly less than did estradiol[60]. Using a different approach, genistein and genistin were both found to have an anabolic effect on femoral metaphyseal tissues of elderly rats, causing a significant increase in alkaline phosphatase activity, DNA and calcium content in metaphyseal tissues[61]. Zinc enhanced the effect of genistein.

Virtually all of the human studies are short-term, although several long-term studies are under way. In one six-month study of 66 postmenopausal women who ingested either 55.6 mg/day or 90 mg/day, dual-energy x-ray absorptiometry revealed a significant increase in bone mineral density and content in the lumbar spine for the 90 mg soy-supplemented group compared with controls[62]. Another randomized, placebo-controlled study of 30 postmenopausal women without osteoporosis found that those taking 60 g/day of soy protein experienced lower bone turnover (as measured by both D-pyridinoline and N-telopeptides) over the three months of investigation[63].

The anticipated benefits of isoflavones on bone health led to the synthesis in 1969 of ipriflavone (7-isopropoxy-3-phenyl-4H-1-benzopyran-4-one), a synthetic isoflavone that is relatively tissue-specific for bone with minimal effect on breast and uterus. The large body of data showing the potential benefits of ipriflavone on bone health[64] is believed to be largely based on the extensive intestinal bacterial biotransformation to many metabolites, including daidzein[65], that act as anti-resorptive agents. The usual dosages are 400–600 mg/day. The data are derived from a number of animal studies[66] and human

studies in which ipriflavone has prevented significant bone resorption in premenopausal women treated with gonadotropin releasing hormone-agonist for fibroids[67], in women following oophorectomy[68] and in the rapid bone-losing phase of early menopause[69].

In summary, the data available thus far suggest that natural and synthetic isoflavones are favorable for bone health. Owing to their relative lack of adverse effects, soy and their isoflavones warrant strong consideration in women who either cannot or will not consider HRT.

Heart health

Although the average woman in America is more worried about dying from breast cancer, nearly ten times as many will die of heart disease. Once again, diet plays an important role[70]. As with the other clinical conditions described in this article, epidemiological evidence from Asia suggests that soy greatly contributes to reducing the risk of cardiovascular heart disease. Animal[71] and clinical[72] trials support these observations.

Soy protein has been associated with an approximately 10% reduction in total cholesterol, 12.9% reduction in low-density lipoprotein cholesterol (LDL-C) and 10.5% reduction in triglycerides. High-density lipoprotein cholesterol (HDL-C) levels are reported to be either unchanged or increased slightly. Individuals with elevated cholesterol levels often see greater effects on cholesterol than those with normal values. The data are sufficiently compelling that the US Food and Drug Administration in October 1999 approved the health claim that a dietary intake of at least 25 g/day of soy protein is capable of lowering cholesterol if taken in conjunction with a healthy lifestyle and a diet low in saturated fat. Some[73,74] but not all studies have shown that isoflavones also favorably affect cholesterol levels. More studies are needed to verify a cholesterol-lowering claim for isoflavones.

Other cardiovascular effects include a possible role in blood pressure. Soy has been found to lower high blood pressure in salt-loaded hypertensive mice[75] but not in humans with high-normal blood pressure[76]. However, diastolic blood pressure was significantly decreased when a soy supplement was given twice daily to 51 normotensive perimenopausal women[77].

In three-year studies in ovariectomized rats, soy containing its isoflavones, but not soy with the isoflavones extracted, significantly reduced atherosclerotic plaque[78] and genistein was found to possess antiangiogenesis and antithrombolytic qualities[79]. Relatively low doses of isoflavones have also been found to possess antioxidative capabilities, protecting LDL-C from oxidation[80].

Soy isoflavones may also benefit the cardiovascular system by increasing arterial compliance[81]. Soy isoflavones (80 mg/day for 5 to 10 weeks) administered to 21 women aged 46–67 improved systemic arterial compliance by 26% compared with placebo. These results are quite similar to results found in postmenopausal women treated with long-term HRT[82] and build on parallel findings observed in primate studies[83]. This has led to the intriguing suggestion that soy isoflavones be considered as a potential alternative to progestins for women with an intact uterus taking estrogen for HRT[84].

How to estimate isoflavone intake

Soy can be consumed in a variety of forms including roasted soybeans, soy flour, soy isolate powder, tempeh (fermented soybean), tofu (congealed soy milk) and supplements. Whole foods may be the best form of soy to consume between 25 and 60 g daily because they provide all the components of soy (Table 1). Nevertheless, many Americans will not eat soy regularly owing to its unfamiliar taste and consistency. For this reason, isoflavone supplements provide a reasonable alternative for obtaining many of soy's benefits. Consumers should read labels and look for approximately equal levels of genistein and daidzein for a total daily consumption of 50 mg and not exceeding 100 mg (Table 2).

Table 1 Isoflavone content of food

Food	mg isoflavone/100 g food
Soybeans, green, raw	151.17
Soy flour	148.61
Soy protein isolate	97.43
Soy protein concentrate (alcohol extraction)	12.47
Miso soup, dry	60.39
Tofu (Mori-Nu) silken, firm	31.32
Tofu (Azumaya) extra firm, steamed	22.70
Tofu yogurt	16.30
Soy milk	9.65
Vegetable burgers, prepared (Green Giant Harvest Burger)	8.22
Soy sauce (from hydrolyzed vegetable protein)	0.10

Source: United States Department of Agriculture–Iowa State University

Table 2 Suggested isoflavone intake

For cardiovascular health	approx. 50 mg/day isoflavones found in approximately 25 g/day soy protein (based on health claims allowed by the FDA) for arterial compliance, 40–80 mg/day isoflavones for antioxidant effects on lipids, 10 mg/day
For bone health	approx. 50 mg/day isoflavones
For hot flashes	40–80 mg/day isoflavones

Modified from Consensus Opinion, North American Menopause Society

Doing so will maintain levels within normal dietary intake.

The argument for increasing soy intake in menopause

Over the next decade, I believe the consumption of soy and soy supplements will be as common as taking calcium is today. This may be true for women who both do and do not take estrogen. The benefits for hot flashes, bone health and cardiovascular health are all important reasons. A further reason was nicely summarized in an article by Birge[85] and has to do with soy's potential benefit as a selective estrogen receptor modulator (SERM). Soy phytoestrogens primarily exhibit ER-β activity whereas breast tissue is largely ER-α[86]. Recent data suggest that selective activation of the ER-β pathway may inhibit the ER-α pathway[87], making the breast less responsive to estrogen. As such, soy could differ greatly over the two most commonly used SERMs, tamoxifen and raloxifene.

Review of the Tamoxifen Breast Cancer Prevention Trial data reveals that 3.6/1000 women treated five years or less were prevented from developing invasive breast cancer but 3.9/1000 additional treatment-related cases of invasive endometrial cancer, stroke or pulmonary embolism occurred. Women treated with tamoxifen for more than five years developed more breast cancer recurrence and mortality than those receiving tamoxifen for five years or less or placebo[88]. These findings create a concern that tamoxifen specifically or antiestrogens *per se* might preferentially convert ER-positive tumors to more malignant ER-negative tumors[88]. As Birge suggests[85], estrogen might increase the expression of breast cancer but reduce long-term mortality from it. This would be achieved by selectively expressing the less malignant ER-positive tumors and may explain why women who take estrogen for more than five years experience a reduction in breast cancer mortality[89,90], even if they have a positive family history of breast cancer[91].

Could SERMs have a negative role on brain function[92]? Estrogen appears to play an important role in delaying brain aging and Alzheimer's disease[93,94]. In contrast, up to 70% of women treated with tamoxifen experience problems with memory and an increased incidence of depression[95], and the incidence of hot flashes is increased in women taking raloxifene. Both of these suggest an antiestrogen effect. Soy isoflavones have been shown to improve working memory in ovariectomized retired breeder female rats and do not antagonize the beneficial effects of estradiol on the working memory of these rats[48]. This latter finding must be verified in light of an observational study reporting cognitive decline in men over age 70 linked to eating tofu more than four times per week compared with those who almost never ate it[96]. An editorial in the same issue cited difficulties assigning the findings only to tofu[97].

Conclusion

Given soy's protective role on the endometrium and other beneficial effects, soy or soy isoflavones might evolve into an alternative to progestins for postmenopausal women with an intact uterus, or an adjunct for those choosing a SERM such as raloxifene. Concerns related to the breast and cognition must be weighed against the apparent benefits of soy on the cardiovascular system, skeletal system and hot flashes. Soy is not equivalent to HRT. But for peri- and postmenopausal women who either cannot or will not take estrogen, soy and soy isoflavones provide an excellent alternative choice.

Acknowledgement

Financial support as a consultant to Inverness Medical, Inc. is acknowledged.

References

1. Ravnikar VA. Compliance with hormone therapy. *Am J Obstet Gynecol* 1987;156:1332–4
2. Eldridge A, Kwolek WF. Soybean isoflavones: effect of environment and variety on composition. *J Agric Food Chem* 1983;31:394–6
3. Wang H-J, Murphy PA. Isoflavone composition of American and Japanese soybeans in Iowa: effects of variety, crop year, and location. *J Agric Food Chem* 1994;42:1674–7
4. Rackis JJ, Sessa DJ, Steggerda FR, *et al.* Soybean factors relating to gas production by intestinal bacteria. *J Food Sci* 1970;35:634–9
5. Anderson RI, Rackis JJ, Tallent WH. Biologically active substances in soy products. In

Wilcke HL, Hopkins DT, Waggle DH, eds. *Soy Protein and Human Nutrition*, New York: Academic Press, 1979

6. Messina MJ. Legumes and soybeans: overview of their nutritional profiles and health effects. *Am J Clin Nutr* 1999;70(Suppl):439s–50s

7. Adlercreutz H, Hamalainen E, Gorbach S, *et al.* Dietary phyto-oestrogens and the menopause in Japan. *Lancet* 1992;339:1233

8. Markiewicz L, Garey J, Adlercreutz H, *et al.* In vitro bioassays of non-steroidal phytoestrogens. *J Steroid Biochem Mol Biol* 1993;45:399–405

9. Makela SI, Pylkkanen LH, Santti RSS, *et al.* Dietary soybean may be antiestrogenic in male mice. *J Nutr* 1995;125:437–45

10. Cassidy A, Bingham S, Setchell KDR. Biological effects of a diet of soy protein rich in isoflavones on the menstrual cycle of premenopausal women. *Am J Clin Nutr* 1994;60:333–40

11. Haines CJ, Chung TKH, Leung DHY. A prospective study of the frequency of acute menopausal symptoms in Hog Dong Chinese women. *Maturitas* 1994;18:175–81

12. Murkies AL, Lombard C, Strauss BJD, *et al.* Dietary flour supplementation decreases postmenopausal hot flushes: Effect of soy and wheat. *Maturitas* 1995;21:189–96

13. Brzezinski A, Adlercreutz H, Shaoul R, *et al.* Short-term effects of phytoestrogen-rich diet on postmenopausal women. *Menopause* 1997;4:89–94

14. Albertazzi P, Pansini F, Bonaccorsi G, *et al.* The effect of dietary soy supplementation on hot flushes. *Obstet Gynecol* 1998;91:6–11

15. Scambia G, Mango D, Signorile PG, *et al.* Clinical effects of a standardized soy extract in postmenopausal women: A pilot study. *Menopause* 2000;7:105–11

16. Upmalis DH, Lobo R, Bradley L, *et al.* Vasomotor symptom relief by soy isoflavone extract tablets in postmenopausal women: A multicenter, double-blind, randomized, placebo-controlled study. *Menopause* 2000;7:236–42

17. Quella SK, Loprinzi CL, Barton DL, *et al.* Evaluation of soy phytoestrogens for the treatment of hot flashes in breast cancer survivors: A North Central Cancer Treatment Group Trial. *J Clin Oncol* 2000;18:1068–74

18. Shaver JLF, Giblin E, Pauslen V. Sleep quality subtypes in midlife women. *Sleep* 1991;14:18–23

19. Rose DP, Boyar AP, Wynder EL. International comparison of mortality rates for cancer of the breast, ovary, prostate, and colon, and per capita food consumption. *Cancer* 1986;58:2363–71

20. Fraser GE. Associations between diet and cancer, ischemic heart disease, and all-cause mortality in non-Hispanic white California Seventh-day Adventists. *Am J Clin Nutr* 1999;70(Suppl):532s–538s

21. Adlercreutz H. Phytoestrogens: Epidemiology and a possible role in cancer protection. *Environ Health Perspect* 1995;103(Suppl 7):103–12

22. Messina M, Persky V, Setchell KDR, *et al.* Soy intake and cancer risk: a review of the *in vitro* and *in vivo* data. *Nutr Cancer* 1994;21:113–31

23. Messina M, Barnes S. The role of soy products in reducing risk of cancer. *J Natl Cancer Inst* 1991;83:541–6

24. Li D, Yee JA, McGuire MH, *et al.* Soybean isoflavones reduce experimental metastasis in mice. *J Nutr* 1999;129:1075–8

25. Kennedy AR. The evidence for soybean products as cancer preventive agents. *M Nutr* 1995;125:S733–43

26. Adlercreutz H, Mazur W. Phyto-oestrogens and western diseases. *Annals Med* 1997;29:95–120

27. Shimizu H, Ross RK, Bernstein L, *et al.* Cancers of the prostate and breast among Japanese and white immigrants in Los Angeles County. *Br J Cancer* 1991;63:963–6

28. Lee HP, Gourley L, Duffy SW, *et al.* Dietary effects on breast-cancer risk in Singapore. *Lancet* 1991;337:1197–200

29. Zheng W, Dai Q, Custer LJ, *et al.* Urinary excretion of isoflavonoids and the risk of breast cancer. *Cancer Epidemiol Biomarkers Prev* 1999;8(1):35–40

30. Yuan JM, Wang QS, Ross RK, *et al.* Diet and breast cancer in Shanghai and Tianjin, China. *Br J Cancer* 1995;71:1353–8

31. Adlercreutz CHT, Goldin BR, Gorbach SL, *et al.* Soybean phytoestrogen intake and cancer risk. *J Nutr* 1995;125:757s–70s

32. Murkies A, Dalais FS, Briganti EM, *et al.* Phytoestrogens and breast cancer in postmenopausal women: a case controlled study. *Menopause* 2000;7:289–96

33. Ingram D, Sanders K, Kolybaba M, *et al.* Case-controlled study of phyto-oestrogens and breast cancer. *Lancet* 1997;350:990–4

34. Murrill WB, Brown NM, Zhang J-X. Prepubertal genistein exposure suppresses mammary

cancer and enhances gland differentiation in rats. *Carcinogenesis* 1996;17:1451–7

35. Duncan AM, Merz BE, Xu X, *et al*. Soy isoflavones exert modest hormonal effects in premenopausal women. *J Clin Endocrinol Metab* 1999;84:192–7

36. Treolar AE, Boynton RE, Behn BG, *et al*. Variation of human menstrual cycle through reproductive life. *Int J Fertil* 1970;12:77–126

37. Henderson BE, Ross RK, Judd HL, *et al*. Do regular ovulatory cycles increase breast cancer risk? *Cancer* 1985;56:1206–8

38. Hawrylewicz EJ, Huang HH, Blair WH. Dietary soybean isolate and methionine supplementation affect mammary tumor progression in rats. *J Nutr* 1991;121:1693–8

39. Lamartiniere CA, Murrill WB, Manzolillo PA. Genistein alters the ontogeny of mammary gland development and protects against chemically-induced mammary cancer in rats. *Proc Soc Exp Biol Med* 1998;217:358–64

40. Schairer C, Lubin J, Troisi R, *et al*. Menopausal estrogen and estrogen-progestin replacement therapy and breast cancer risk. *JAMA* 2000; 283:485–91

41. Hsieh CY, Santell RC, Haslam SZ, *et al*. Estrogenic effects of genistein on the growth of estrogen receptor-positive human breast cancer (MCF-7) cells *in vitro* and *in vivo*. *Cancer Res* 1998;58: 3833–8

42. Wang C, Kurzer MS. Effects of phytoestrogens on DNA synthesis in MCF-7 cells in the presence of estradiol or growth factors. *Nutr Cancer* 1998;31:90–100

43. McMichael-Phillips DF, Harding DF, Morton M, *et al*. Effects of soy-protein supplementation on epithelial proliferation in the histologically normal human breast. *Am J Clin Nutr* 1998; 68:1431s–1435s

44. Hargreaves DF, Potten CS, Harding C, *et al*. Two-week dietary soy supplementation has an estrogenic effect on normal premenopausal breast. *J Clin Endocrinol Metab* 1999;84:4017–24

45. Consensus Opinion. The role of isoflavones in menopausal health: Consensus opinion of the North American Menopause Society. *Menopause* 2000;7:215–29

46. Parkin DM. Cancers of the breast, endometrium and ovary: geographic correlations. *Eur J Cancer Clin Oncol* 1989;25:1917–25

47. Safe SH. Environmental and dietary estrogens and human health: is there a problem? *Environ Health Perspect* 1995;103:346–51

48. Pan Y, Anthony M, Watson S, *et al*. Soy phytoestrogens improve radial arm maze performance in ovariectomized retired breeder rats and do not attenuate benefits of 17-β estradiol treatment. *Menopause* 2000;7:230–5

49. Tang BY, Adams NR. Effect of equol on estrogen receptors and on synthesis of DNA and protein in immature rat uterus. *J Endocrinol* 1980;85:291–7

50. Foth D, Cline JM. Effects of mammalian and plant estrogens on mammary glands and uteri of macaques. *Am J Clin Nutr* 1998;68:1413s–17s

51. Scambia G, Mango D, Signorile PG, *et al*. Clinical effects of standardized soy extract in postmenopausal women: A pilot study. *Menopause* 2000;7:105–11

52. Wilcox G, Wahlqvist MS, Burger HG, *et al*. Oestrogenic effects of plant foods in postmenopausal women. *Br J Med* 1990;301:905–6

53. Baird DD, Umbach DM, Lansdell L, *et al*. Dietary intervention study to assess estrogenicity of dietary soy among postmenopausal women. *J Clin Endocrinol Metab* 1995;80: 1685–90

54. Scheiber MD, Rebar RW. Isoflavones and postmenopausal bone health: a viable alternative to estrogen therapy? *Menopause* 1999;6:233–41

55. Fujita T, Fukase M. Comparison of osteoporosis and calcium intake between Japan and the United States. *Proc Soc Exp Biol Med* 1992; 200:149–52

56. Ross PD, Fujuwara S, Huang C, *et al*. Vertebral fracture prevalence in women in Hiroshima compared to Caucasians or Japanese in the US. *Int J Epidemiol* 1995;24:1171–7

57. Anderson JJ, Ambrose WW, Garner SC. Biphasic effects of genistein on bone tissue in the ovariectomized, lactating rat model. *Proc Soc Exp Biol Med* 1998;217:345–50

58. Blair HC, Jordan E, Peterson TG, *et al*. Variable effects of tyrosine kinase inhibitors on avian osteoclastic activity and reduction of bone loss in ovariectomized rats. *J Cell Biochem* 1996;61:629–37

59. Ishida H, Uesugi T, Hirai K. Preventive effects of the plant isoflavones, daidzin and genistin, on bone loss in ovariectomized rats fed a calcium-deficient diet. *Biol Pharm Bull* 1998; 21:62–6

60. Arjmandi BH, Alekel L, Hollis BW, *et al*. Dietary soybean protein prevents bone loss in an ovariectomized rat model of osteoporosis. *J Nutr* 1996;126:161–7

61. Yamaguchi M, Gao YH. Anabolic effect of genistein and genistin on bone metabolism in the femoral-metaphyseal tissues of elderly rats: the genistein effect is enhanced by zinc. *Mol Cell Biochem* 1998;178:377–82

62. Potter SM, Baum JA, Teng H, *et al.* Soy protein and isoflavones: their effects on blood lipids and bone density in postmenopausal women. *Am J Clin Nutr* 1998;68(Suppl 6):1375s–9s

63. Bonaccorsi G, Albertazzi P, Constantino D. Soy phytoestrogens and bone. Presented at the *North American Menopause Society Meeting* 1997; abstr. 44

64. Yoshida K, Tsukamoto T, Torii H. Metabolism of ipriflavone (TC-80) in rats. *Radioisotopes* 1985;34:61–7

65. Cecchini MG, Fleisch H, Muhlbauer RC. Ipriflavone inhibits bone resorption in intact and ovariectomized rats. *Calcif Tissue Int* 1997;61: S9–S11

66. Notoya K, Yoshida K, Tsukuda R, *et al.* Increase in femoral bone mass by ipriflavone alone and in combination with 1α-hydroxyvitamin D3 in growing rats with skeletal unloading. *Calcif Tissue Int* 1996;58:88–94

67. Gambacciani M, Cappagli B, Piaggesi L, *et al.* Ipriflavone prevents the loss of bone mass in pharmacological menopause induced by GnRH-agonists. *Calcif Tissue Int* 1997;61: S15–S18

68. Gambacciani M, Spinetti A, Cappagli B, *et al.* Effects of ipriflavone administration on bone mass and metabolism in ovariectomized women. *J Endocrinol Invest* 1993;16:333–7

69. Melis GB, Paoletti AM, Cagnacci A. Ipriflavone prevents bone loss in postmenopausal women. *Menopause* 1996;3:27–32

70. Seibel MM. The role of nutrition and nutritional supplements in women's health. *Fertil Steril* 1999;72:579–91

71. Anthony MS, Clarkson TB, Bullock BC, *et al.* Soy protein versus soy phytoestrogens in the prevention of diet-induced coronary artery atherosclerosis of male cynomolgus monkeys. *Arterioscler Thromb Vasc Biol* 1997;17:2524–31

72. Anderson JW, Johnstone BM, Cook-Newell ML. Meta-analysis of the effects of soy protein intake on serum lipids. *N Engl J Med* 1995; 333:276–82

73. Wangen KE, Duncan AM, Xu Xia, *et al.* Soy isoflavones improve plasma lipids in normocholesterolemic and mildly hypercholesterolemic postmenopausal women. *Am J Clin Nutr* 2001;73:225–31

74. Baber R, Clifton Bligh P, Fulcher G, *et al.* The effect of an isoflavone dietary supplement (P-081) on serum lipids, forearm bone density and endometrial thickness in postmenopausal women (Abstr. 27). *Menopause* 1999;6:326

75. Fang Z, Chen YF, Oparil S, *et al.* Induction of dietary NaCl-sensitive hypertension in female spontaneously hypertensive rats: role of estrogen (abstract). *Hypertension* 1999;34:336

76. Hodgson JM, Puddey IB, Beilin IJ, *et al.* Effects of isoflavonoids on blood pressure in subjects with high-normal ambulatory blood pressure levels: a randomized controlled trial. *Am J Hypertens* 1999;12:47–53

77. Washburn S, Burke GL, Morgan T, *et al.* Effect of soy protein supplementation on serum lipoproteins, blood pressure, and menopausal symptoms in perimenopausal women. *Menopause* 1999;6:7–13

78. Anthony MS, Clarkson TB. Comparison of soy phytoestrogens and conjugated equine estrogens on atherosclerosis progression in postmenopausal monkeys (abstract). *Circulation* 1998;97:829

79. Kapiotis S, Hermann M, Held I, *et al.* Genistein, the dietary-derived angiogenesis inhibitor, prevents LDL oxidation and protects endothelial cells from damage by atherogenic LDL. *Arterioscler Thromb Vasc Biol* 1997

80. Tikkanen MJ, Wahala K, Ojala S, *et al.* Effect of soybean phytoestrogen intake on low density lipoprotein oxidation resistance. *Proc Natl Acad Sci USA* 1998;95:3106–10

81. Nestel PJ, Yamashita T, Sasahara T, *et al.* Soy isoflavones improve systemic arterial compliance but not plasma lipids in menopausal and perimenopausal women. *Arterioscler Thromb Vasc Biol* 1997;17:3392–8

82. McGrath BP, Liang YL, Teede H, *et al.* Age-related deterioration in arterial structure and function in postmenopausal women: impact of hormone replacement therapy. *Arterioscler Thromb Vasc Biol* 1998;18:1149–56

83. Honore EK, Williams JK, Anthony MS, *et al.* Soy isoflavones enhance coronary vascular reactivity in atherosclerotic female macaques. *Fertil Steril* 1997;67:148–64

84. Clarkson TB. Soy phytoestrogens: What will be their role in postmenopausal hormone replacement therapy? *Menopause* 2000;7:71–5

85. Birge SJ. Soy phytoestrogens: An adjunct to hormone replacement therapy? *Menopause* 2000;7:209–12

86. Kuiper GG, Carlsson B, Grandien K, *et al.* Comparison of the ligand binding specificity and tanscript tissue distribution of estrogen receptors 34 α and 36 β. *Endocrinology* 1997; 138:863–70

87. Hall JM, McDonnell DP. The estrogen receptor beta-isoform (ERβ) of the human estrogen receptor modulates ERα transcriptional activity and is a key regulator of the cellular response to estrogens and antiestrogens. *Endocrinology* 1999;140(12):5566–78

88. Fisher B, Dignam J, Bryant J, *et al.* Five versus more than five years of tamoxifen therapy for breast cancer patients with negative lymph nodes and estrogen receptor positive tumors. *J Natl Cancer Inst* 1997;88(21):1529–42

89. Henderson BE, Paganini-Hill Z, Ross RK. Decreased mortality in users of estrogen replacement therapy. *Arch Intern Med* 1991; 151(1):75–8

90. Grodstein F, Stampfer MJ, Colditz GA, *et al.* Postmenopausal hormone therapy and mortality. *N Engl J Med* 1997;336(25):1769–75

91. Sellers TA, Mink PJ, Cerhan JR, *et al.* The role of hormone replacement therapy in the risk for breast cancer and total mortality in women with a family history of breast cancer. *Ann Intern Med* 1997;127(11):973–80

92. Mathews K, Cauley J, Yaffe K, *et al.* Estrogen replacement therapy and cognitive decline in older women. *J Am Geriatr Soc* 1999;47:518–23

93. Jacobs D, Tang MX, Stern Y, *et al.* Cognitive function in nondemented older women who took estrogen after menopause. *Neurology* 1998;50:368–93

94. Birge SJ. Practical strategies for the diagnosis and treatment of Alzheimer's disease. *Clin Geriatr* 1999;7:56–74

95. Cathcart CK, Jones SE, Pumroy CS, *et al.* Clinical recognition and management of depression in node negative breast cancer patients treated with tamoxifen. *Breast Cancer Res Treat* 1993; 27:277–81

96. White LR, Petrovitch H, Ross GW, *et al.* Brain aging and midlife tofu consumption. *J Am Coll Nutr* 2000;19(2):242–55

97. Grodstein F, Mayeux R, Stampfer MJ. Tofu and cognitive function: food for thought. *J Am Coll Nutr* 2000;19(2):207–9

The validity of diagnostic tests for adnexal mass: a critical analysis

43

T. Gürgan and Z. S. Tuncer

Introduction

The uterine adnexal of gynecologic origin consist of the ovaries, the Fallopian tubes and the uterine ligaments. Although adnexal mass often involves the pathology of the ovaries, contiguous tissues of non-gynecologic origin may also rarely be involved (Table 1). One of the major goals of the evaluation of adnexal mass is to rule out ovarian malignancy.

Approximately 5–10% of women will undergo surgery for adnexal mass in their lifetime, and 13–21% of them will be found to have ovarian malignancy[1]. Furthermore, adnexal mass is one of the leading causes of hospitalization at gynecology clinics[2]. While benign or non-neoplastic lesions require a conservative approach, malignant lesions should be subjected to surgical staging, usually followed by adjuvant chemotherapy. Thus, differential diagnosis between benign and malignant pathology represents a real challenge for both the gynecologist and the patient. Clinical features, as well as the specialized diagnostic tests, are used for the evaluation of the adnexal mass (Table 2).

Clinical features

The age of the patient, the size of the mass and findings at pelvic examination have been found to be valuable clinical diagnostic features. Age is an independent risk factor for malignancy of an adnexal mass. An adnexal mass in the premenarchal and postmenopausal periods is considered to be highly abnormal[3,4]. The incidence of malignant neoplasm significantly increases after age 50 years[5].

Table 1 Classification of the adnexal mass

Gynecologic origin (non-neoplastic)
  ovarian
    physiologic cyst
    follicular cyst
    corpus luteum cyst
    theca lutein cyst
    luteoma of pregnancy
    polycystic ovary
    inflammatory cyst
  non-ovarian
    ectopic pregnancy
    embryologic remnants
    pyosalpinx
    hydrosalpinx
Gynecologic origin (neoplastic)
  ovarian cancer
  leiomyoma
  paraovarian cyst
  tubal carcinoma
Non-gynecologic origin (non-neoplastic)
  appendiceal abscess
  diverticulosis
  adhesions of bowel and omentum
  peritoneal cyst
  pelvic kidney
Non-gynecologic origin (neoplastic)
  sigmoid carcinoma
  appendix carcinoma
  bladder carcinoma
  presacral teratoma

In an evaluation of women of all ages, 3% of masses smaller than 5 cm and 7% of masses 5 to 10 cm in diameter were found to be malignant. The incidence of malignancy for masses larger than 10 cm was 13%[6]. Clinical findings at pelvic examination are often helpful in differentiating a malignant mass from a

Table 2 Special diagnostic procedures for the evaluation of an adnexal mass

Non-operative (non-invasive)
  imaging
    ultrasonography
    computed tomography
    magnetic resonance imaging
    intravenous pyelography
    barium enema
  tumor markers
    CA 125
    human chorionic gonadotropin
Non-operative (invasive)
  culdocentesis
  hysterosalpingography
  arteriography
Operative (non-invasive)
  examination under anesthesia
Operative (invasive)
  laparoscopy
  laparotomy

Table 3 Ultrasound characteristics of adnexal mass

Benign pattern
Simple cyst without internal echoes
Simple cyst with scattered echoes
Polycystic echoes
Polycystic echoes with thick septum
Sessile or polypoid smooth mural echoes
Central dense round echoes
Thin or thick multiple linear echoes
Thin or thick linear echoes with dense part
Malignant pattern
Cystic echoes with papillary or indented mural part
Polycystic echoes with irregularly thick septum
  and solid part
Solid pattern (> 50%) heterogenous component
  with irregular cystic part
Completely solid with homogenous component
Low impedance to flow (color Doppler)

benign neoplasm. A bilateral, solid, irregular, fixed and rapidly growing adnexal mass is suspicious for malignancy[7]. Cul-de-sac nodules and ascites are the other significant pelvic findings in malignant ovarian tumors.

Ultrasonography

Transabdominal and transvaginal ultrasonography, Doppler ultrasonography, three-dimensional sonography, computed tomography and magnetic resonance are the imaging modalities that can be used for differential diagnosis of the adnexal mass. Several characteristic features on ultrasonography have been observed to identify malignant neoplasms (Table 3). Collected data from studies of ultrasound accuracy in prediction of malignancy have an average positive predictive value of 74% and an average sensitivity of 88%[6,8–13]. Intramural blood vessels consistently demonstrated low impedance to flow with a pulastility index below 1 : 16 in women with malignant tumors. The sensitivity and specificity of the pulsatility index in detecting malignant tumors were 94% and 97%, respectively [14,15].

Tumor markers

Serum CA 125 levels have been shown to be useful in distinguishing malignant from benign pelvic masses[16]. CA 125 is increased in approximately 80% of patients with ovarian carcinoma. Although levels of CA 125 are increased in most cases with advanced-stage carcinoma, only 50% of patients with stage I ovarian carcinoma will have elevated levels[1,7,16,17]. After the age of 50 years, an elevated CA 125 level is associated with ovarian carcinoma in 80% of patients, whereas this figure is less than 50% in patients younger than the 50 years[16]. Pelvic inflammatory disease, pregnancy, endometriosis, uterine myomata, hepatitis, heart failure, liver disease and renal disease are the non-malignant conditions that may elevate CA 125 levels[7]. Decreased specificity may be improved with the detection of multiple serum tumor markers[18].

Laparoscopy

An increasing number of reports support laparoscopic management of a pelvic mass. The sensitivity, specificity and positive predictive value of laparoscopy in diagnosing ovarian cancer are 94%, 98% and 44%, respectively[19–23]. The incidence of removing a benign-appearing mass that proved to be malignant at pathologic examination is approximately 1 : 1000[19-23]. Although laparoscopy is reliable in diagnosing malignant cases, an increase in substage with tumor spillage and treatment delay are still unsolved problems. To have the lowest possible risk, the patient should meet the following criteria[7]:

(1) No personal or family history of cancer;

(2) Reproductive age (premenopausal);

(3) Mass smaller than 5 cm;

(4) Ultrasonography showing a unilateral mass that is unilocular, has a smooth border and has no excrescences;

(5) Normal tumor markers.

Intraoperative frozen section has a sensitivity of 93% and a specificity of 99% for diagnosing malignant adnexal mass[24].

Conclusion

The overwhelming majority of adnexal masses are benign and it is extremely important to determine preoperatively whether a patient is at a high risk for ovarian malignancy, in order to minimize the number of operative procedures performed for self-limiting processes. Management of adnexal mass depends on a combination of many predictive factors, including clinical features, imaging modalities and tumor markers.

References

1. Disaia PJ, Creasman WT. *Clinical Gynecologic Oncology*. St. Louis: Mosby Year-Book Inc., 1997:253

2. Velebil P, Wingo PA, Xia A, *et al.* Rate of hospitalization for gynecologic disorders among reproductive-age women in the United States. *Obstet Gynecol* 1995;86:764–9

3. Van Winter JT, Simmons PS, Podratz KC. Surgically treated adnexal masses in infancy, childhood and adolescence. *Am J Obstet Gynecol* 1994;170:1780–6

4. Rulin MC, Preston AL. Adnexal masses in postmenopuasal women. *Obstet Gynecol* 1987;70:578–81

5. Ries LAG, Miller BA, Hankey BF, *et al. SEER Cancer Statistics Review, 1973–1991, Tables and Graphs*. Bethesda, MD: NIH Publ. No. 94-2789, 1994

6. Sassone AM, Timor-Tritsch IE, Artner A, *et al.* Transvaginal sonographic characterization of ovarian disease: evaluation of a new scoring system to predict ovarian malignancy. *Obstet Gynecol* 1991;78:70–6

7. Rock JA, Thampson JD. *TeLinde's Operative Gynecology*. Philadelphia: Lippincott-Raven Publishers, 1997:628–31

8. Kobayashi M. Use of diagnostic ultrasound in trophoblastic neoplasms and ovarian tumors. *Cancer* 1976;38:441–52

9. Meire HB, Farrant P, Guha T. Distinction of benign from malignant ovarian cysts by ultrasound. *Br J Obstet Gynaecol* 1978;85:893–9

10. Herrmann UJ Jr, Locher GW, Goldhirsch A. Sonographic patterns of ovarian tumors: prediction of malignancy. *Obstet Gynecol* 1987;69:777–81

11. Finkler NJ, Benacerraf B, Lavin PT, *et al.* Comparison of serum CA 125, clinical impression, and ultrasound in the postoperative evaluation of ovarian masses. *Obstet Gynecol* 1988;72:659–64

12. Benacerraf BR, Finkler NJ, Wojciechowski C, *et al.* Sonographic accuracy in the diagnosis of ovarian masses. *J Reprod Med* 1990;35:491–5

13. Granberg S, Wikland M, Jansson I. Macroscopic characterization of ovarian tumors and relation to the histologic diagnosis. Criteria to be used for ultrasound evaluation. *Gynecol Oncol* 1989;35:139–44

14. Kurjak A, Predanic M, Kupesic Urek S, *et al.* Transvaginal color and pulsed Doppler assessment of adnexal tumor vascularity. *Gynecol Oncol* 1993;50:3–9

15. Weiner Z, Thaler I, Beck D, *et al.* Differentiating malignant from benign ovarian tumors with transvaginal color flow imaging. *Obstet Gynecol* 1992;79:159–62

16. Malkasian GD, Knapp RC, Lavin PT, *et al.* Preoperative evaluation of serum CA 125 levels in premenopausal and postmenopausal patients with pelvic masses: discrimination of benign from malignant disease. *Am J Obstet Gynecol* 1988;159:341–6

17. Jacobs I, Bast RC. The Ca 125 tumor-associated antigen: a review of the literature. *Hum Reprod* 1989;4:1–12

18. Soper JT, Hunter VJ, Daly L, *et al*. Preoperative serum tumor-associated antigen levels in women with pelvic masses. *Obstet Gynecol* 1990;75:249–54

19. Hulka JF, Peterson HB, Phillips JM, *et al*. Operative laparoscopy. American Association of Gynecologic Laparoscopists 1991 Membership Survey. *J Reprod Med* 1993;38:569–71

20. Nezhat F, Nezhat C, Welander C, *et al*. Four ovarian cancers diagnosed during laparoscopic management of 1011 women with adnexal masses. *Am J Obstet Gynecol* 1992;167:790–6

21. Maiman M, Seltzer V, Boyce J. Laparoscopic excision of ovarian neoplasms subsequently found to be malignant. *Obstet Gynecol* 1991;77:563–5

22. Seltzer V. Laparoscopic surgery for ovarian lesions: potential pitfalls. *Clin Obstet Gynecol* 1993;36:402–12

23. Seltzer V, Maiman M, Boyce J. Laparoscopic survey in the management of ovarian cysts. *Female Patient* 1992;17:19–24

24. Usubutun A, Altinok G, Küçükali T. The value of intraoperative consultation (frozen section) in the diagnosis of ovarian neoplasms. *Acta Obstet Gynecol Scand* 1998;77:1013–6

The secretion of inhibin-related molecules by ovarian tumors

44

H. G. Burger, P. J. Fuller, S. Chu, P. Mamers,
A. Drummond and D. M. Robertson

Introduction

The earliest studies of the secretion of inhibin-related molecules by ovarian tumors were those in which patients with granulosa cell tumors were shown to have elevated immunoreactive inhibin levels in a panel of stored sera[1]. This was consistent with the knowledge that the ovarian granulosa cell is the source of secretion both of inhibin A and inhibin B. Subsequent studies established that inhibin secretion is also a characteristic of other types of ovarian tumor[2]. The present report summarizes current knowledge of inhibin as an ovarian tumor marker, reviews the evidence for inhibin synthesis by ovarian tumors and comments on the application of inhibin immunohistochemistry in ovarian tumor pathology. Finally, current studies of the molecular pathogenesis of ovarian tumors, particularly relating to inhibin secretion, are reviewed.

Ovarian cancer

Ovarian cancer is the most common fatal gynecological malignancy and can be classified into three major types: epithelial – the most common variety, stromal and germ cell. Australian women have a one in 90 lifetime risk of developing the disease and in the majority, the tumor is well advanced by the time the diagnosis is made. It would thus be of considerable interest to develop markers that can be used for earlier diagnosis.

Types of inhibin assay used in ovarian cancer research

The earlier reports on elevated inhibin levels in patients with ovarian tumors utilized the original 'Monash assay'[3], which detects α-subunit-related peptides, including free α-subunit, which has no inhibin-like activity on follicle-stimulating hormone (FSH) secretion. This assay and subsequent assays using antisera directed to epitopes on the α-subunit have proven to be the most useful in ovarian tumor detection[4]. The specific assays for inhibin A and B, which detect the biologically active dimeric forms, have been applied in limited studies[5]. Work is ongoing in the authors' laboratory to develop new α-subunit-directed assays that would allow lower limits of assay detection.

Inhibin concentrations in patients with ovarian tumors

The authors have studied sera from women with ovarian tumors of defined histology and compared values obtained with various assays with results in normal postmenopausal women[5]. Granulosa cell tumors ($n = 9$–11) were always detected using the Monash assay and the specific inhibin B enzyme-linked immunosorbent assay (ELISA), and were detected in 90% of cases using the pro-α_C ELISA and in 77% using the inhibin A assay. Sera from patients with mucinous tumors were positive in 70% using the Monash assay and in 60% by the inhibin B ELISA. Pro-α_C assay gave a 55% positivity rate, but the inhibin A assay only a 20% rate. Patients with serous tumors had elevated levels in the Monash assay in 35% of cases, but were positive in less than 15% using the other assays. Miscellaneous tumors including endometrioid, mixed Mullerian, pseudomyxomas, etc. were detected in the Monash assay in 41% of cases, but in less than 30% using the other assays.

The best-known tumor marker in ovarian cancer is CA125, which is positive in the majority of patients with serous and miscellaneous tumors, but less frequently positive in patients with mucinous and granulosa cell tumors. On the other hand, as indicated, the inhibin assay gives positive results in the majority of mucinous tumors and in virtually all granulosa cell tumors. The authors therefore examined the utility of combining a CA125 assay with an assay directed against the α-subunit, in this case a modified immunofluorimetric assay[6]. These were applied to a bank of ovarian cancer sera. The CA125 assay was positive in 94% of serous tumors, 65% of mucinous, 57% of granulosa cell tumors and 82% of the miscellaneous group. The inhibin α-subunit directed assay was positive in 44% of serous tumors and 47% of the miscellaneous group, and in all sera from mucinous and granulosa cell tumors. Using both assays together, therefore, the detection rate, at 90% specificity, for all ovarian tumors was 93% compared with 84% for CA125 alone and 56% for the inhibin assay. Thus, the combination of CA125 and inhibin measurements has potential for ovarian cancer screening. New α-subunit assays are currently being developed.

Synthesis of inhibin by ovarian tumors

A recent report from the authors' laboratory[7] described mRNA levels for the inhibin subunits in 16 primary ovarian tumors, using reverse transcriptase–polymerase chain reaction (RT-PCR). Gene-specific primers were used and the products were analyzed by Southern blot analysis with gene-specific ^{32}P-labeled probes. Abundant expression of the inhibin α-subunit gene was found in granulosa cell tumors, and to a lesser degree in mucinous and serous tumors, whilst granulosa cell tumors also expressed the β-subunits, which were found to a lesser degree in the other tumor types. Both the activin type II receptor gene and the follistatin genes were detected. The expression of the inhibin subunit genes in ovarian tumors confirms them as a source of the increased inhibin seen in the circulation. The presence of both the activin receptor and follistatin genes suggests that activin may have a paracrine role in such tumors, modulated by follistatin.

Immunohistochemistry of the inhibin subunits in ovarian tumors

In 1995, Gurusinghe et al.[8] reported on the immunohistochemical detection of dimeric inhibin and the inhibin α and βA subunits in a series of tumors where fresh frozen sections were stained. Both polyclonal and monoclonal antibodies were used. In mucinous tumors in particular, clear-out staining of the epithelial cells was noted. Subsequent reports used the R1 antibody generated by Groome and O'Brien[9], an antibody directed at the N-terminus of the inhibin α-subunit. When this antiserum was used to stain paraffin-fixed sections, scattered staining was noted in the stroma of mucinous and other tumors, but not in the epithelial cells. We have undertaken studies to attempt to resolve this paradox. When sections from the same tumor were examined using both fresh frozen and paraffin-embedded material, the R1 antibody and other α-subunit-directed antibodies showed only epithelial staining in the fresh frozen sections and only stromal staining in the paraffin-fixed tissues. No explanation for this paradoxical observation is currently available. In our recent studies in collaboration with Dr Nigel Groome, new antisera directed against epitopes in the middle of the α_C-subunit and at its C-terminal end have been examined. The C-terminally directed antibody shows little staining in ovarian tumors, but the mid-section antibodies stain both the epithelium and the stroma of paraffin-fixed sections of mucinous tumors. This work is ongoing.

The molecular pathogenesis of ovarian granulosa cell tumors

The major observations suggesting that inhibin may be involved in the pathogenesis of ovarian tumors was reported by Matzuk et al.[10], who showed that mice transgenic for deletion of the inhibin α-subunit developed sex-cord stromal tumors, and, if they survived, later adrenal tumors. The authors concluded that the α-subunit gene is a tumor suppressor gene. In further studies, they showed that the mechanism did not involve an effect of activin through the activin RII receptor, though their study did not exclude a possible action via activin RIIB. The actions of FSH did not appear to be a direct cause of the tumors[11]. Paradoxically, human granulosa cell tumors abundantly express the α-subunit. Loss of heterozygosity at the α-subunit locus has not been found in granulosa cell tumors[12].

Studies in the authors' laboratory have explored possible activating mutations of the FSH receptor[13], or of the G-proteins[14] to attempt to explain the excessive secretion of inhibin, but no such mutations have been found. In contrast, high levels of estrogen

receptor ERβ expression in granulosa cell tumors has been reported[15]. A series of studies has been undertaken to examine genes involved in granulosa cell proliferation. Positive findings have included that of elevated levels of the luteinizing hormone (LH) responsive gene cyclin D2, whilst the LH receptor is expressed at lower levels than in the normal ovary. The profile of gene expression suggests a molecular phenotype of granulosa cell tumors similar to the late preovulatory granulosa cell in the normal ovary. The pattern is similar to that seen with FSH stimulation, but without progression to expression of markers or genes involved in luteinization and differentiation. Interestingly, levels of the possible inhibin receptors betaglycan[16] and p120[17] were normal or elevated in these tumors, thus providing no evidence to support the proposal that a defect in inhibin signaling may be involved in tumor pathogenesis.

Conclusions

The assay of inhibin α-subunit peptides is of value in the diagnosis and monitoring of patients with ovarian granulosa cell tumors. Combined assays for inhibin and CA125 represent a promising dual diagnostic tool for ovarian cancer. Inhibin α-subunit immunohistochemistry is of potential application in diagnostic pathology, and the molecular pathogenesis of ovarian granulosa cell tumors is gradually being elucidated.

References

1. Lappöhn RE, Burger HG, Bouma J, et al. Inhibins as a marker for granulosa cell tumors. N Engl J Med 1989;321:790–3
2. Healy DL, Burger HG, Mamers P, et al. Elevated serum inhibin concentrations in postmenopausal women with ovarian tumours. N Engl J Med 1993;329:1539–42
3. McLachlan RI, Robertson DM, Healy DL, et al. Circulating immunoreactive inhibin levels during the normal human menstrual cycle. J Clin Endocrinol Metab 1987;65:954–61
4. Burger HG. Inhibin as a tumour marker. Commentary. Clin Endocrinol 1994;4:151–3
5. Robertson DM, Cahir N, Burger HG, et al. Inhibin forms in serum from postmenopausal women with ovarian cancers. Clin Endocrinol 1999;50:381–6

6. Robertson DM, Cahir N, Burger HG, *et al.* Combined inhibin and CA125 assays in the detection of ovarian cancer. *Clin Chem* 1999;45:651–8

7. Fuller PJ, Chu S, Jobling T, *et al.* Inhibin subunit gene expression in ovarian cancer. *Gynecol Oncol* 1999;73:273–9

8. Gurusinghe CJ, Healy DL, Jobling T, *et al.* Inhibin and activin are demonstrable by immunohistochemistry in ovarian tumor tissue. *Gynecol Oncol* 1995;57:27–32

9. Groome NP, O'Brien M. Two-site immunoassays for inhibin and its subunits. Further applications of the Synthetic peptide approach. *J Immunol Methods* 1993;165:167–76

10. Matzuk MM, Finegold M, Su JG, *et al.* α-inhibin is a tumor-suppressor gene with gonadal specificity in mice. *Nature* 1992;360:313–9

11. Kumar TR, Palapattv G, Klang P, *et al.* Transgenic models to study gonadotropin function: the role of follicle-stimulating hormone in gonadal growth and tumorigenesis. *Mol Endocrinol* 1999;13:851–65

12. Watson RH, Roy WJ Jr, Davis M, *et al.* Loss of heterozygosity at the α-inhibin locus on chromosome 2q is not a feature of human granulosa cell tumors. *Gynecol Oncol* 1997;165:387–90

13. Fuller PJ, Verity K, Shen Y, *et al.* No evidence for a role for mutations or polymorphisms of the follicle stimulating hormone receptor in ovarian granulosa cell tumors. *J Clin Endocrinol Metab* 1998;83:274–9

14. Shen Y, Mamers M, Jobling T, *et al.* Absence of the previously reported G protein oncogene (gip2) in ovarian granulosa cell tumors. *J Clin Endocrinol Metab* 1996;81:4159–61

15. Chu S, Burger HG, Mamers P, *et al.* Estrogen receptor isoform gene expression in ovarian stromal and epithelial tumors. *J Clin Endocrinol Metab* 2000;85:1200–5

16. Lewis KA, Gray PC, Blound AL, *et al.* Betaglycan binds inhibin and can mediate functional antagonism of activin signalling. *Nature* 2000;404:411–4

17. Chong H, Pangas SA, Bernard DJ, *et al.* Structure and expression of a membrane component of the inhibin receptor system. *Endocrinology* 2000:2600–7

Inhibin-related proteins and endometrium 45

L. Cobellis, P. Florio, F. Arcuri, P. Ciarmela, S. Luisi, C. Mangani,
C. Bocchi, M. G. Ricci, M. Cintorino and F. Petraglia

Introduction

Inhibin-related proteins (inhibins and activins) are dimeric glycoproteins belonging to the transforming growth factor-β (TGF-β) superfamily. Inhibins are heterodimers of a unique α subunit with one of two β subunits, βA or βB, and the two circulating forms known are inhibin A (α, βA) and inhibin B (α, βB). Three forms of activins, consisting of β subunits only, have been isolated: activin A (βA, βA), activin AB (βA, βB) and activin B (βB, βB)[1]. Inhibin-related proteins are multifunctional molecules, originally isolated from the gonads and found to be involved in the control of gonadotropin secretion, and later studied in follicular development, placental function and spermatogenesis. Several studies have demonstrated that inhibin-related proteins are widely expressed in different tissues and act as growth factors influencing cell proliferation and differentiation[2].

Inhibin receptors have not yet been identified, but several effects of inhibins are associated with antagonism of activin. Activins act on activin type I and type II receptors, which contain an extracellular domain, a transmembrane region and a serine/threonine kinase intracellular domain. Some of activin's biological functions are not antagonized by inhibin. This might indicate the existence of a specific inhibin receptor, expressed in most but not all target tissues. Inhibin binds to the type II activin receptor. The inhibin-related proteins have been investigated in male and female reproductive functions, and the expression and fluctuation in serum levels during the different menstrual phases, throughout gestation in physiological and pathological pregnancy and in the presence of gonadal tumors are well known[3].

Healthy endometrium

The human endometrium is a complex structure composed of luminal surface epithelium, simple and tortuous glands, and stroma containing different cell types. The expression of specific mRNA for inhibin and activin subunits and for activin type II receptor has been demonstrated in normal human endometrial stromal and epithelial cells, and medium collected from cultured normal epithelial and stromal cells contains discrete amounts of inhibin A, inhibin B and activin A (Figure 1)[4]. Leung et al.[5] showed the immunohistochemical expression of αC/αN subunits of inhibin in the luminal epithelium, glands, endometrial stroma and vascular endothelium, without significant cyclical differences during the menstrual cycle. Proliferative and secretory endometrium showed βA subunit staining, which was raised in the secretory phase in the glandular and luminal epithelium. βB subunit was less expressed[5].

Otani et al.[6] were not able to detect α subunit of inhibin expression in human endometrium during the menstrual cycle and in decidual tissues in early pregnancy. The βA subunit and activin A were strongly stained in endometrial glands during the various phases of the menstrual cycle and in initial decidual expression; conversely, in the endometrial stroma the staining was weak. Recently, Jones

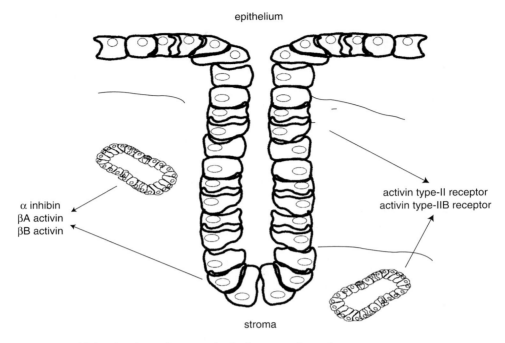

epithelium

α inhibin
βA activin
βB activin

activin type-II receptor
activin type-IIB receptor

stroma

Figure 1 Inhibin-related protein expression by human endometrium

et al.[7] showed that all three subunits of inhibin are expressed in normal endometrium, in glandular epithelium, during the proliferative phase of the menstrual cycle, whereas the luteal phase and the onset of decidualization are characterized by an elevated expression of endometrial stromal compounds.

The human decidua contains and synthesizes inhibin α, βA, and βB subunits. Immunohistochemical data have shown that decidual cells can be stained with both inhibin α and βB antisera, showing a similar localization. These results suggest that decidua may be a further source of inhibin-related proteins during pregnancy and emphasize the endocrine competence of human decidua[8].

Endometrial cells, both epithelial and stromal, undergo cyclical proliferation, differentiation and shedding throughout the menstrual cycle. These mechanisms are regulated by the concurrent variations of estrogen and progesterone serum levels, which are the main regulators of endometrial function. Moreover, the endometrium is able to synthesize cytokines and growth factors, derived directly from endometrial or inflammatory cells, which play a role in modulation, proliferation and differentiation of endometrium in combination with sex steroid hormones. Sex steroid hormones, cytokines and growth factors constitute a complex pool of substances that interact and form the basis for autocrine, paracrine and endocrine regulation in endometrial cells[9]. Several observations have linked the activin system to the modulation of the acute-phase reaction and inflammation. Activin A, like TGF-β, suppresses T cell activation and is an antagonist of interleukin (IL)-6 and IL-1 actions. The demonstration of these properties confirms the possibility that activin acts as an anti-inflammatory agent both locally and peripherally. In fact, an increased expression of activin is demonstrated in cutaneous wound repair[10], in inflammatory bowel disease[11], in liver injury and cirrhosis[12], in repair of the vasculature[13] and in inflammatory arthropathies[14].

Endometriosis

Inhibin A, inhibin B and activin A serum levels in women with endometriosis are not significantly different to healthy controls[15]. The concentrations of inhibin-related proteins measured in peritoneal fluid are higher than in serum. Women with endometriosis have similar peritoneal fluid inhibin A, inhibin B and activin A levels to healthy women, which are independent of the stage of disease and/or the menstrual phase. Indeed, the expression of inhibin and activin subunit mRNA was demonstrated in ectopic endometrial tissue and in peritoneal specimens from healthy women and from patients with endometriosis[15]. Ovarian endometriotic cyst fluid contains higher amounts of inhibin A and activin A than serum and peritoneal fluid. Inhibin α, βA and βB subunits, demonstrated by reverse transcription polymerase chain reaction (RT-PCR), are strongly expressed in epithelial and stromal components of ovarian endometrioma, and the immunohistochemical staining of the subunits of these proteins confirm, once again, a local production of inhibin-related proteins[16]. A putative role of these proteins in local modulation and differentiation, and a possible interaction in the immune regulation of endometriosis, can be hypothesized.

Endometrial adenocarcinoma

Patients with endometrial adenocarcinoma have higher serum levels of activin A with respect to healthy controls, and which are significantly decreased when measured 1 month after surgical removal of the tumor[4]. No significant difference in inhibin A and inhibin B concentrations was demonstrated in endometrial cancer patients. Higer concentrations of activin A in uterine fluid collected from patients with endometrial adenocarcinoma with respect to healthy controls suggest a local secretion[4]. Moreover the detection of these proteins in culture medium of two endometrial adenocarcinoma cell lines, HEC 1A and HEC 1B, confirms the secretion and production from endometrial tissue. The α, βA and βB subunits of inhibin and activin, and activin type II receptor (RII/RIIB) mRNA subunits demonstrated by RT-PCR in malignant endometrial tissue indicate a putative role of inhibin-related proteins in endometrial carcinogenesis[4].

Conclusion

In conclusion, the expression of inhibin-related proteins in human endometrium, stained in various physiological and pathological conditions, underlies a role in proliferation and differentiation of endometrial tissue. The endometrium can be considered as not only a source but also a target of inhibin-related proteins, and the interaction of these proteins with the immune system cell components may modulate the endometrial ectopic cell response. A role in regulation of endometrial tumorigenesis as well in the implantation process can be postulated.

References

1. Vale W, Rivier C, Hsueh A, *et al.* Chemical and biological characterization of the inhibin family of protein hormones. *Recent Prog Horm Res* 1988;44:1–34
2. Knight PG. Roles of inhibins, activins and follistatin in the female reproductive system. *Front Neuroendocrinol* 1996;17:476–509
3. Petraglia F, Zanin E, Faletti A, *et al.* Inhibins: paracrine and endocrine effects in female reproductive function. *Curr Opin Obstet Gynecol* 1999;11:241–7
4. Petraglia F, Florio P, Luisi S, *et al.* Expression and secretion of inhibin and activin in normal and neoplastic uterine tissues. High levels of

serum activin A in women with endometrial and cervical carcinoma. *J Clin Endocrinol Metab* 1998;83:1194–200

5. Leung PHY, Salamonsen LA, Findlay JK. Immunolocalization of inhibin and activin α subunits in human endometrium across the menstrual cycle. *Hum Reprod* 1998;13:3469–77

6. Otani T, Minami S, Kokawa K, *et al.* Immunohistochemical localization of activin A in human endometrial tissues during the menstrual cycle and in early pregnancy. *Obstet Gynecol* 1998;91:685–92

7. Jones RL, Salamonsen LA, Critchley HO, *et al.* Inhibin and activin subunits are differentially expressed in endometrial cells and leukocytes during the menstrual cycle, in early pregnancy and in women using progestin-only contraception. *Mol Hum Reprod* 2000;6:1107–17

8. Petraglia F, Calza L, Garuti GC, *et al.* Presence and synthesis of inhibin subunits in human decidua. *J Clin Endocrinol Metab* 1990;71:487–92

9. Giudice LC. Growth factors and growth modulators in human uterine endometrium: their potential relevance to production medicine. *Fertil Steril* 1994;61:1–17

10. Hubner G, Hu Q, Smola H, *et al.* Strong induction of activin expression after injury suggests an important role of activin in wound repair. *Developmental Biology* 1996;173:490–8

11. Hubner G, Brauchle M, Gregor M, *et al.* Activin A: a novel player and inflammatory marker in inflammatory bowel disease? *Lab Invest* 1997;4:311–18

12. Sugiyama M, Ichida T, Sato T, *et al.* Expression of activin A is increased in cirrhotic and fibrotic livers. *Gastroenterology* 1998;114:550–8

13. Pawlosky JE, Taylor DS, Valentine M, *et al.* Stimulation of activin α A expression in rat aortic smooth muscle cells by thrombin and angiotensin II correlates with neointimal formation *in vivo. J Clin Invest* 1997;100:639–648

14. Yu EW, Dolter KE, Shao LE, *et al.* Suppression of IL-6 biological activities by activin α A and implication for inflammatory arthropathies. *Clin Exper Immunol* 1998;112:126–132

15. Florio P, Luisi S, Vigano P, *et al.* Healthy women and patients with endometriosis show high concentrations of inhibin A, inhibin B, and activin A in peritoneal fluid throughout the menstrual cycle. *Hum Reprod* 1998;13:2606–11

16. Reis FM, Di Blasio AM, Florio P, *et al.* Evidence for local production of inhibin A and activin A in patients with ovarian endometriosis. *Fertil Steril* 2001;75:367–73

Somatostatin receptors and vascular endothelial growth factor in human breast cancer

46

C. Casini Raggi, M. Pazzagli, C. Orlando, C. Tricarico, S. Gelmini,
L. Cataliotti, V. Distante, M. Maggi, D. Amadori and M. Serio

Introduction

Somatostatin regulates multiple cellular activities. In particular, it regulates secretion and proliferation through a family of G-protein-coupled receptor subtypes (sst)[1]. The mechanism of the antiproliferative effect of somatostatin is partly through suppression of the effects of mitogenic hormones and growth factors, and partly by a direct action on cell growth. The study of the antiproliferative action of somatostatin is relevant not only for understanding the regulation of neuroendocrine tumors expressing sst receptors, but also the regulation of non-endocrine tumors expressing these receptors.

Effects of somatostatin in breast cancer cell lines

Breast cancer cell lines are extensively studied as models to elucidate the mechanisms involved in the antiproliferative action of somatostatin. The antiproliferative action of somatostatin on some breast cancer cell lines (MCF7 and T47D) is characterized by apoptosis (cytotoxic effect) or cell cycle arrest (cytostatic effect)[2-6]. An arrest in the G1 phase of the cell cycle requires inhibition of a cycline-dependent kinase, and increase in the retinoblastoma gene product RB, while apoptosis requires induction of the BAX gene. The BAX gene is induced by p53, which in the absence of growth factors stimulates apoptosis, while in the presence of growth factors produces only G1 arrest.

It has been demonstrated that somatostatin induces apoptosis through the sst3 receptor, while it provokes G1 arrest via a stimulation of the subtypes 5 and 2, 4 and 1 (sst5 > sst2 > sst4 > sst1)[5]. The latter effect seems to be due to the induction of the retinoblastoma gene product RB in its hypophosphorylated form, as well as of cycline-dependent kinase inhibitors of the p21 family[5].

On the other hand, the activation of tyrosine phosphatase SHP-1 induces both cytotoxic and cytostatic effects in MCF7 and T47D. The cytostatic effect is in part due to a reduction in MAP kinase activity. In other breast cancer cell lines (MDA, MB231), the cytotoxic effect of SHP-1 has not been observed[5].

In some breast cancer cell lines (T47D and ZR75-1), the interaction of sst receptors with estrogen receptors has been studied[7]. The sst2 receptor is clearly up-regulated in these cell lines by estrogen, via a nuclear receptor, because the increase in sst2 induced by the 17β-estradiol can be reduced by tamoxifen.

Clinical application of the antiproliferative effects of somatostatin in breast cancer

The clinical applications of the aforementioned *in vitro* studies have yielded surprising results. Although a clear cytotoxic and cytostatic effect of somatostatin has been demonstrated *in vitro* in human breast cancer, a controlled trial[8] in estrogen-receptor positive, postmenopausal women with advanced breast cancer showed no improvement in the arm treated with octreotide plus tamoxifen versus tamoxifen alone.

Table 1 Somatostatin receptor subtype mRNAs in human breast tumors[9]

| | Receptor subtype – mRNA in situ hybridization | | | |
Patient	sst1	sst2	sst3	sst5
01/245	+	+	+	−
02/111	+	+	+	−
03/648	+	+	+	−
04/312	−	+	−	+
05/468	−	+	−	+
06/323	−	+	+	−
07/379	−	+	+	−
08/724	−	+	+	−
09/247	−	+	+	−
10/619	+	+	−	−
11/582	+	+	−	−
12/115	−	+	−	−
13/099	−	+	−	−
14/114	−	+	−	−
15/813	−	+	−	−
16/282	+	−	−	−
17/248	−	−	+	−
18/235	−	−	−	−
19/307	−	−	−	−
20/597	−	−	−	−
21/409	−	−	−	−
22/462	−	−	−	−

Table 2 Somatostatin receptor subtype sst2 mRNA expression in breast cancer ($n = 102$)

Ratio tumor/ normal tissue	sst2 mRNA expression	n	Percentage
< 1	Expression in tumor tissue lower than in normal tissue	35	34.3
< 4	Expression in tumor tissue 1–4-fold higher than in normal tissue	22	21.6
> 4	Expression in tumor tissue 4-fold higher than in normal tissue	45	44.1

Table 3 Vascular endothelial growth factor (VEGF) mRNA expression in breast cancer ($n = 88$)

Ratio tumor/ normal tissue	VEGF mRNA expression	n	Percentage
< 1	Expression in tumor tissue lower than in normal tissue	35	34.3
< 4	Expression in tumor tissue 1–4-fold higher than in normal tissue	22	21.6
> 4	Expression in tumor tissue 4-fold higher than in normal tissue	45	44.1

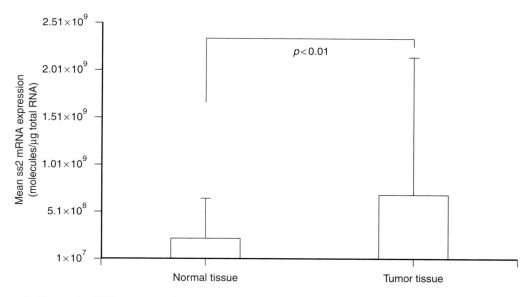

Figure 1 Mean sst2 mRNA expression in breast cancer tissue and corresponding normal tissue

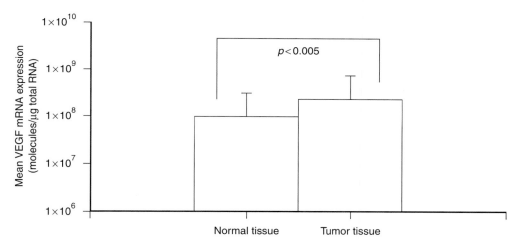

Figure 2 Vascular endothelial growth factor (VEGF) mRNA expression in breast cancer tissue and corresponding normal tissue ($n = 88$)

To attempt to elucidate the reasons for such disagreement between *in vitro* studies and clinical results, we used real time reverse transcriptase–polymerase chain reaction (RT-PCR) to measure the sst2 mRNA expression in both cancerous and normal breast tissue of the same subject, in 102 postmenopausal women affected by breast cancer. We chose the sst2 receptor, since previous studies have clearly demonstrated that this receptor subtype is the most prevalent in human breast cancer (Table 1)[9]. The amount of sst2 receptor mRNA was higher ($p < 0.01$) in breast cancer ($6.49 \times 10^8 \pm 1.53 \times 10^9$ molecules/μg of total RNA) than in normal tissue ($1.91 \times 10^8 \pm 5.40 \times 10^8$ molecules/μg of total RNA) (Figure 1). However, we observed very large interindividual variations in the sst2 mRNA ratio in tumor versus normal tissue. Some patients showed a ratio of less than 1, some a ratio of between 1 and 4, and a large number of patients showed a tumor/normal ratio of more than 4 (Table 2). In addition, sst2 levels in these tumors did not correlate with estrogen and progesterone receptors status.

In conclusion, breast cancers are largely dishomogeneous in terms of sst2 levels. These results could explain the poor effect of octreotide in the randomized trial discussed above.[8] The selection of patients with high levels of sst2 receptors could improve the antiproliferative effects of somatostatin analogs in clinical studies. In addition, since sst2 levels do not correlate with the number of estrogen receptors, a double arm with somatostatin analogs plus antiestrogens (or aromatase inhibitors) appears to be a rational approach.

VEGF in breast cancer

Vascular endothelial growth factor (VEGF) has been studied in human breast cancer and has been shown to correlate with prognosis[10]. Because an antiangiogenetic activity of somatostatin has been reported, we measured mRNA of VEGF, one of the most potent angiogenetic molecules, in the same tumors using the same experimental approach as described above (breast cancer tissue versus normal tissue of the same subjects). For our study, we used competitive RT-PCR, as previously described, and found that the expression of VEGF in the tumor was higher than in normal tissue ($2.37 \times 10^8 \pm 3.9 \times 10^8$ vs. $9 \times 10^7 \pm 1.7 \times 10^8$ molecules/µg of total RNA) (Figure 2). However, even in this case the interindividual variability was high (Table 3). The mRNA expression of VEGF correlated with that of sst2.

Conclusions

The study of somatostatin's antiproliferative action on cancer cell lines should give useful information on the biochemical mechanisms underlying the cytotoxic or cytostatic effects of the hormone. However, cancer cell lines are frequently different in terms of expression of receptor subtypes, as well as in terms of antiproliferative response. For instance, somatostatin stimulation by SHP-1 induces apoptosis in some breast cancer cell lines (MCF7 and T47D), but not in other cell lines (MPH, MB231).

The results obtained in tumor cell lines *in vitro* cannot be extrapolated to human tumors, which are largely heterogeneous in terms of receptor subtype expression, as well as receptor concentration. It remains to be established whether targeting the tumors on the basis of sst2 or VEGF concentrations could improve the clinical response in an individual.

References

1. Patel YC, Srikant C. Somatostatin receptors. *Trends Endocrinol Metab* 1997;8:398–405
2. Sharma K, Srikant CB. Induction of wild type p53, Bax and acidic endonuclease during somatostatin-signaled apoptosis in MCF-7 human breast cancer cells. *Int J Cancer* 1998;76:259–66
3. Thangaraju M, Sharma K, Liu D, *et al*. Interdependent regulation of intracellular acidification and SHP-1 in apoptosis. *Cancer Res* 1999; 59:1649–54
4. Sellers LA, Feniuk W, Humphrey PPA, *et al*. Activated G protein-coupled receptor induces tyrosine phosphorylation of STAT3 and agonist-selective serine phosphorylation via sustained stimulation of mitogen-activated protein kinase. *J Biol Chem* 1999;274:16423–30
5. Sharma K, Patel YC, Srikant CB. C-terminal region of human somatostatin receptor 5 is required for induction of Rb and G_1 cell cycle arrest. *Mol Endocrinol* 1999;13:82–90

6. Thangaraju M, Sharma K, Leber B, *et al*. Regulation of acidification and apoptosis by SHP-1 and Bcl-2. *J Biol Chem* 1999;274: 29549–57

7. Xu Y, Song J, Berelowitz M, *et al*. Estrogen regulates somatostatin receptor subtype 2 messenger ribonucleic acid expression in human breast cancer cells. *Endocrinology* 1995;136:5070–5

8. Ingle JN, Suman VJ, Kardinal CG, *et al*. A randomised trial of tamoxifen alone or combined with octreotide in the treatment of women with metastatic breast carcinoma. *Cancer* 1999;85:1284–92

9. Shaer J-C, Waser B, Mengod G, *et al*. Somatostatin receptor subtypes sst1, sst2, sst3 and sst5 expression in human pituitary gastroentero-pancreatic and mammary tumors: comparison of mRNA analysis with receptor autoradiography. *Int J Cancer* 1997; 70:530–7

10. Linderholm B, Grankvist K, Wilking N, *et al*. Correlation of vascular endothelial growth factor content with recurrences, survival and first relapse site in primary node-positive breast carcinoma after adjuvant treatment. *J Clin Oncol* 2000;18:1423–31

Index